Violence in Mental
Health Settings

Violence in Mental Health Settings

Causes, Consequences, Management

Edited by

Dirk Richter
Westphalian Hospital Münster and
University of Münster
Münster, Germany

and

Richard Whittington
University of Liverpool
Liverpool, England

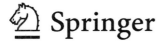 Springer

Dirk Richter, PhD
Institute of Sociology
Westphalian Hospital Münster
PO Box 200 252
D-48103 Münster
Germany
e-mail: dirk.richter@uni-muenster.de

Richard Whittington, PhD
School of Health Sciences
University of Liverpool
Liverpool L69 3GB
United Kingdom
e-mail: whitting@liverpool.ad.uk

Library of Congress Control Number: 2006926439

ISBN-10: 0-387-33964-7   e-ISBN-10: 0-387-33965-7
ISBN-13: 978-0387-33964-1   e-ISBN-13: 978-0387-33965-8

Printed on acid-free paper.

9 8 7 6 5 4 3 2 1

springer.com

About the Editors

Dirk Richter, PhD, a nurse (with working experience in mental health) and sociologist, is currently researcher and quality manager at Westphalian Hospital in Münster, Germany, and associate professor (*Privatdozent*) at the Institute of Sociology, University of Münster. In German, he has authored and edited three books on violence in health care. He has co-authored a widely distributed booklet on conflict management in psychiatric settings and has written several research papers and book chapters on the topic. He has also published in fields such as social psychiatry, evaluation and quality management, medical philosophy, nursing science, social theory, and nationalism research. His latest book on the sociology of mental disorders in the era of life sciences was published in 2003 (in German).

Richard Whittington, PhD, is a reader in the School of Health Sciences, University of Liverpool, and an honorary research fellow with the Merseycare NHS Trust in Liverpool, United Kingdom. He is a psychologist and researcher with a background as a mental health nurse in intensive care and general acute psychiatric settings. He has published widely on psychological and social aspects of violence in both institutional and community settings, with a particular focus on the role of threat and fear in the generation of aggression. Topics include risk assessment, coercive interventions for managing aggression, traumatic and other responses among care staff following assaults, and the provision of workplace counseling services. His other interests include exploration of research methods, international comparisons between mental health services, psychological responses to the diagnosis of physical illness, and self-harm.

Contributors

Christoph Abderhalden, Nursing Researcher, University of Berne Psychiatric Services, Berne, Switzerland

Roger Almvik, Senior Researcher, St. Olav's Hospital, Regional Secure Unit Bröset, Trondheim, Norway

Eric Baskind, Senior Lecturer, School of Law, Liverpool John Moores University, Liverpool, United Kingdom

Anna Björkdahl, Nursing Researcher, Department of Psychiatry, Karolinska University Hospital Huddinge, Stockholm, Sweden

Stål Bjørkly, Clinical Psychologist and Professor, Faculty of Health and Social Sciences of Molde University College, Norway, and Research Consultant, Centre for Research and Education in Forensic Psychiatry, Ullevål University Hospital, Oslo, Norway

Yvonne D. B. Bonner, Clinical Psychologist, Reggio Emilia Mental Health Trust, Reggio Emilia, Italy

Seamus Cowman, Professor and Head of Nursing, Royal College of Surgeons in Ireland, Dublin, Ireland

Athanassios Douzenis, Assistant Professor of Forensic Psychiatry, Athens Medical School, Athens, Greece

Joy Duxbury, Divisional Leader for Mental Health, Department of Nursing, University of Central Lancashire, Preston, Lancashire, United Kingdom

Toine C. G. Egberts, Professor, Utrecht University, Faculty of Science, Utrecht Institute for Pharmaceutical Sciences, Division of Pharmacoepidemiology & Pharmacotherapy, Utrecht, The Netherlands; Hospital Pharmacy Midden-Brabant, Tweesteden and St Elisabeth Hospital, Tilburg, The Netherlands

Gian Maria Galeazzi, Clinical Psychiatrist, Department of Neuroscience TCR, Section of Psychiatry, University of Modena and Reggio Emilia, Modena, Italy

Laurette E. Goedhard, Physician, Altrecht Institute for Mental Health Care, Den Dolder, The Netherlands; Utrecht University, Faculty of Science, Utrecht Institute for Pharmaceutical Sciences, Division of Pharmacoepidemiology and Pharmacotherapy, Utrecht, The Netherlands

Sabine Hahn, Lecturer/Researcher in Health Applied Research, Bern University of Applied Science, Switzerland

Trond Hatling, Senior Research Scientist, SINTEF Health, Department of Mental Health, Trondheim, Norway

Eibert R. Heerdink, Assistant Professor of pharmacoepidemiology, Utrecht University, Faculty of Science, Utrecht Institute for Pharmaceutical Sciences, Division of Pharmacoepidemiology and Pharmacotherapy, Utrecht, The Netherlands

Sheena Johnson, Research Assistant, School of Psychology, University of Liverpool, United Kingdom

Stefan Kunz, Nursing Researcher, University of Applied Sciences, Fribourg, Switzerland

Jim Maguire, Lecturer in mental health nursing, Athlone Institute of Technology, Athlone, Ireland

Kevin J. McKenna, Lecturer in mental health nursing, Dundalk Institute of Technology, Dundalk, Ireland

Ian Needham, Nursing Researcher and Head of Research, University of Applied Sciences, Department of Health, St. Gallen, Switzerland

Henk L. I. Nijman, Professor of forensic psychology, Radboud University of Nijmegen, the Netherlands; Senior Researcher Kijvelanden Forensic Psychiatric Hospital, Portugal, the Netherlands; visiting professor, City University, London, United Kingdom

Berend Olivier, Professor, Utrecht University, Faculty of Science, Department of Pharmaceutical Sciences, Division Psychopharmacology, Utrecht, The Netherlands; Department of Pharmacology and Anatomy, Section Behavioral Genomics, Rudolf Magnus Institute of Neuroscience, Utrecht University; Department of Psychiatry, Yale University School of Medicine, New Haven, Connecticut, USA

Nico E. Oud, Nursing Researcher and Consultant, Oud Consultancy, Amsterdam, The Netherlands

Tom Palmstierna, Psychiatrist and Head of the dependency disorders section St Göran Hospital, Stockholm, Sweden, Associate Professor, Forensic psychiatry section, Department of Clinical Neurosciences, Karolinska Institute, Stockholm, Sweden; Assistant Professor St. Olav's Hospital, Forensic Department and Research Centre, Brøset, Norwegian University of Science and Technology, Trondheim, Norway

Brodie Paterson, Lecturer, School of Nursing & Midwifery, University of Stirling, Scotland, United Kingdom

Dirk Richter, Researcher and Quality Manager, Westphalian Hospital Munster, Munster, Germany; Associate Professor (*Privatdozent*), Institute of Sociology, University of Munster, Germany

Tilman Steinert, Clinical Psychiatrist and Professor, Centre of Psychiatry Weissenau, Department Psychiatry I, University of Ulm, Ravensburg–Weissenau, Germany

Joost Jan Stolker, Psychiatrist, Medical Director of the Division for Forensic Psychiatry, Altrecht Institute for Mental Health Care, Den Dolder, The Netherlands; Senior Researcher, Utrecht University, Faculty of Science, Utrecht Institute for Pharmaceutical Sciences, Division of Pharmacoepidemiology and Pharmacotherapy, Utrecht, The Netherlands

Richard Whittington, Psychologist and Reader, School of Health Sciences, University of Liverpool, United Kingdom; Honorary Research Fellow Merseycare Mental Health NHS Trust, Liverpool, United Kingdom

Contents

IV IMPROVING STAFF SKILLS IN HANDLING MANAGEMENT

10 Aggression Management Training Programs: Contents, Implementation, and Organization 193
Nico E. Oud

11 The Effects of Aggression Management Training for Mental Health Care and Disability Care Staff: A Systematic Review 211
Dirk Richter, Ian Needham, and Stefan Kunz

V THE ORGANIZATIONAL CONTEXT

12 Locating Training Within a Strategic Organizational Response to Aggression and Violence 231
Kevin J. McKenna and Brodie Paterson

13 Safety and Security in Psychiatric Clinical Environments 253
Seamus Cowman

14 Ward Culture and Atmosphere 273
Joy A. Duxbury, Anna Björkdahl, and Sheena Johnson

VI CONSEQUENCES: HANDLING THE AFTERMATH

VII CONCLUSIONS

Introduction

RICHARD WHITTINGTON AND DIRK RICHTER

1 INTRODUCTION

Although, often enough, patients and staff in mental health settings disagree on clinical issues, they certainly agree on the fact that violence still poses a large problem in the delivery of effective modern services. Even after several decades of mental health care reforms and deinstitutionalization initiatives, violence has by no means disappeared from the wards. Early assumptions about the benefits of community psychiatry were that deinstitutionalization and effective outpatient services would lead to fewer involuntary admissions and, hence, to less violence on the wards. It is clear now that these assumptions were wrong. Today, we have to acknowledge that the rate of involuntary and revolving-door admissions is still high and these are important elements of the problem.

It is really no great surprise that many staff and patients alike feel that violence is one of the biggest problems affecting contemporary psychiatric institutions. Surveys which ask mental health staff about the amount of violence they have experienced in their careers have found that up to 100% of nurses on acute wards have been assaulted during their work (e.g., Menckel & Viitisaara, 2002). Certainly, nurses who work more directly with patients experience more physical violence than doctors who do not have this amount of face-to-face contact with patients. Verbal threats, sexual harassment, and stalking are also important concerns for many mental health staff (Sandberg, McNiel, & Binder, 2002). It is widely acknowledged that high rates of aggression and violence lead to mental health problems in affected staff, ranging from depression and burn-out to post-traumatic stress disorders. On the other hand, many patients admitted to wards worry about the potential for violence from the other, unknown, patients around them, and so they lose the sense of safety and security which is the bedrock of effective asylum. In addition, patients who end up being subjected to the coercive practices used to manage potential violence, such as restraint can, in turn, experience it themselves as a form of institutional aggression.

At the same time the practice of compulsory admissions and coercive measures on the ward have recently become the focus of significant research efforts. In the UK, for example, there has been a passionate medical, legal, and political debate on the use of coercion in psychiatry following the death of a particular patient while being physically restrained (Department of Health, 2005) and in Germany there has recently been a discussion on the apparent increase in the rates of compulsory admissions into psychiatric hospitals.

What is different today, compared to the old days, is that talking about violence and coercion is no longer taboo among service providers and the professional communities, and that it is now possible to draw on a huge amount of research literature on this topic if one intends to set up some prevention initiatives. Interestingly enough, this literature deals with nearly all aspects of violence in mental health care settings in terms of causes, consequences, and management of the problem. There is a large body of research which aims to analyze the contributing factors that increase the risk of aggression and violence of patients against staff. More and more studies are carried out which try to find out what works to prevent violence and minimize coercion. National and regional guidelines on the management of violent patients have been launched by political bodies or professional societies in many countries around the world. It is, therefore, certainly timely to take stock of where we have got to after more than two decades of sustained attention to the problem.

One feature of this period has been a shift toward an increasingly strident "rights"-based discourse where two, largely incompatible, sets of rights are placed in opposition to each other. From one perspective, that of the staff, violence by patients in mental health care settings is part of the wider problem of work-related violence. Increasingly, staff and their employers have come to think of the risk as job-related and unacceptable, with all the managerial and legal consequences that such an interpretation entails, including, for instance, Zero Tolerance initiatives (considered below in Chapter 13). From another perspective, that of "the aggressive patient," violence can be felt to be an understandable, even legitimate, response to a problem caused, or at least exacerbated, by the service itself. Here, coercion by staff and oppressive institutional practices are seen as the root of the problem to which aggression by the patient is simply the response. Both of these perspectives have their proponents and have generated extensive political debate and calls for action (Szasz, 2002; WHO, 2002). While written by, and targeted at, professionals, this book attempts to include consideration of both of these perspectives because it seems obvious that prevention and management programs must take both perspectives into account if they are to be effective. We aim to move this polarized debate forward, away from an emphasis on violence *by* people with mental disorder toward an emphasis on violence *in* mental health settings; from concern with the violent individual to a focus on the violent incident, a social interaction involving two or more actors enacting complementary and multiple roles.

The book covers three main aspects of the problem: causes, consequences, and management. Obviously, violence is a very complex phenomenon and the causes or facilitators of violence in mental health care settings are very varied. They range from personal predispositions rooted in genetic makeup, to broad social and environmental factors, and several of the chapters here address the issue of causation in various ways. In addition, all violence has consequences for both the assaulted person and for the perpetrator. The effects for the assaulted person can range from physical injury, and psychological distress, to social and occupational effects. For the perpetrator, the consequences can include restraint, seclusion, and a restricted environment. Again, some consideration of these various consequences is given below in a range of chapters. Since violence has such serious consequences there must be efforts to improve our management of the problem. Management here, again, ranges broadly from biological and pharmacological treatment, through psychological, to social and organizational change, and all of these approaches are considered below. Only improvements on all of these levels will reduce the scale of the problem and make the experience of giving and receiving, mental health care more palatable for staff and patients alike.

One of our aims here is to integrate theoretical explanations, empirical findings, and practical solutions from many countries and from different professional contexts in order to provide a state-of-the-art overview of the contexts, causes, treatment, and prevention of violence in mental health settings. Much of the discussion below is concerned with practical and applied guidance to employees and others but, where possible, this is based on a clear understanding of conceptual and theoretical issues. The book is intended to be of interest to all those who work in mental health care settings and have direct clinical contact with mentally disordered people, whatever specific discipline they are from, and whatever the specific setting in which they work. While the emphasis here is on hospital in-patient units, there is much that can be related to community and outpatient work, as well as care homes for people with a learning disability, nursing homes, specialist departments of general hospitals (e.g., emergency treatment), and ambulance personnel. The geographical reach of the book is also intended to be wide. All the authors are based in Europe and represent some of the key authorities in this area, but each has written with a much wider remit attempting to capture at least the flavor of research on this topic from around the world. In addition, the emphasis here is also very much on multidisciplinarity. All the main professions which work in this area are represented, since each discipline has something to offer in understanding and managing the problem, and only a multilevel approach in research and practice can deal with the complexity of the problem.

Some aspects of terminology need to be cleared up from the start. Firstly, we have not asked our contributors to stick to a policy on the use of the term patient or service user. There is of course, disagreement about which term to use and also about the value of worrying about which term to use. We don't believe there is unanimity among the recipients of mental health services about which term they prefer, and each term has advantages, and disadvantages, for those to whom it is applied. Ultimately, anybody receiving mental health care is both a patient and a service user at one and the same time, though their ownership of each identity at any one moment will fluctuate according to the circumstances. Related to this, there is no explicit "service user perspective" here in the sense of one or more chapters written by service users. Instead, an awareness of this perspective is inherent in most chapters and in some places there is an explicit consideration of what has been said by service users (e.g., on involuntary commitment and coercive measures) via published research. Thirdly the term "victim" is sometimes used below to refer exclusively to the staff member who is injured by a patient. This term is again controversial, with its inherent implication that the staff member is the innocent party and their injury represents some end point in the interaction with the patient. In fact, many patients will feel, sometimes legitimately, that they are a victim either of the entire mental health system, or of an attack by an individual staff member. Equally, both staff and patients affected by aggression may eschew the victim label with its intimations of powerlessness and passivity. So here, the use of the term victim is a shorthand which should not be taken to suggest that all violence in care systems is by patients against staff.

We have planned and organized the book from a particular perspective, and with specific aims which we intend to be of use to those delivering and managing mental health services. The emphasis here is on surveying the current state of research and practice at this point, early in the 21st century, after at least two decades of sustained attention to the problem of violence. Where possible, the best available evidence has been considered and used as a basis for practical recommendations. Several chapters (those on pharmacological management, staff training, and the impact of exposure to violence) are based on full systematic review principles. We have attempted to balance practice with theory in the belief that effective improvements will only occur when these two aspects are combined. So, while the ultimate purpose is to improve things in the real world of mental health services, our conviction is that such improvement can only occur when a clear theoretical understanding of the relevant processes at all levels (biological, psychological, sociological) is achieved. Research on this topic was pioneered by nurses and doctors in the 1970s, driven by a desire to do something about problems which they encountered in their everyday work, and there was an early emphasis on individualistic, even biological, explanations. We are ready now for the next stage, where this clinical problem is understood within the wider frameworks available from psychology and sociology, and we aim to provide a platform for these ideas here.

It is worth noting that most of the authors here have collaborated for some time in the European Violence in Psychiatry Research Group (EViPRG, www.liv.ac.uk/eviprg), a network of researchers and clinicians with backgrounds in nursing, psychology, psychiatric medicine and education which was founded in 1997. The book, to some extent, reflects debates and discussions within the group on the best way forward. Such multidisciplinary and international collaborations are becoming more common in this area (e.g., Salize & Dressing, 2004) and they represent the best opportunity we have to share, and thus improve, practice across services in different countries. Having said this, one has also to acknowledge that the current practice for dealing with violence, and the use of coercion, in different countries still reflects national historical developments. A major revelation early on in the activities of EViPRG was the discovery that different countries, even those neighboring each other, have adopted very different policies, usually reflecting their unique legal traditions. For example, the use of specific compulsory measures against violent patients in one country is regarded as barbaric in others. Such diversity within the relatively small area of the European region is likely to be magnified when comparing mental health systems around the world. Some legal traditions do not allow mechanical restraint of patients while others pose legal barriers against compulsory medication. Generally, however, all of these clinical and legal practices have not been tested empirically against others. Thus, it is still not known whether mechanically restraining or sedating patients is preferable in terms of their safety, security, or acceptability. In our culture of evidence-based practice, one has to admit that this is a major failure by the psychiatric community given that the use of coercion is clearly one of the biggest infringements of a patient's personal rights. In addition, the comparison of different practices and legal positions might also be an incentive to review local or national policies and, at the very least, we are convinced that every country can learn a lot from the experience of those in other countries.

The book is organized along five themes, each relating to a different aspect of the problem to be faced. The first task is to establish the scale of violence in mental health care settings and the patterns of cause and effect which surround its occurrence. While, as already mentioned, there is huge cultural diversity, mental health services around the world face the same basic problem of hostility and conflict when providing front-line care and treatment to some people, so there is much to be gained by measuring the problem systematically and internationally. Risk assessment of violent individuals has, in the past decade, moved forward rapidly in this way, but the movement toward standardized measurement of violent incidents is in its infancy. Effective risk prediction can only be achieved on the basis of effective risk outcome measurement. In the first Chapter Henk Nijman and his colleagues examine the robustness of a range of pragmatic instruments for capturing key aspects of a violent incident and consider the benefits of a shift toward the standardized use of a single instrument (the SOAS-R) across different countries.

The second theme is concerned with providing a theoretical context for thinking about violent incidents. While human aggression has a clear biological basis, this approach has been over-emphasized in the violence—mental disorder equation over recent years, leading to an unhelpful focus on violent individuals rather than violent situations. The three chapters in this section attempt to redress this balance a little by considering psychological, sociological, and user-focused perspectives. Firstly, Stal Bjørkly provides an overview of three psychological approaches to understanding human aggression (psychoanalytic, drive, and social learning theories), and links each of these perspectives to the practical clinical situation within mental health services. Our own chapter then attempts to draw on a range of other theoretical concepts from psychology and sociology to construct an integrated approach toward the specific problem of reactive aggression on psychiatric wards in which the "provoking" environment and reciprocal aversive stimulation lead from escalation to outright violence. Both of these chapters examine the meaning of the violent incident for both staff and patients but work from "official" theoretical perspectives. Christoph Abderhalden and his colleagues move beyond these professional perspectives and complete this section by examining research into service users' perceptions of violence and their experiences of psychiatric coercion. From this perspective, physical coercion by staff is experienced as a form of aggression which may cause more problems than it solves, a theme which recurs in several places throughout this volume.

The next section moves on from attempts to theoretically understand the problem toward examining effective ways of predicting when violence is likely to occur and managing it when it does take place. Such management takes place within a legal framework which is considered firstly by Trond Hatling and his colleagues, in an attempt to establish what might be considered to be the core legal arrangements for managing dangerousness shared by most European countries, and that which is specific to individual jurisdictions. These findings may then be compared to frameworks in other countries beyond Europe to examine whether any sort of global consensus exists, or is possible to achieve in the future. Practical management starts with effective risk assessment, a rapidly developing field in terms of mental disorder and violence, and Tilman Steinert provides a comprehensive overview of the current status of research in this area. We then have three chapters which examine the evidence relating to various steps in the hierarchy of coercive interventions. De-escalation should always be a core component and the first step in managing potential violence, and yet it is surprising how little research is available to support effective interventions of this type. Dirk Richter considers some of this research and draws on other related topics, such as conflict management, to begin building a more sophisticated understanding of the processes operating when staff attempt to calm an angry and aroused patient. Richard Whittington and his colleagues then examine the issues and dilemmas surrounding the next step when coercive interventions, such as seclusion and restraint, are used, and note the growing attempts around the world to develop less repressive alternatives, such as enhanced observation. Pharmacological interventions and tranquillization are options in some, otherwise uncontrollable situations, and to complete this section, Laurette Goedhard and her colleagues provide some recommendations for best practice, based on a recently completed systematic review.

A constant theme here is the need to improve our understanding and management of violence in mental health settings and the belief that positive change can be introduced at both individual and organizational levels. At the individual level, improved staff training in incident management is often seen as the fundamental building block for improved practice, and the next section has two chapters concerned with this issue. Nico Oud examines various aspects of best practice with regard to training, including ideals with regard to course aims, content, and the process of training the trainers. Dirk Richter and his colleagues then go on to examine the evidence base for the effectiveness of training by conducting a systematic review of the available literature, and making recommendations for "what works" in this vital area.

One of the most important new developments in this area is the attempt to move from focusing on the individual interaction or member of staff, to consideration of the organizational context in which violence occurs, and this is the theme of the next section of the book. Kevin McKenna and Brodie Paterson provide the link from the previous section by considering how staff training fits within a total organizational response to violent incidents. Seamus Cowman then examines the balancing act which is needed when attempting to provide an environment which is both safe (i.e., well-controlled) on the one hand, but which is at the same time, therapeutic, enabling, and caring. Joy Duxbury and her colleagues then conclude this section by considering the concept of the ward as a mini-organization, and ways of developing a positive and facilitating culture for patients and staff as a key element of any violence minimization program.

Despite all our best efforts at improving prediction and management, we must accept that violence in mental health settings will always be a possibility, and that those exposed to it will be affected in a variety of ways. Some of these effects will be quite disabling and Ian Needham provides some ideas for improving the support and post-incident care offered to assaulted staff, based on a systematic review of current knowledge on the full range of potential responses to violence. Finally, our conclusions section tries to give the reader some "take-home messages" from each of the preceding chapters.

We believe each chapter has important practical implications built, wherever possible, on current research and theory. If the reader is planning to start his or her own prevention efforts as an individual or as a manager from zero, each chapter, and the entire book, taken together should provide enough suggestions to enable such a project to get off the ground.

REFERENCES

Department of Health (2005). *Delivering race equality in mental health care: An action plan for reform inside and outside services and the Government's response to the Independent inquiry into the death of David Bennett*. London: Department of Health.

Menckel, E., & Viitisaara, E. (2002). Threats and violence in Swedish care and welfare–magnitude of the problem and impact on municipal personnel. *Scandinavian Journal of Caring Sciences, 16*(4), 376–85.

Salize, H., & Dressing, H. (2004). Epidemiology of involuntary placement of mentally ill people across the European Union. *British Journal of Psychiatry, 184,* 163–168.

Sandberg, D. A., McNiel, D. E., & Binder, R. L. (2002). Stalking, threatening, and harassing behavior by psychiatric patients toward clinicians. *The Journal of the American Academy of Psychiatry and the Law, 30*(2), 221–9.

Szasz, T. (2002). *Liberation by oppression: A comparative study of slavery and psychiatry*. Somerset, New Jersey, USA: Transaction Publishers.

World Health Organization (2002). *World report on violence and health*. Geneva: WHO.

I

MEASUREMENT AND EPIDEMIOLOGY

1

Assessing Aggression of Psychiatric Patients: Methods of Measurement and Its Prevalence

HENK NIJMAN, STÅL BJØRKLY, TOM PALMSTIERNA, AND ROGER ALMVIK

1 INTRODUCTION

Inpatient aggression threatens the safety and well being of staff members and fellow patients. Nursing staff in particular appear to be at risk of being assaulted by their patients, e.g., Carmel and Hunter (1989), Nijman, Allertz, Merckelbach, à Campo, and Ravelli (1997), and Tamm, Engelsmann, and Fugere (1996). In a recent survey among 148 psychiatric nurses in East London (Nijman, Bowers, Oud, & Jansen, 2005), almost one out of every six nurses (16%) claimed to have experienced, over the last year, severe physical violence during their work. A little over one in five nurses (22%) revealed they have called in sick in connection with workplace violence. Sick nurses stayed at home for an average of 5.2 days per nurse (range 1–23 days). In other words, violence from psychiatric patients not only has considerable physical and psychological consequences, but is also very likely to have substantial financial implications. This is underlined by a much cited study of Hunter and Carmel (1992) in which an annual total of 134 serious injuries for a 973-bed forensic psychiatric hospital was reported. The average costs per injury were conservatively estimated to be $5719, making the total annual loss $766,290.

Figures like this illustrate the (potential) magnitude of the problem. It should be noted though that the nurses from the anonymous survey in East London (Nijman, Bowers, et al., 2005) may have overexaggerated or overestimated the prevalence of workplace violence. Furthermore, severely victimized caregivers may have been more inclined to respond to a survey about patient violence. As the overall response rate to the survey was 39%, it remains unclear whether or not the other 61% of nurses had similar experiences to the ones who replied.

Such obvious limitations of survey instruments, i.e., recall and selection bias, stress the necessity for the continuous monitoring of aggressive occurrences on psychiatric wards. Reliable and time-efficient methods of recording aggression need to be in place on psychiatric wards in order to get complete and factual information on the magnitude of the problem of aggression. Continuous monitoring of incidents on the ward may also be helpful in detecting typical precipitants and triggers of violent behavior. Presumably, options to intervene will increase with more knowledge of when and why patients are most likely to engage in aggressive behavior. This chapter addresses a number of methods for measuring the aggressiveness of psychiatric patients. Firstly the use of, and problems with, self-report questionnaires for measuring aggression, anger, and hostility of psychiatric (in)patients are briefly discussed. Following this, staff observation scales designed to observe aggressive behavior of patients on psychiatric wards are addressed. Finally, the prevalence of inpatient aggression in psychiatric institutions is illustrated, on the basis of the results of such aggression observation tools.

2   ASSESSING THE AGGRESSION OF PSYCHIATRIC PATIENTS WITH SELF-REPORT QUESTIONNAIRES

The most frequently used methods for assessing the aggression of psychiatric patients can be roughly divided into self-rating and observer aggression scales (Bech, 1994). A well-known, self-rating questionnaire with a long history, the Buss–Durkee Hostility Inventory (BDHI), is used for measuring hostility and anger (Buss & Durkee, 1957). Research over the years on the psychometric qualities of BDHI items has led to adapted versions of the BDHI, such as the Aggression Questionnaire (AQ) (Buss & Perry, 1992).

On the basis of the literature, Bjørkly (1995) noted that the BDHI's "predictive value for adult psychiatric patients has not been convincing so far" (Bjørkly, p. 49). Indeed, much of the research on the psychometric properties of aggression self-report measures has traditionally been done in normal subjects (see Yudofsky, Silver, Jackson, Endicott, & Williams, 1986), such as that on psychology students, but this seems to be changing rapidly, e.g., Novaco and Taylor (2004). One of the problems with aggression self-reports may be that patients with (severe) psychiatric disorders, e.g., antisocial personality disorder or schizophrenia, lack insight into their own role in (creating) conflicts. Furthermore, self-reports of aggressive behavior rely heavily on the honesty of respondents about their tendency to become angry and behave aggressively. Yudofsky et al. noted, about aggression self-reports in general, that: "many patients are not angry between aggressive episodes, and do not reliably recall or admit to past violent events" (Yudofsky et al., 1986, p. 35).

Especially in forensic psychiatric samples, in which release from custody may be connected to the psychiatric condition, the inclination to provide socially desirable answers may pose large problems for the validity of self-reported symptoms, among which is aggressiveness. This seems to be illustrated by a Dutch study by Hornsveld, van Dam-Baggen, Lammers, Nijman, and Kraaimaat (2004). These researchers found that forensic patients sentenced to one of the Dutch "TBS" hospitals reported lower aggression and hostility scores than forensic outpatients outside a TBS hospital. In Dutch, TBS stands for "Ter Beschikking Stelling," which may be translated best as being "placed at the disposal" of the government in one of the specialized maximum security institutions for forensic psychiatric care, i.e., TBS hospitals. On the basis of the severe, violent, and criminal histories of TBS-patients rather the opposite would be expected. Possibly, outpatients' answers were more honest because high hostility scores in this group could not lead to longer admission periods, whereas for the sample of incarcerated TBS patients, a judge has to decide every two years on either the continuation or termination of the TBS sentence. In other words, apart from a lack of insight into one's own behavior, one problem with aggression self-reports may be that certain subgroups have a strong interest in minimizing their impulse control problems.

On the other hand, several recent studies can be found that present evidence for the predictive validity of self-reports of feelings of anger and aggressiveness, even in (forensic) psychiatric patient samples. To give an example, Novaco and Taylor (2004) measured aggressiveness and anger among 129 male forensic patients with intellectual disabilities by means of modified versions of the Novaco Anger Scale (NAS) (Novaco, 1994) and the Spielberger State-Trait Anger Expression Inventory (STAXI) (Spielberger, 1996). In this study, significant correlations were found between the STAXI "Trait Anger" and "Anger Expression" subscales on the one hand, and hospital physical assaults on the other (correlations of 0.34 and 0.37, respectively). The correlation between hospital assaults and the NAS total score was 0.43 (Novaco & Taylor).

It should be further noted that aggression self-report questionnaires are, generally, designed to assess the tendencies of individuals to react in a hostile or angry way. Aggression self-report scales rarely ask to record discrete aggressive incidents, and therefore they are not designed to provide information on the prevalence of aggressive incidents on specific wards or institutions. For this reason, much of the scientific literature on the prevalence, as well as on the prevention of aggressive behavior on psychiatric wards has relied on the use of aggression observation scales. With aggression observation scales the aggressive behavior of psychiatric patients is generally recorded by the ward staff after the aggressive incident has occurred. In other words, in contrast to aggression self-report questionnaires, the majority of observer aggression instruments aim at measuring discrete, separate incidents. In the next paragraph, several reliable—but easy-to-use—observer-based instruments for recording aggressive incidents of psychiatric inpatients are discussed.

3 ASSESSING THE AGGRESSION OF PSYCHIATRIC PATIENTS WITH OBSERVATION SCALES

As discussed earlier, aggression observation instruments may avoid many problems that a lack of insight, or a tendency to give socially desirable answers in patients, may give. One could argue, however, that ward staff themselves are also part of the interaction that leads to aggressive incidents on psychiatric wards, e.g., see Whittington and Wykes (1996), which also may affect the objectivity of the ratings. One way to avoid this may be to videotape ward activity, e.g., see Crowner, Stepcic, Peric, and Czobor (1994), so that conflicts on the ward can be rated by independent observers later on. Due to practical and ethical problems, however, this approach is not in use in clinical practice.

For prevention of aggression in inpatient facilities, however, recording discrete incidents separately, directly after they occur may have advantages. For instance, it seems to provide more opportunities to investigate the specific circumstances and times that are connected to violent outbursts, e.g., Nijman et al. (1997). The registration of aggressive behavior directly after each incident is possibly also beneficent in creating more insight into aggression-eliciting factors (see Nilsson, Palmstierna, & Wistedt, 1988; but also see De Niet, Hutschemaekers, & Lendemeijer, 2005 for a critical discussion).

Well-known examples of aggression observations scales that are meant to be completed after an incident has occurred are:

- The Overt Aggression Scale (OAS) (see Silver & Yudofsky, 1991; Yudofsky et al., 1986).
- The Modified version of the OAS (MOAS) (Kay, Wolkenfield, & Murril, 1988).
- The Staff Observation Aggression Scale (SOAS) (Palmstierna & Wistedt, 1987).
- The revised version of the SOAS (SOAS-R) (Nijman et al., 1999).
- The Report Form for Aggressive Episodes (REFA) (Bjørkly, 1996).
- The Attempted and Actual Assault Scale (ATTACKS) (Bowers, Nijman, & Palmstierna, 2005; Bowers, Nijman, Palmstierna, & Crowhurst, in press).

One of the disadvantages of "incident-based" scales is that they may not become part of ward routines easily (see Sjöstrom, Eder, Malm, & Beskow, 2001), particularly when the target behavior is rare. That is to say, the reliability of an incident-based registration method relies heavily on the preparedness of ward staff to record all aggressive incidents. "Period-based" aggression observation scales, targeting at rating aggressive behavior at predetermined times, may be less likely to be "forgotten." Examples of specific period-based aggression observation tools are the Social Dysfunction and Aggression Scale, or SDAS (Wistedt et al., 1990), and the Ward Anger Rating Scale (WARS) (Novaco, 1994). Such period-based aggression observation scales may, however, provide less information about specific circumstances leading to incidents on the ward. Therefore, for researching the effects of potential aggression reducing interventions a combination of "incident-based" and "period-based" aggression observation scales may be advisable.

One thing the incident-based aggression observation scales such as the MOAS, SOAS-R, REFA, and ATTACKS all have in common is that, to a large extent, they are made out of predefined answering options, which makes them time-efficient, as well as easy to use. In other words, the registration of aggression can be performed by marking options that apply to the observed aggressive conduct. The easier and more time-efficient these scales are to complete, the more likely it will be that ward staff will record all the incidents they encounter (ranging from mild to severe). Below, the MOAS, SOAS(-R), REFA, and ATTACKS will be briefly outlined. Following the presentation of these incident-based aggression observation instruments, the prevalence of aggression on psychiatric wards will be addressed in more detail. This will be done by summarizing aggression frequencies reported in the scientific literature.

3.1   The Modified Overt Aggression Scale (MOAS)

The MOAS is an aggression observation instrument that divides aggression into four main categories: verbal aggression, aggression against property, autoaggression, and physical aggression (Kay et al., 1988). Each of these four types of aggression is specified in five subcategories that reflect the severity of the behavior (severity scores ranging from zero to four points for each category).

In order to calculate the overall severity of an incident, aggression against property scores are multiplied by a factor of two, autoaggression scores by a factor of three, and physical aggression scores by a factor of four, and then added to the verbal aggression score. In other words, the scores of the categories are weighted in a way that the physical aggression score is the most important in calculating the overall severity. In this way, the total MOAS severity scores can theoretically range from zero, no aggression, to 40, most severe aggression.

The interrater reliability of MOAS, based on the total severity scores of two independent raters has been found to be good (Pearson's rs of 0.85 and 0.94; see Kay et al., 1988). In a recent Italian validation study (Margari et al., 2005), again the reliability, as well as the validity of the MOAS, were found to be high, and on the basis of its psychometric properties the instrument was judged to be more suitable for the assessment of aggression than the Nurses' Observation Scale for In-patient Evaluation (NOSIE).

3.2   The Staff Observation Aggression Scale (SOAS)

The SOAS (Palmstierna & Wistedt, 1987) is aimed at measuring verbal and physical aggression against objects, patients, or staff. The SOAS comprises five columns pertaining to specific aspects of aggressive behavior, i.e., the provocation of the aggression, the means used during the aggression, the target of the aggression, the consequences of the behavior, and the measures taken to stop aggression.

Every time a staff member witnesses aggression by one of his or her patients, a SOAS form is to be completed. The first column of the SOAS-R in particular, concerning what seems to have provoked or triggered the aggression, has been assumed to increase staff members' sensitivity to risk factors in specific patients (see Nilsson et al., 1988; and also De Niet et al., 2005, for a critical discussion of this notion).

Since 1999, a revised version of the SOAS, i.e., the SOAS-R[1] (Nijman et al., 1999) has been in use. This adapted version has a validated, more finely tuned severity scoring system, which may increase the possibilities of comparing aggression rates between wards. In the original SOAS severity scoring system, a maximum score of 12 indicated the most severe incident. The revised SOAS-R severity score ranges from 0 to 22 points with higher scores, again, indicating greater severity. The rationale behind this revised severity scoring system was that the severity of aggressive behavior depends on an array of features with some, such as the consequences for victims, being more important than others, e.g., means used by the aggressive patient, in calculating the overall severity of incidents. With regression techniques a severity scoring system was developed in which separate features are weighted in a way that they make a differential contribution to the overall aggression severity score (Nijman et al.).

Studies addressing the concurrent validity of SOAS and SOAS-R severity scores with other measures of aggression severity yielded significant results, i.e., correlations with other methods for assessing the severity of aggressive behavior varied between 0.38 and 0.81 (see Nijman, Palmstierna, Stolker, & Almvik, 2005). Cross-validations with clinical estimates of severity provided by staff members, who had experienced aggression, indicated that the revised SOAS-R severity scores approximate the general opinion of ward staff of the severity of incidents better than those from the original SOAS (Dias Marques & Cruz Mendes, 2003; Nijman et al., 1999; Nijman, Evers, Merckelbach, & Palmstierna, 2002).

Study results indicate fair to good interrater reliability for SOAS scores. On the basis of the four incidents described, Palmstierna and Wistedt (1987) initially found an intraclass correlation of 0.96 between total SOAS scores from independent raters. Later studies, conducted in clinical practice, supported an acceptable interrater reliability for the scale, with Cohen's κs being 0.61 and 0.74 (Nijman et al., 1997; Steinert, Woefle, & Gebhart, 1999, 2000) and a Pearson's r between independent raters of 0.87 (Nijman et al.). However, none of these studies examined the reliability between raters of the decision of when, or when not, to complete a SOAS(-R) form. As mentioned earlier, the reliability of all incident-based aggression observation methods relies on the preparedness of ward staff to complete a form after each aggressive occurrence. Aggression on the SOAS-R is defined as:

"Any verbal, non-verbal, or physical behavior that was threatening (to self, others or property), or physical behavior that actually did harm (to self, others, or property)" (Morrison, 1990, p. 67).

[1]For more information on the SOAS-R contact: Henk Nijman: hennij@kijvelanden.nl or Tom Palmstierna: tom.palmstierna@mailbox.euromail.se.

Particularly in cases of "mild" aggressive behavior, inconsistency between raters could exist on whether or not a SOAS-R form should be used to report the observed behavior.

3.3   Report Form for Aggressive Episodes (REFA)

The REFA[2] is a behavioral rating scale which measures aggressive behavior toward other persons (Bjørkly, 1996). The REFA was specifically designed for the diagnostic purpose of mapping the situations that provoke aggressive behavior in each patient. In other words, even more so than with the SOAS-R, the focus of the REFA is on detecting (situational) triggers of aggression. Aggression on the REFA is understood as a personality characteristic manifesting itself as a function of the triggering qualities of each situation or interaction. A situation is defined as the actual situation is perceived, interpreted, and assigned meaning (Magnusson, 1981). Situational vulnerability is defined as increased probability of behaving aggressively toward others, given certain classes of interactions. By using REFA, a patient's profile of situational vulnerability may be obtained. This aspect of the instrument corresponds to approaches from behavioral analysis and cognitive therapy that advocate analysis of stimulus control factors (Foreyt & Rathjen, 1978; Marlatt & Gordon, 1985).

The form consists of a list of 30 situations or interactions that could have triggered aggression, grouped in the following seven main categories:

- Physical contact (4 items).
- Limit setting (6 items).
- Problems of communication (3 items).
- Changes/readjustments (6 items).
- Persons (6 items).
- High-risk contact (2 items).
- Drugs/stimulants (3 items).
- Open category for additional situations or interactions.

Next to the precipitants of aggression, there are six vertical sections for the recording of characteristics of aggressive episodes: one for verbal threats, one for physical threats, and four sections for physical assaults. Verbal and physical threats are operationally defined as: Verbal and nonverbal communication conveying a clear intention to inflict physical injury upon another person. Physical assaults are defined as the intended infliction of bodily injury upon another person. As is the case with the SOAS-R, the nurse who observed the event must record the aggressive incident on the form as soon as possible after the aggressive incident has taken place. However, for the REFA, at least one other staff member must also be consulted for a second opinion on the precipitants and the characteristics of the actual aggressive incident. After patients have calmed down, they are asked to provide information that may be of relevance to the accurate recording of the incident.

[2]For more information on the REFA contact Stål Bjørkly: Stal.Bjorkly@hiMolde.no.

Two studies on the interrater reliability of the REFA have been conducted. One study dealt with individual ratings and involved personnel from an acute psychiatric admission ward and a special secure ward for forensic patients ($N = 48$) (Bjørkly, 2000). Results showed that interrater agreement and reliability were high. (Correct classification of both precipitant and type of aggression = 83%, precipitants = 94%, and type of aggression = 89%; Kuder-Richardson coefficient = 0.71; $k = 0.84$; k max = 0.93, $N = 480$ ratings). The purpose of the second investigation was to study levels of interrater reliability based on joint ratings (Bjørkly, 1998). This study involved staff from a 12-bed admissions ward ($N = 20$). Again, results were positive (Precipitant and type of aggression = 96%; precipitant = 98%, type of aggression = 98%; Subkoviak index of decision consistency = 0.87; CI for the probability of obtaining 100% correct ratings = 0.961, 0.999; significance level for the probability of obtaining 100% correct ratings: $z = 3.77$, $p = <0.0001$, one tailed).

Fifteen years of clinical application indicate that the REFA has three clear assets: accurate operational criteria for the definition of aggression, adequate emphasis on assessing situational variables, and that nurses find this instrument clinically useful. Finally, clinical experience indicates that REFA recordings are easily integrated in the planning and implementation of coping interventions, and secure preventive measures, in the clinical setting. This is supported by nurses reporting that they find this approach to measurement of aggression useful and motivating in their clinical work.

However, the REFA also has several limitations (1) it does not distinguish between serious and less serious physical assaults; (2) it does not provide information on whether the actual aggressive behavior has resulted in physical injury; (3) it does not provide information on what kind of measures were required to stop the aggressive behavior; and (4) it has limited applicability concerning patients with very low rates of aggressive behavior.

3.4   The Attempted and Actual Assault Scale: The Attacks

The ATTACKS[3] is a more recently designed instrument (Bowers et al., 2002, in press), that exclusively seeks to measure physical violence towards a person, but aims to do this in great detail. Again, the Attacks is to be completed by staff members witnessing aggression, directly after a violent incident has taken place on their ward.

The center table is the most important and innovative part of the scale (Bowers et al., in press). In this table, all physically violent actions that have been witnessed during an (attempted) assault are to be recorded. More specifically, all means and weapons used, e.g., sharp objects, hot liquids, spitting, poking, etc., are to be noted down in combination with the targets at which they are aimed, e.g., head, limbs, torso, etc. The frequencies of the separate physical actions are also to be estimated, as it can be assumed that striking more than once increases the capacity of violence to cause serious harm.

---

[3]For more information on the ATTACKS contact: Len Bowers: L.Bowers@city.ac.uk.

After the rater has broken down the witnessed assault into the separate components of action, they are also asked to judge the commitment of the assailant to cause harm by using a Visual Analogue Scale, and to provide a judgment of the overall injury potential of the assault. In calculating the overall severity of an assault on the basis of a completed ATTACKS form, it is the combination of the weapon(s) chosen by the assailant, the parts of the victim's body that were aimed at, whether one or multiple blows or strikes were used, the commitment of the assailant to cause harm, and the injury potential of the assault, that determines the overall severity of the assault.

One of the preliminary tests of the reliability and validity of the ATTACKS (Bowers et al., in press) was done by means of a videotape of interpersonal assaults, compiled from regular television broadcasts. During a meeting of the European Violence in Psychiatry Research Group (EVIPRG), 22 members from 14 different countries were instructed to rate the videotaped assaults on both the MOAS and the Attacks. It was found that the intra class correlation coefficient of the Attacks severity scores was 0.70, and higher than that of the MOAS in this specific exercise. In other words, the interrater reliability of Attacks severity appears to be promising. Yet, it should be noted that all incidents used in this videotape study concerned interpersonal physical violence, whereas the MOAS is not specifically designed for exclusively rating this type of behavior. This factor is likely to have negatively influenced the reliability results for the MOAS in this specific test. As mentioned earlier, the interrater reliability of MOAS has been found to be good (Pearson's rs of 0.85 and 0.94; see Kay et al., 1988) in earlier studies.

The raters were also asked to provide their judgments of the severity of the assaults shown on the tape. The connections between the Attacks severity scores with the overall judgment of severity of the assaults was 0.70 (Spearman's ρ). These results indicate that the Attacks scale may be a useful addition to scales already available for aggression research, but further research on the use of the scale in clinical practice is needed to confirm the first findings.

4 THE PREVALENCE OF INPATIENT AGGRESSION

Reviews on the prevalence of aggressive behavior of psychiatric patients reveal that about 10% of hospitalized psychiatric patients (Bjørkly, 1995; Tardiff, 1992) have engaged in violence prior to admission. Reliance on hospitalized samples may lead to an overestimation of the prevalence of aggressive behavior in the psychiatric population as a whole (Monahan & Shah, 1989). Yet, for psychiatric outpatients also, the empirical data make "a convincing preliminary case for an association between mental illness and community violence" (Mulvey, 1994; p. 664). As violence is one of the major selection criteria for (involuntary) psychiatric hospitalization, e.g., Fuller Torrey (1994), the frequency of aggressive acts among psychiatric inpatients can be assumed to be higher than those found in community samples. On the basis of the literature, Bjørkly estimated in 1995 that 15–30% of hospitalized psychiatric patients are involved in physical assaults. In descriptive studies, the prevalence of aggressive behavior ranges considerably, from as low as 0.15 assaults per bed, per year (Fottrell, 1980) to as high as 88.8 incidents per bed, per year, on a specialized high security ward (Brizer, Convit, Krakowski, & Volavka, 1987). These differences will be largely due to the selection of patients studied. Apart from that, criteria used to define and measure aggressive behavior deviates considerably across the studies, thereby adding to the inconsistency of the results. Bowers (1999, 2000) noted that the comparison of aggression frequencies between different wards and hospitals has been severely hand-icapped by a failure to uniformly express incidents rates in the past.

However, as relatively many researchers have reported SOAS or SOAS-R results over the last few years (for a review see Nijman, Palmstierna, et al., 2005), there could be an opportunity to make a more significant comparison of aggression frequencies across countries and types of wards, as many studies have used an iden-tical or very similar method for monitoring aggression. A review of the reported SOAS(-R) frequencies at the ward or subgroup level ($n = 54$ separate observations; Nijman, Palmstierna, et al.) yielded a median value for all reports of a little under eight incidents per psychiatric patient per year. This figure would mean that, on a 15-bed psychiatric ward, a SOAS-R form is, on average, to be completed once every three days. However, the reported annual number of SOAS(-R) incidents per psy-chiatric patient still varied considerably across studies from as low as 0.4 to as high as 59.9 incidents per year, depending on the type of ward and country involved.

When the annual number of SOAS(-R) incidents per patient was studied sepa-rately for acute admission wards taking care of adult patients ($n = 38$ separate obser-vations), a mean of 9.3 incidents per bed, per year, was found. Remarkably, several studies on aggression in psychogeriatric samples, conducted in Sweden and the UK, reported a high prevalence of aggression (more than 15 incidents per patient, per year, with a maximum of 59.9), but there is some indication that the severity of the incidents, in terms of physical consequences, on average is low on such wards. In general, the proportion of incidents leading to physical consequences, e.g., pain, bruises, welts, etc., ranges from 10 to 20% of the total number of SOAS(-R) assess-ments (Nijman, Palmstierna, et al., 2005). Even more severe assaults for which victims require somatic treatment, constitute about 1–5% of all SOAS(-R) reports.

As could be expected, high SOAS(-R)-frequencies of incidents were also found on wards providing care to selected groups of high-risk patients, e.g., 40.2 and 29.2 in selections of violent schizophrenic patients in Finland, and 31.2 in a selection of young, high-risk, Dutch patients who required involuntary admission at a young age. With the REFA, Bjørkly (1999) also found high aggression frequencies on special-ized wards, such as a 19-bed Norwegian special secure unit for dangerous psychotic patients. In a ten-year prospective study, a total of 2021 incidents of aggressive behavior were recorded. Equivalent values of rates of aggression per patient, per year, were: 25.9 (total of aggressive episodes), 13.5 (verbal threats), 6.5 (physical threats), and 5.9 (physical assaults). Four patients accounted for 1,558 (77%) of the aggressive episodes that occurred during the study period. Interestingly, in this REFA study, a comparison between rates of aggression in the first five-year period and in the last five-year period yielded a 60% reduction over the study period (Bjørkly).

Several SOAS(-R) studies also reported reductions in aggression reports over time (but were concerned with shorter time periods in these studies). Nilsson et al. (1988) have speculated that this "reduction phenomenon" could be:

> "Caused by a learning process from the ordinary nursing staff, who during a study of this kind are forced to systematize their observation of their patients" (p. 174).

Alternatively, the "spontaneous" decrease of the registration of incidents over time could have something to do with changes in the way aggression observation scales are completed as time progresses, e.g., see De Niet et al. (2005), Shah (1999), and Sival, Albronda, Haffmans, Saltet, and Schellekens (2000).

The preliminary evidence from the SOAS(-R) review (Nijman, Palmstierna et al., 2005), carefully suggested there may be differences in the prevalence rates in various European countries. The mean number of incidents per patient, per year, from Dutch acute admission wards, for instance, was high when compared to the mean number of incidents from other countries, e.g., the UK, Germany, Norway, and Denmark (see Nijman, Palmstierna et al.), but the relatively low number of studies per country does not allow us to draw very firm conclusions on this finding. However, the fact that standardized aggression report forms from scientific literature have come to be used more and more in psychiatric institutions across Europe is likely to improve the comparability of aggression frequencies between wards, hospitals, and countries in the future. Possibly, some interesting cross-national differences may emerge when aggression frequencies can be compared on a larger scale.

REFERENCES

Bech, P. (1994). Measurement by observations of aggressive behavior and activities in clinical situations. *Criminal Behaviour and Mental Health, 4*, 290–302.

Bjørkly, S. (1995). Prediction of aggression in psychiatric patients. A review of prospective prediction studies. *Clinical Psychology Review, 15*, 475–502.

Bjørkly, S. (1996). Report form for aggressive episodes: Preliminary report. *Perceptual and Motor Skills, 83*, 1139–1152.

Bjørkly, S. (1998). Inter rater reliability of the report form for aggressive episodes in group ratings. *Perceptual and Motor Skills, 87*, 1405–1406.

Bjørkly, S. (1999). A ten-year prospective study of aggression in a special secure unit for dangerous patients. *Scandinavian Journal of Psychology, 40*, 57–65.

Bjørkly, S. (2000). The inter rater reliability of the report form for aggressive episodes. *Journal of Family Violence, 15*, 269–279.

Bowers, L. (1999). A critical appraisal of violent incident measures. *Journal of Mental Health, 8*, 335–345.

Bowers, L. (2000). The expression and comparison of ward incident rates. *Issues in Mental Health Nursing, 21*, 365–386.

Bowers, L., Nijman, H., & Palmstierna, T. (in press). The Attempted and Actual Assault Scale (Attacks). *The International Journal of Methods in Psychiatric Research.*

Bowers, L., Nijman, H., Palmstierna, T., & Crowhurst, N. (2002). Issues in the measurement of violent incidents and the introduction of a new scale: The Attacks (Attempted and Actual Assault Scale). *Acta Psychiatrica Scandinavica, 106* (Suppl. 412), 106–109.

Brizer, D. S., Convit, A., Krakowski, A., & Volavka, J. (1987). A rating scale for reporting violence on psychiatric wards. *Hospital & Community Psychiatry, 38,* 769–770.

Buss, A. H., & Durkee, A. (1957). An inventory for assessing different kinds of hostility. *Journal of Consulting Psychology, 21,* 343–349.

Buss, A. H., & Perry, M. (1992). The aggression questionnaire. *Journal of Personality and Social Psychology, 63,* 452–459.

Carmel, H., & Hunter, M. (1989). Staff injuries from inpatient violence. *Hospital & Community Psychiatry, 40,* 41–46.

Crowner, M. L., Stepcic, F., Peric, G., & Czobor, P. (1994). Typology of patient–patient assaults detected by video cameras. *American Journal of Psychiatry, 151,* 1669–1672.

De Niet, G. J., Hutschemaekers, G. J. M., & Lendemeijer, B. H. H. G. (2005). Is the reducing effect of the Staff Observation Aggression Scale owing to a learning effect? An explorative study. *Journal of Psychiatric and Mental Health Nursing, 12,* 687–694.

Dias Marques, M. I., & Cruz Mendes, A. (2003). Violence in psychiatry: An exploratory study in the Coimbra Psychiatric Services. In *European violence in psychiatry research group dissemination project. Report to the European Commission on behalf of the EVIPRG (EVIPACOM, QLAM-2000-00011).* City University, London.

Foreyt, J. P., & Rathjen, D. (1978). *Cognitive behavior therapy—Research and application.* New York: Plenum Press.

Fottrell, E. (1980). A study of violent behaviour among patients in psychiatric hospitals. *The British Journal of Psychiatry, 136,* 216–221.

Fuller Torrey, E. (1994). Violent behavior by individuals with serious mental illness. *Hospital and Community Psychiatry, 45,* 653–662.

Hornsveld, R. H. J., van Dam-Baggen, C. M. J., Lammers, S. M. M., Nijman, H. L. I., & Kraaimaat, F. W. (2004). Forensische patiënten met geweldsdelicten: Persoonlijkheidskenmerken en gedrag. *Tijdschrift voor Psychiatrie, 46,* 133–143.

Hunter, M., & Carmel, H. (1992). The cost of staff injuries from inpatient violence. *Hospital & Community Psychiatry, 43,* 586–588.

Kay, S. R., Wolkenfield, F., & Murril, L. (1988). Profiles of aggression among psychiatric patients. I: Nature and prevalence. *The Journal of Nervous and Mental Disease, 176,* 539–546.

Magnusson, D. (1981). *Toward a psychology of situations. An interactional perspective.* Hillsdale, New Jersey: Lawrence Erlbaum Associates.

Margari, F. Matarazzo, R., Casacchia, M., Roncone, R., Dieci, M., Safran, S., et al and the EPICA Study Group (2005). Italian validation of MOAS and NOSIE: A useful package for psychiatric assessment and monitoring of aggressive behavior. *International Journal of Methods in Psychiatric Research, 14,* 109–118.

Marlatt, G. A., & Gordon, J. R. (Eds.) (1985). *Relapse prevention.* New York: Guilford.

Monahan, J., & Shah, S.A. (1989). Dangerousness and commitment of the mentally disordered in the United States. *Schizophrenia Bulletin, 15,* 541–553.

Morrison, E. F. (1990). Violent psychiatric inpatients in a public hospital. *Scholarly Inquiry for Nursing Practice: An International Journal, 4,* 65–82.

Mulvey, E. P. (1994). Assessing the evidence of a link between mental illness and violence. *Hospital & Community Psychiatry, 45,* 663–668.

Nijman, H. L. I., Allertz, W. W. F., Merckelbach, H., à Campo, J., & Ravelli, D. (1997). Aggressive behavior on an acute psychiatric admissions ward. *European Psychiatry : The Journal of the Association of European Psychiatrists, 11,* 106–114.

Nijman, H. L. I., Bowers, L., Oud, N., & Jansen, G. (2005). Psychiatric nurses' experiences with inpatient aggression. *Aggressive Behavior, 31,* 217–227.

Nijman, H., Evers, C., Merckelbach, H. L. G. J., & Palmstierna, T. (2002). Assessing aggression severity with the revised Staff Observation Aggression Scale (SOAS-R). *Journal of Nervous and Mental Disease, 190,* 198–200.

Nijman, H. L. I., Muris, P., Merckelbach, H. L. G. J., Palmstierna, T., Wistedt, B., Vos, A. M., et al. (1999). The Staff Observation Aggression Scale—Revised (SOAS-R). *Aggressive Behavior, 25,* 197–209.

Nijman, H., Palmstierna, T., Almvik, R., & Stolker, J. (2005). Fifteen years of research with the Staff Observation Aggression Scale. A review. *Acta Psychiatrica Scandinavica, 111,* 12–21.

Nilsson, K., Palmstierna, T., & Wistedt, B. (1988). Aggressive behavior in hospitalized psychogeriatric patients. *Acta Psychiatrica Scandinavica, 78,* 172–175.

Novaco, R.W. (1994). Anger as a risk factor for violence among the mentally disordered. In: J. Monahan & H. J. Steadman (Eds.), *Violence and mental disorder* (pp. 21–59), Chicago: University of Chicago Press.

Novaco, R.W., & Taylor, J. L. (2004). Assessment of anger and aggression in male offenders with developmental disabilities. *Psychological Assessment, 16,* 42–50.

Palmstierna, T., & Wistedt, B. (1987). Staff observation aggression scale. Presentation and evaluation. *Acta Psychiatrica Scandinavica, 76,* 657–663.

Shah, A. (1999). Some methodological issues in using aggression rating scales in intervention studies among institutionalized elderly. *International Psychogeriatrics, 11,* 439–444.

Silver, J. M., & Yudofsky, S. C. (1991). The Overt Aggression Scale. *Journal of Neuropsychiatry, 3,* 22–29.

Sival, R. C., Albronda, T., Haffmans, P. M. J., Saltet, M. L., & Schellekens, C. M. (2000). Is aggressive behavior influenced by the use of a behavior rating scale in patients in a psychogeriatric nursing home? *International Journal of Geriatric Psychiatry, 15,* 108–111.

Sjöstrom N., Eder, D. N., Malm, U., & Beskow, J. (2001). Violence and its prediction at a psychiatric hospital. *European Psychiatry : The Journal of the Association of European Psychiatrists, 16,* 459–465.

Spielberger, C. D. (1996). *State-Trait anger expression inventory professional manual.* Odessa, USA: Psychological Assessment Resources.

Steinert, T., Woefle, M., & Gebhardt, R. P. (1999). No correlation of serum cholesterol levels with measures of violence in patients with schizophrenia and non-psychotic disorders. *European Psychiatry: The Journal of the Association of European Psychiatrists, 14,* 80–81.

Steinert, T., Wölfle, M., & Gebhardt, R. P. (2000). Measurement of violence during in-patient treatment and association with psychopathology. *Acta Psychiatrica Scandinavica, 102,* 107–112.

Tamm, E., Engelsmann, F., & Fugere, R. (1996). Patterns of violent incidents by patients on a general hospital psychiatric facility. *Psychiatric Services, 47,* 86–88.

Tardiff, K. (1992). The current state of psychiatry in the treatment of violent patients. *Archives of General Psychiatry, 49,* 493–498.

Whittington, R., & Wykes, T. (1996). Aversive stimulation by staff and violence by psychiatric patients. *British Journal of Clinical Psychology, 35,* 11–20.

Wistedt, B., Rasmussen, A., Pedersen, L., Malm, U., Träskman-Bendz, L., Wakelin, J., et al. (1990). The development of an observer-scale for measuring social dysfunction and aggression. *Pharmacopsychiatry, 23,* 249–252.

Yudofsky, S. C., Silver, J. M., Jackson, W., Endicott, J., & Williams, D. (1986). The overt aggression scale for the objective rating of verbal and physical aggression. *The American Journal of Psychiatry, 143,* 35–39.

II

THE PSYCHOLOGY AND SOCIOLOGY OF THE VIOLENT INCIDENT

2

Psychological Theories of Aggression: Principles and Application to Practice

STÅL BJØRKLY

ABSTRACT

Aggression and violence are studied in a variety of disciplines. However, it is difficult to study human aggression directly, because it occurs sporadically and people often have reasons for not acknowledging or reporting it. This methodological complexity is probably reflected in the fact that each scientific discipline has its own level of analysis and develops its own set of theories and methods to explain aggression. This chapter deals with theoretical issues related to psychological approaches to aggression. Three main groups of aggression theories are examined: Psychoanalytic, drive and learning theory. The reciprocal relationship between theory, definition of aggression and study method is addressed in this chapter. Another aim is to give a critical review of definitional, methodological and theoretical strengths and shortcomings pertaining to the three historically dominant theories of aggression presented here. A final scope is to discuss the current clinical relevance of the individual theory concerning the treatment of violent mentally ill patients.

1   INTRODUCTION

Aggression, violence, and related behaviors have been studied in a wide range of disciplines including anthropology, biology, economy, political science, communication research, history, and sociology. In the present chapter, however, the primary focus is on psychological theories of human aggression. Elements from other disciplines, e.g., biology, sociology, etc., are only addressed provided they constitute naturally integrated parts of the actual psychological theory of aggression. Important issues such as the mutual relationship between genetics and psychosocial factors, gender and age differences, and measurement issues are not dealt with unless such topics are emphasized in the individual theory.

It is well known that human aggression is not an easy field to study. In this respect, the heterogeneous nature of the term "aggression" constitutes a major complicating factor. Bandura (1973) claimed that conducting research in this field was like entering a semantic jungle of ideas that span an ample range of phenomena and activities. A study in a Dutch psychiatric hospital illustrates the clinical relevance of Bandura's point very well (Finnema, Dassen, & Halfens, 1994). Finnema and co-workers interviewed nurses working in a psychiatric hospital to find out more of how they perceived and characterized patient aggression. Most of the nurses acknowledged positive as well as negative aspects of aggressive behavior. However, the descriptions of aggression varied considerably and the authors concluded that "it was not possible to formulate a general definition of aggression on the basis of the results of the study" (Finnema et al., p. 1088). One may question how the nurses managed to plan and coordinate treatment interventions in relation to aggressive incidents when they apparently were unable to share a common definition of the phenomenon. It is claimed here that the definitional issue described above illustrates a situation representative of state of the art in a majority of clinical practice settings, and that this is closely related to the low status of theories of aggression in clinical practice. In sharp contrast to this, it is generally acknowledged that a sound theoretical grounding is at the core of efficient clinical practice. Taken together, these assumptions contribute to justify the focus on theories of aggression in this chapter.

The primary aims of this chapter are:

1. To give a brief introduction to three basic psychological theories of aggression;
2. To address their relevance to clinical psychiatric practice.

Contributions from the following main theories of aggression are presented:

- Psychoanalytic theory
- Drive theory
- Social learning theory

Naturally, limitations of space allow neither for detailed presentations and analysis nor for an outline of more than one theory from each theoretical perspective. The selection of perspectives is based on a search in the literature that yielded 140 works on theories of aggression (Bjørkly, 2001). At least one of the following criteria had to be met to be included here:

- Early theories of historical significance and/or of relevance to recent theories of aggression

- Current theories of aggression that are distinguishable from other theories
- Theories based on empirical research, including clinical research.

The presentation of the individual theory is arranged in the following way (1) theoretical main points, (2) definition and study design, (3) limitations and shortcomings, and (4) relevance to current clinical treatment of violent mentally ill patients.

2 PSYCHOANALYTIC THEORY

In approaching the topic of aggression from the perspective of psychoanalysis it is important to recognize that contemporary psychoanalysis is not a unified theory. As the original theory has been modified and expanded, it has gradually developed into several distinctive approaches. A basic disagreement exists between structural theorists, who tend to see aggression as an innate drive or instinct, and self-psychologists, who tend to view aggression as secondary to narcissistic injury. For a more detailed discussion of the various psychoanalytic views, the reader is referred to other literature, e.g., Buss (1961) and Pedder (1992). This chapter is confined to a brief review of Sigmund Freud's theory of aggression as an instinctual drive.

2.1 Theory of Aggression

Freud initially sought to derive all manifestations of human behavior from one basic life instinct, designated as Eros. Conceived of as a force, this life instinct was referred to as libido which functioned to enhance, prolong, and reproduce life. Freud showed very little interest in aggression, as such, in his early writings. In 1920, however, he proposed a dual-instinct theory in which the life instinct was matched by a death instinct, termed Thanatos (Freud, 1920). This instinct was conceived of as a force urging the disintegration of the individual and human life at large. The relationship between the life and death instinct is polarized and any destructive or non-destructive activity can be construed as the specific interaction of the antagonistic forces. Freud also claimed that feelings of anger and hostility result in conflict and unconscious guilt in the same manner that sexual wishes do, and that these effects initiate defensive activity. Further, he observed that many impulses contain both sexual and aggressive components, and that many clinical manifestations, including sadism, masochism, and ambivalence, can be explained in terms of varying degrees of conflict between these drives or their fusion. In Freud's view, the death instinct forces the individual to direct aggressive acts against the social and physical environment in order to save themselves from self-destruction. Displacement and sublimation were introduced as central dynamic agents in the conversion of the potential attack on the self into an outward redirection. This inner dynamic process was instrumental to very different behavioral outcomes, such as coping, creativity, self-destruction, and aggression toward inanimate objects and living beings. According to the dual drive-theory, if the aggressive impulses are not combined with or adequately "bound" or fused with love, then increased aggression and destructiveness can be expected. Deprivation, object loss, or child abuse are all traumas that can interfere with attachment and the normative fusion of love and aggression. In case of such failures, destructive energy will accumulate and, in its primitive form, result in destructive behavior. Freud entertained the notion of catharsis or tension reduction in connection with destructive energy. Catharsis refers to a process in which the affective, nondestructive display or hostile and aggressive inclinations can discharge destructive energy and thereby reduce the strength of these inclinations.

2.2 Definition and Study Design

Aggression is defined as an intrapsychological phenomenon. The death instinct is its basic source of energy, but this energy can also result in creativity, coping, or self-injurious behavior. The definition of aggression is wide and different human behavior and emotions such as sarcastic language, passive–aggressive responses, and murder are understood to be expressions of one unifying concept. The definition is process oriented and of an intuitive nature.

Because psychoanalysis is built on the foundation of the patient's narrative, psychoanalytic research differs from research in other areas of psychology. The traditional study design is founded on therapy material (the patients' contribution) and therapy interventions (the therapists' contribution). Psychoanalysis is also the preferred method to detect the causes of individual aggression. Scientifically valid analysis rests on psychoanalytic interpretations of psychological data and the assumption that there exists one underlying order in the universe that the phenomenon under study represents. Freud was the first to adopt the causality principle to the study of personality (psychological determinism). One of the main aims in psychoanalytic treatment of aggression is to help the patient gain insight into the intrapsychological mechanisms behind the aggressive drive. A move from unconscious to conscious motivation is basic to this process. In line with this, the emphasis on the role of intrapsychic mechanisms in aggression is reflected in the wide psychoanalytical definition of aggression.

2.3 Limitations and Shortcomings

Freud's death instinct is perhaps the most controversial element of psychoanalytic theory. Some authors are very harsh in their criticism of Freud's contribution to the theoretical understanding of human aggression:

> "The basic concepts of Freud's theories are metaphorical and do not yield testable hypotheses." (Tedeschi & Felson, 1994, p. 39)

Other serious objections to Freud's theory of aggression are (1) Is it really possible to understand aggression, which is a highly complex phenomenon, by means of a single explanatory factor, the death instinct? (e.g., Okey, 1992). (2) Freud's stance that aggression is of a primary (instinctual) nature, held up against strong empirical evidence of its reactive (secondary) character (Pedder, 1992). (3) Lack of empirical documentation of the biological origins of aggression as a drive (Brenner, 1971). (4) According to Freud, the never-ceasing self-destructive impulses of the death instinct have to be transformed continuously into outwardly directed hostility and aggression to ward off the lasting threat of discontinuation of life. Aggression is thus inevitable, and attempts to control and eliminate it can only be temporary (e.g., Bandura, 1973). (5) Finally, Freud's reasoning on catharsis has been questioned: Is the reduction of tension a matter of seconds, minutes, days, or months? Does it happen quickly or very slowly? And, how is it possible to treat catharsis as an unquestionable mechanism in spite of strong negative research evidence on this point? (e.g., Zillman, 1979).

2.4   Relevance to Current Clinical Practice

The psychoanalytical model of aggression has undergone considerable changes over time. According to Akhtar (1995) there are two extreme positions concerning the nature and origins of aggression. Sigmund Freud is found at one extreme, one that holds to the concept of death instinct and that aggression is a destructive outward deflection of this instinct. The other extreme is represented by Suttie, Fairbairn, Guntrip, and Kohut whose view holds that aggression is a reactive and interactional phenomenon that definitely does not have an instinctual basis.

Apart from some articles on the role of countertransference reactions to violent patients, e.g., Dubin (1989) and Lion and Pasternak (1973), there is a paucity of publications on specified treatment approaches based on Freud's theory of aggression. On the other hand, there are a growing number of publications that focus on the clinical application of the Rorschach method for diagnostic purposes in the assessment of violent psychiatric patients. The scope of this diagnostic procedure is to provide information about implicit motives and underlying personality dimensions that the patient may be unaware of, or does not want to reveal (e.g., Bornstein, 2001; Gacono, Meloy, & Bridges, 2000). In particular, these studies have addressed the option of differentiating between psychopathy and other antisocial disorders, and the difference between violent and nonviolent offender groups.

Inspired by Fairbairn, John Bowlby developed the attachment theory, located at the other extreme of psychoanalytical theories of aggression. Within this perspective, humans are essentially social animals who need relationships for survival, and whose first relationships with parental figures have unique characteristics (Bowlby, 1989). The child's expression of distress normally elicits a helpful response from the caregiver. A consequence of this is that the child will most likely develop and generalize a strategy of seeking proximity to the caregiver when distressed. Conversely, when the child's expression of distress results in further rejection or conflict, the child's most adaptive strategy is to control the distress by either attempting to inhibit it, or by amplifying and exaggerating it. Attachment theory further assumes that cognitive strategies (internal working models) developed early in life will come to regulate how internal stimuli are attended to and interpreted, the nature of the emotional experiences triggered, and the memories that are retrieved in adulthood. There are numerous methods for assessing adult attachment. Mary Main's Adult Attachment Interview (AAI) has been subject to the most rigorous evaluation, and its psychometric properties are well demonstrated (e.g., Bakermans-Kranenburg & van Ijzendoorn, 1993). The classification has four attachment categories: secure, avoidant, ambivalent, and disorganized. Although several studies indicate an increased risk of aggression stemming from avoidant attachment patterns, the strongest evidence of aggression risk pertains to the disorganized category. The term disorganized refers to the apparent lack, or collapse of, a consistent strategy for organizing responses to the need for comfort and security when under stress. Disorganized behavior increases under attachment-relevant family risk conditions such as maternal alcohol consumption, maternal depression, adolescent parenthood, or multiproblem family status.

The contributions of Paul G. Nestor and Peter Fonagy may illustrate the growing number of clinically relevant publications on relation-focused psychodynamic perspectives pertaining to mental disorder and violence. Nestor (2002) mapped clinical risk factors for violence onto four fundamental personality dimensions resulting from early attachment relationships and interaction with significant others. Two were related to regulatory functions of impulse control and affect regulation, and two to the personality surface traits of narcissism and paranoid cognitive personality style. Nestor also presented empirical evidence for, and recommendations of, measurement methods with very good psychometric properties. This kind of assessment may prove to be a highly relevant contribution to improve the quality of milieu treatment approaches. Fonagy (2003) delineated a developmental understanding of violence in the mentally ill. He emphasized that the key to the understanding of the development of violence and its treatment may be found in a thorough analysis of the individual's attachment patterns. Attachment enables the mastery of aggression through the process of mentalization. According to Fonagy, mentalization refers to our capacity to understand others' subjective experiences. Although he argues for early intervention, the main point of creating strong attachment relationships to enhance mentalization is highly relevant to clinical practice with adult psychiatric patients as well.

In sum, psychoanalytic understanding of aggression has moved from a medically and psychiatrically dominated strategy with a focus on the individual child and his or her pathology to include social interactionist perspectives on the etiology and treatment of aggression. A social, interactionist approach is critical to the view that aggression is "pushed out" or "compelled" by inner forces such as death instinct or aggressive energy. At present, attachment theory forms the dominant psychoanalytic contribution to clinical research on aggression. This represents a major change from an instinctually based understanding to an interactional understanding of the nature and origins of aggression. Methodologically, this has resulted in a change from Freud's narrative research method to quantitative measurement by means of structured interviews and observation of social interactions. The current standing of

Sigmund Freud's theory of aggression in clinical practice outside the classical analyst context seems to be of a historic nature.

3 DRIVE THEORY

As described above, Freud's theory of aggression was heavily attacked by contemporary psychoanalysts and psychologists. In particular, the notion of spontaneity in aggression; that is, the endogenous build-up of aggressive energy, has been dismissed. Still, in the late 1930s the energy concept was re-labeled "the drive concept" by the Yale researchers Dollard, Doob, Miller, Mowrer, and Sears (1939) in their formulation of the frustration–aggression hypothesis. This was motivated by a wish to translate the Freudian instinct propositions into more objective behavioral terms which could be put to empirical test.

3.1 Theory of Aggression

The original hypothesis first posited that any interference with an individual's goal-directed activities causes frustration. In the frustration–aggression hypothesis, not only those factors that will determine how frustrated an individual will become was specified, but also how and when aggression will be expressed. One may wonder why this approach to the understanding of aggression was termed a hypothesis. Obviously, it was more distinct and open to empirical testing than Freud's original approach. Maybe this formulation was chosen because Dollard and collaborators meant that they were actually only expanding on Freud's theory. Thus the premise of the frustration–aggression hypothesis is that when people become frustrated (thwarting of goals) they respond aggressively. This is clearly highlighted by Dollard and coworkers in their original work:

> "The occurrence of aggressive behavior always presupposes the existence of frustration and, contrariwise, that the existence of frustration always leads to some form of aggression" (Dollard et al., 1939, p. 11).

Thus, although aggressive behavior emanates from an aggressive drive, this drive is not of an instinctive nature. The drive is only initiated due to perceptions of frustrating external stimuli. Accordingly, this represents a breach with Freud's instinctual understanding by the fact that aggression is understood as a reactive phenomenon. The blocking of an ongoing goal response leads to a build-up of aggressive energy within the organism. This energy is noxious and must be released by the organism in the form of aggressive behavior. Any response that releases this aggressive energy is an instance of aggression. The strength of the instigation to aggression (e.g., the aggressive drive) varies according to three factors:

1. The amount of frustration.
2. The degree of interference with a goal-seeking response.
3. The number of frustrated responses experienced by the individual.

Aggressive responses are considered self-reinforcing within the hydraulic model adopted by frustration–aggression theorists. Thus, the association between frustration and a particular aggressive response is strengthened by reinforcement associated with drive reduction. Still, the performance of the same behavior again requires a new build-up of drive for activation. Dominant aggressive responses may be weakened through punishment. This type of learned inhibition results, in effect, in the lowering of a dominant response in the hierarchy of aggressive responses. One possible consequence of this is that the organism will subsequently exhibit a different aggressive response. The aggressive drive has found a new outlet by means of displacement. However, Dollard et al. (1939) did not propose that frustration always leads immediately or directly to aggression. Learned inhibitions may dam up the drive until some later frustrating event occurs.

Although the potential for an aggressive drive is claimed to be inborn, frustrating stimuli must also be present to initiate its development. Both biological and social factors appear equally important in the development of aggressive behavior and, as a result, the frustration–aggression hypothesis implies no clear primacy of either genetics or environment in the etiology of individual aggressive behavior.

3.2 Definition and Study Design

Aggression is defined as the "sequence of behavior, the goal-response to which is the injury of the person toward whom it is directed" (Dollard et al., 1939, p. 9). The connection between frustration and the build-up of aggressive energy or drive was postulated to be innate. Aggressive drive serves to energize available aggressive responses. This is basically a process-oriented and intuitive definition, but the theory's focus on frustration is also consistent with trigger-mechanism definitions.

Social psychological laboratory design represents the dominant study setting. While many different methods for investigating aggression in laboratory settings have been devised, most seem to fall into one of four major categories, involving (1) verbal assaults against others; (2) attacks against inanimate objects; (3) "safe" noninjurious assaults against live victims; and (4) ostensibly harmful attacks against such persons. The low threshold for behavior to be defined as aggression in drive theory is probably influenced by two factors: (1) the inheritance from the psychoanalytic founding of drive theory and (2) ethical limitations pertaining to the study of human aggression within the laboratory context.

3.3 Limitations and Shortcomings

Perhaps one of the strongest assets of the frustration–aggression hypothesis was the specifications of those factors which determine not only how frustrated an individual may become, but also how and when aggression will be expressed. The focus on these causative variables gave researchers the opportunity to test specific premises of the hypothesis empirically, resulting in intensive scientific scrutiny of the building blocks of the hypothesis. As a consequence, several specific predictions that were made from this hypothesis were validated (for reviews, see Bandura, 1973; Feshbach, 1970; Parke & Slaby, 1983). In particular, the formulation that frustration was a necessary precipitant of aggression was questioned by a substantial number of researchers (e.g., Buss, 1963; Pastore, 1952). Bandura criticized the drive (and instinct) theory because the internal determinants were inferred from the behavior they caused. He pinpointed this by applying the term pseudoexplanations on this process of circularity and clarified his position by stating that:

> "It should be emphasized here that it is not the existence of motivated behavior that is being questioned, but rather whether such behavior is at all explained by ascribing it to the action of drives or other inner forces." (Bandura, 1973, p. 40).

In sum, without an independent ability to observe and measure the presence, accumulation, and release of aggressive energy, it is not possible to identify responses as aggression (Tedeschi, 1983). The assumption that an organism is programmed so that frustration always creates an instigation to aggress, and that this remains until it is discharged by aggressive behavior has been contradicted by two lines of evidence. Firstly, efforts to provide empirical support have failed to do so and, more fundamentally, biologists have found that an organism is simply not capable of storing energy or of cumulating energy over time.

In a midway point on the continuum of critics, Leonard Berkowitz (e.g., Berkowitz, 1993) emerged as a proponent of both support to, and criticism of, the original formulation. He reformulated the hypothesis by lending increased emphasis to the impact of social context and social judgment. By this he more or less discarded the original linear stimulus-drive conceptualization. One of his theoretical building blocks was to comprehend frustration to be an aversive event that generates aggression only to the extent that it produces negative affect.

The attractiveness of the actual goal, the character of associated cognitions and situational cues have an important influence on the strength of the instigation to aggression and the reader is referred, for example, to Tedeschi and Felson (1994) for a critical review of Berkowitz's theory of aggression. In sum, the frustration—aggression theory was sufficiently accurate to allow for experimental disconfirmations as well as support for the theory. Thus, as is the case with all good scientific theories, it produced evidence of its own limitations.

3.4   Relevance to Current Clinical Practice

Because drive theory of aggression attributes such behavior to the presence of specific environmental conditions, i.e., frustrating events, and not only to innate tendencies toward violence, it is somewhat more optimistic with respect to prevention, control, and treatment than Freud's instinct theory. That is, it seems to suggest that the removal of all external sources of frustration from the environment would go a long way toward eliminating human aggression. Unfortunately, though, frustration is probably such a frequent and commonplace occurrence for most individuals that its total elimination seems quite unfeasible.

The impact of frustration as a precursor to intrainstitutional aggressive behavior in psychiatric patients clearly demonstrates this point. Clinical studies on the exact nature of patient–staff interactions that may increase the risk of violence in psychiatric wards are steadily growing in number (e.g., Nijman, Merkelbach, Allert, & a Campo, 1997). A strong relationship between problems of communication in staff–patient interactions and the increased risk of violence is documented in several studies (Owen, Tarantello, Jones, & Tenant, 1998; Whittington & Wykes, 1996). Shah, Fineberg, and James (1991) argued that authoritarian staff attitudes and lack of communication between staff and patient may elicit violence. Earlier studies have reached similar conclusions (e.g., Katz & Kirkland, 1990; Rice, Harris, Varney, & Quincey, 1989). In their studies, Blair (1991) and Flannery, Hanson, Penk, and Flannery (1996) found that inflexible attitudes among staff members and lack of consistency in setting limits may induce violence. Still another study concluded that experienced staff were significantly more competent in helping patients control their anxiety, more ready to ask for help and less reluctant to admit that they were anxious in certain limit-setting interactions (Perregaard & Bartels, 1992). The authors hypothesize that such characteristics explain the disproportionately low number of violent encounters experienced nurses were involved in, compared to those with less experience.

It is quite well documented that limit-setting situations are frequent precipitants of violence in psychiatric wards. Efforts to reduce the number of limit-setting interactions may be one evident consequence of these findings. However, limit setting is an integrated part of a structured treatment approach that has been demonstrated to be superior to an unstructured approach in the treatment of potentially violent, psychiatric patients (e.g., Aquilina, 1991; Flannery et al., 1996; Friis & Helldin, 1994; Katz & Kirkland, 1990). It is argued here that efforts to better nurses' ability to identify escalating situations, together with measures taken to improve the quality of staff communication in limit-setting interactions, may reduce both rates of violence and the number of limit-setting episodes. Empirical evidence for the efficacy of staff training programs is steadily growing. Using a therapeutic management protocol, Kalogjera and associates obtained a 64% reduction in seclusions and restraints on three wards (Kalogjera, Bedi, Watson, & Meyer, 1989). Their protocol gives detailed suggestions about how staff members should react to patients' disruptive behavior at an early stage. To reduce the individual patient's level of frustration is basic to this procedure. To my knowledge, a study by Nijman and coworkers (1997) is one of the first studies of staff training programs that include control conditions. This study failed to find a strong effect of staff training on rates of aggression, mainly because there was a marked reduction in frequencies of aggressive behavior in both experimental (about 60%) and control wards (about 40%). Nijman and coworkers conclude that standardized reporting, by staff, of aggressive episodes may, in itself, reduce rates of aggression. Similar findings have been reported in other studies (e.g., Nilson, Palmstierna, & Wistedt, 1988). There are reasons to believe that one positive effect of accurate recording of aggressive incidents is to obtain an improved overview of frustrating factors and interactions for the individual patient.

Apparently, there is a need for further research to improve the content and clinical implementation of such standardized staff training programs. Such programs should primarily focus warning signs and situational antecedents of violence, in addition to communication styles aimed at conflict resolution and calming down in limit-setting interactions to minimize frustration.

Since violence rarely erupts without warning, staff guidelines for optimal timing of, and preplanned criteria for, when to set limits for patients are important factors in an optimal staff intervention procedure. Monitoring of early warning signs in the individual patient may allow for early interventions while the level of frustration is still low in both patient and staff (Tardiff, 1989). There appears to be good empirical evidence for the fact that recidivist patients generally show warning signs prior to violent acts in psychiatric wards (Linaker & Busch-Iversen, 1995; Powell, Caan, & Crowe, 1994).

Very few procedures and forms developed to measure violence in psychiatric patients give prominence to situational factors in their structures (Bjørkly, 1996). Referring to findings from studies within the drive theory tradition, it is claimed here that effective treatment and prevention of violence on psychiatric wards may profit from a more comprehensive and accurate monitoring of frustrating situational precipitants of violence (Bjørkly, 1999).

4   SOCIAL LEARNING THEORY

Learning theory was the dominant scientific approach to psychology in the first half of the twentieth century. The development and application of these theories to aggressive behavior has been led by Arnold Buss and Albert Bandura. In sharp contrast to the instinct or drive views of aggression, which suggest that aggression stems from one or a limited number of crucial factors, the social learning framework holds that it may actually be elicited and established by a large and varied range of conditions. Buss's theory represented a transition by its emphasis on personality and social factors as variables affecting aggressive behavior. Still, Bandura's theory is the most influential learning theory of aggression, and a natural first choice for presentation here.

4.1   Theory of Aggression

According to Bandura (1973), a comprehensive analysis of aggressive behavior requires careful attention to three issues (1) the ways such actions are acquired ("Origins of aggression"), (2) the factors that instigate their occurrence ("Instigators of aggression"), and (3) the conditions that maintain their performance ("Regulators of aggression"). In short, to understand aggressive behavior, we need exactly the same kind of analyses that would be required for any other kind of behavior. A wide variety of reinforcers appear to play a role ("Origins of aggression") (1) acquisition of material incentives, (2) social approval or increased status, (3) the alleviation of aversion treatment, and (4) pain and suffering on the part of the victim. Although people sometimes learn aggressive behavior by trial and error, most complex skills are learned vicariously by observing others. According to Bandura, learning by observation involves four interrelated processes. First, one must notice or pay attention to the cues, behavior, and outcomes of the modeled event. Then the observations must be encoded into some form of memory representation. Third, these cognitive processes are transformed into new imitative response patterns. Finally, given the appropriate incentives, the modeled behavior will be performed. The characteristics of the model are important in this process:

> "People are most frequently rewarded for following the behavior of models who are intelligent, who possess certain social and technical competencies, command social power, and who, by their adroitness, occupy high positions in various status hierarchies." (Bandura, 1986, p. 128).

Bandura claims that family members, individual subcultures, and mass media are the three principal sources of aggressive modeling.

Social learning theory distinguishes between two broad classes of motivators of behavior. Biologically based motivators include internal aversive stimulation arising from tissue deficits, and external sources of aversive stimulation that activate behavior through their painful effects. Cognitive representation of future outcomes aiding individuals to generate current motivators of aggression, form the other main group of motivators. Both classes of motivators are closely linked up to modeling of aggressive behavior. There are four processes by which modeling can instigate aggressive behavior ("Instigators of aggression"): A *directive function* of modeling serves to inform the observer about the causal means-ends relations in the situation. By extracting a general principle from observing the model's experience, observers can generalize a causal understanding that, under the same conditions, they will receive the same outcome as the model if they imitate him/her. On the other side, a *disinhibitory function* of a model teaches observers that they can get away with aggressive behavior without being punished for it. Observations of others who engage in aggressive behavior cause *emotional arousal* in the observers. This may increase the likelihood of imitative aggression and even heighten the intensity of aggressive responses. Finally, observations of a model may have *stimulus-enhancing effects* by directing the observers' attention to the aggressive expressions and methods being used. In addition to this, Bandura claims that *instructions* also serve as instigators of aggressive behavior, and that aggression can be triggered by bizarre internal beliefs such as delusions.

Once aggression has been acquired, a number of different factors operate to ensure that it will be maintained ("Regulators of aggression"). Not surprisingly, many of these are similar to the factors that facilitate their initial acquisition. (1) Successful aggression against others often continues to provide aggressors with tangible and social rewards. (2) It also has the potential of alleviating aversive or abusive treatment from others. (3) Self-reinforcement by self-administering praise and approval for the completion of aggressive behavior is yet another regulator of aggression. It is worthwhile noting, however, that in social learning theory a self-system is not a psychic agent that controls aggressive behavior. Rather, it refers to cognitive structures that provide the referential standards against which aggressive and other behavior is judged.

4.2   Definition and Study Design

According to Bandura, aggression is defined as:

> "Behavior that results in personal injury and physical destruction. The injury may be physical, or it may involve psychological impairment through disparagement and abusive exercise of coercive power." (Bandura, 1983, p. 2).

The emphasis on the attribution of personal responsibility and injurious intent to the harm-doer places this definition within the trigger-mechanism group. The important role of various types of reinforcement and punishment as regulators of aggression confirms that this is also a consequence-oriented definition.

Assaults by individuals against inanimate objects are by far the most frequently used study method within the social learning paradigm. Typically, participants are first instigated to aggression through exposure to the actions of an aggressive model, and then provided with an opportunity to kick, punch, or otherwise attack some inanimate object. Aggression is then assessed in terms of the frequency with which they direct such actions against the target. The best-known application of such procedures is found in the "Bobo doll" studies first conducted by Bandura and his colleagues (Bandura, Ross, & Ross, 1963). These procedures have been criticized for only inflicting harm upon an inflatable doll and not upon another living being, as is explicitly included in Bandura's definition of aggression. Bandura has responded to this criticism by calling attention to the distinction between the learning and the performance of aggressive responses. Still, one may question as to what extent Bandura's strong emphasis on subjective judgments of intentions and causality in the definition of aggression is influenced by the preferred study design, and vice versa.

4.3   Limitations and Shortcomings

Bandura's social learning theory has been criticized for not being a specific aggression theory per se (e.g., Pepitone, 1974). This concurs well with Bandura's learning theory position claiming that even though deviant, e.g., aggressive, and constructive, e.g., pro-social, behavior are topographically different, they are established and maintained by the same basic learning principles. Tedeschi and Felson (1994) have focused on two main shortcomings in Bandura's theory of aggression. Firstly, they question the evidence for the role of self-regulation as applied to aggressive behavior. Their main point is that the development of self-regulatory processes do not place all aggressive behavior under self-control:

> "Cognitive reinterpretations can take the form of justifying the aggressive behavior, by minimizing, ignoring, or misconstruing the consequences, or by

dehumanizing or blaming the victim. Such justifications disinhibit behavior that otherwise would be considered reprehensible and would be inhibited by anticipations of self-punishment." (Tedeschi & Felson, 1994, p. 108).

Secondly, they claim that social learning theory ignores the social context within which behavior is learned or performed. More specifically, this relates to limitations set by the laboratory design that has dominated social learning theory studies on aggression. The generalizability or external validity of laboratory findings is questioned by stating that, in spite of the name, the focus of social learning theory is on the individual, and the theory tends to underestimate the reciprocal behavior of people engaged in social interactions. Others have pointed at considerable ambiguity concerning the various mechanisms posited to explain the empirically demonstrated modeling effects in aggressive behavior (e.g., Zillmann, 1979). Exposure to models is a basic element for any kind of model learning. In his research Bandura has addressed important determining factors of this exposure (origins, instigators and regulators of aggression). Yet, basic questions remain unanswered concerning which of the mechanisms proposed is mainly responsible for the modeling effect: What type of model achieves what effect, on what kind of individuals, under what circumstances? The informative function, vicarious conditioning, and changes in the perception of salient features of the individuals involved are confounded: Is it possible to test their involvement or their respective contributions in the modeling process?

Whatever its shortcomings, Bandura's theory is the most sophisticated theory of aggression from a learning perspective. Today, few psychologists question the importance of modeling in the study of human behavior or the view that anticipations of future consequences guide human behavior.

4.4   Relevance to Current Clinical Practice

Although originally not meant to be a model of clinical relevance, principles from social learning theory can be traced to current clinical psychology. In particular, cognitive behavior therapy (CBT) shares basic behavior analytical concepts and explanatory mechanisms with social learning theory. In addition to agreement on how behavior is regulated by external consequences, the understanding of self-regulatory mechanisms constitutes an important point of contact. According to Bandura, people can exercise some influence over their own behavior through self-generated inducements and self-produced consequences. In this self-regulatory process, people adopt through tuition and modeling certain standards of behavior, and respond to their own actions in self-rewarding or self-punishing ways. In social learning theory, a self-system refers to cognitive structures that provide the referential standards against which behavior is judged. Howells and collaborators have described nine types of basic CBT intervention methods for violent offenders (Howells, Watt, Hall, & Baldwin, 1997). Six of these reflect basic elements from Bandura's social learning theory of aggression: identifying and modifying the immediate triggering events, identifying and modifying contextual stressors, changing cognitive inferences and dysfunctional schemata, undermining dysfunctional inferences and schemata by tracing their developmental roots, broadening the repertoire of coping responses, and prevention of escalating social behavior. These interventions all relate to one or more of Bandura's three main components of social learning analysis of aggression: origins, instigators and regulators of aggression.

Dialectical Behavior Therapy (DBT) is a comprehensive cognitive behavioral treatment originally developed for chronically parasuicidal women diagnosed with Borderline Personality Disorder (Linehan, 1993). Over the past decade it has been adapted for many other populations, including violent psychiatric patients (e.g., Berzins & Trestman, 2004). A central component of DBT involves targeting the following four behavioral skills modules (1) mindfulness skills, (2) distress tolerance skills, (3) emotion regulation skills, and (4) interpersonal effectiveness skills. Mindfulness targets lack of self-regulation and confusion by emphasizing self-awareness. Distress tolerance involves distraction and self-soothing techniques. Emotion regulation teaches people how to reduce their vulnerability to negative emotions and how to increase positive emotions. Interpersonal effectiveness teaches them assertiveness and how to deal with conflict situations. There is a striking resemblance between these skill modules and Bandura's component processes in the self-regulation of behavior (1) self-observation (performance dimensions), (2) judgmental process (personal standards, referential performances, valuation of activity, and personal attribution), (3) self-response (self-evaluative reactions, tangible self-applied consequences, and no self-response).

Clinical assessment and interventions based on individual warning signs fit well into Bandura's component processes in the self-regulation of behavior. Some patients isolate themselves, others become overactive, some become physically tense, others glower, some express psychotic symptoms, etc., as indicators of increased violence risk. Recognition and an awareness of these warning signs may help both patients and their environment to implement aggression preventive measures. In both CBT and DBT the recognition of recurrent warning signs as specific individual precursors of violence is emphasized to have an important role in successful treatment and relapse prevention. In spite of this, there appears to be a paucity of instruments available for accurate and clinically useful measurement of warning signs of violence.

Although the influence of principles from social learning theory, to my knowledge, is not outspoken in either the CBT or the DBT tradition, it appears to be present in the basic principles depicted above. No matter what came first of CBT and social learning theory, the clinical relevance of Bandura's theory of aggression appears to be well demonstrated.

5   CONCLUDING REMARKS

By addressing the main theoretical points, this chapter deals with three classical theories of aggression and their definition of aggression, study design, limitations and shortcomings, and relevance to clinical practice. In Table 1, the main theoretical foci of the three theories are depicted. It illustrates the psychoanalytic biological/instinctive position at one extreme, and the cognitive and social interactionist stance of social learning theory at the other.

Still, it is worthwhile to note that one of the hallmarks of modern psychoanalytic theories such as attachment theory is the emphasis put on cognitive functions and social interactions in the understanding of human aggression. In psychological terms, secure attachment relationships allow the developing individual to construct "internal working models," of himself and others. These models are based on the interaction between the individual and the attachment figure, which becomes established as internal cognitive structures. The idea that disrupted social interactions with important others may predispose the individual to disrupted/aggressive cognitive schemata constitute a basic idea in Bandura's theory of aggression. Thus, apparently the last decades have witnessed that psychoanalysis and social learning theory have approached each other concerning the view on the nature and origins of aggression.

Naturally, the main theoretical foci are reflected in the individual theory's preferred definition of aggression as well. Psychoanalysis and drive theory share the process-oriented/intuitive type of definition (Table 2). Social learning theory stands alone as an adherer of a consequence-oriented definition, while it shares the trigger-mechanism element with drive theory.

The psychoanalytical definition does not include reactive aggression and social learning theory does not hold the view that self-injurious behavior is aggression (Table 3). Apart from that, the definitions are surprisingly similar when one takes into consideration that they represent different theoretical positions.

The inclusion of damage to property is controversial in terms of the discriminant validity of the definition of aggression. Discriminant validity involves documenting that a characteristic, e.g., aggression, does not relate to other characteristics, e.g.,

Table 1. Theoretical Main Foci

Theory of Aggression	Biological Perspective	Instinct Perspective	Drive Perspective	Cognitive Functions	Social Interaction
Psychoanalysis	X	X			
Drive theory		X	X		
Social learning theory				X	X

Table 2. Type of Definition of Aggression

Theory of Aggression	Process Oriented/Intuitive	Trigger Mechanism	Consequence Oriented
Psychoanalysis	X		
Drive theory	X	X	
Social learning theory		X	X

Table 3. Definitional Criteria

Theory of Aggression	Physical Damage to			Type of Aggression			
	Verbal	Indirect	Reactive	Property	Self	Other persons	Intension
Psychoanalysis	X	X	X	X	X		(X)[b]
Drive theory	X	X	X	X	X	X	X
Social learning theory	X		X	X	X	X	X

[a]As sufficient criterion in itself.
[b]The motive of the act may be unconscious but the act may still be intentional.

anger, from which it should be independent. In short: What is the rationale behind categorizing damage to property as aggression instead of, let us say, anger? Freud's theory has been criticized for lack of discriminant validity due to the wide array of very different social expressions he asserted to be governed by the death instinct. More precisely, it is not very easy to acknowledge that diametrically opposed behavior such as artistic creativity and homicide stem from the same instinct. Concerning the two other theories of aggression, one may question whether a wide definition of aggression has emerged due to the fact that the great majority of investigations of aggression have been performed within laboratory settings. Naturally, a research design involving damage to property is much more feasible and ethically acceptable than letting participants hurt each other physically. However, in addition to the definitional issue, laboratory research raises a number of potential problems. For example, participants know quite well that they are taking part in a psychological experiment, and once they do they may confirm, refute or ignore predictions of "what the experiment is all about." Social learning theory is the most broadly based, and psychoanalysis the most limited, approach in terms of span of research methods (Table 4). One may question whether sticking to one single research method has deprived psychoanalysis of a more comprehensive external validation of the theory.

At the other end, the fact that social learning theory has been empirically validated within a range of multiple research designs may have strengthened its current position as the leading theory of aggression.

Table 4. Research Methods

Theory of Aggression	Laboratory Trials	Indirect Methods[a]	Information from Victim/ Aggressor	Direct Observation	Field Experiment	Therapy Notes
Psychoanalysis						X
Drive theory	X				X	
Social learning theory	X	X	X	X	X	

[a]Criminal registers, information from collaterals, surveys, etc.

In this chapter, three classical theories of aggression and their relevance to clinical practice have been presented. The main motive for doing this has been to bring attention to the importance of a careful theoretical founding of research on aggression. It is claimed that this is of particular relevance to clinical research and practice pertaining to aggression in people with mental disorders, since atheoretical positions very easily lead into aimless clinical pragmatism. Still, one must always remember that theory is a useful servant, but a useless master.

REFERENCES

Akhtar, S. (1995). Some reflections on the nature of hatred and its emergence in the treatment process—Discussion of Kernberg's chapter "Hatred as a core affect of aggression" In: S. Akhtar, S. Kramer & H. Parens (Eds.), *The birth of hatred. Developmental, clinical, and technical aspects of intense aggression* (pp. 83–103). New Jercy: Jason Aronson Inc.

Aquilina, C. (1991). Violence by psychiatric in-patients. *Medicine, Science, and the Law, 31*, 306–312.

Bakermans-Kranenburg, M. J., & van Ijzendoorn, M. H. (1993). A psychometric study of the Adult Attachment Interview: Reliability and discriminant validity. *Developmental Psychology, 29*, 870–879.

Bandura, A. (1973). *Aggression: A social learning analysis*. Englewood Cliffs, NJ: Prentice Hall.

Bandura, A. (1983). Psychological mechanisms of aggression. In: R. G. Geen & E. I. Donnerstein (Eds.), *Aggression: Theoretical and empirical reviews. (Vol. 1) Theoretical and methodological issues* (pp. 1–40). New York: Academic Press.

Bandura, A. (1986). *Social foundations of thought and action: A social cognitive theory*. Englewood Cliffs, NJ: Prentice Hall.

Bandura, A., Ross, D., & Ross, S. A. (1963). Vicarious reinforcement and imitative learning. *Journal of Abnormal and Social Psychology, 67*, 601–607.

Berkowitz, L. (1993). *Aggression—Its causes, consequences, and control*. New York: McGraw-Hill.

Berzins, L. G., & Trestman, R. L. (2004). The development and implementation of Dialectical Behavior Therapy in forensic settings. *International Journal of Forensic Mental Health, 3*, 93–103.

Bjørkly, S. (1996). Report Form for Aggressive Episodes: Preliminary report. *Perceptual and Motor Skills, 83*, 1139–1152.

Bjørkly, S. (1999). A ten-year prospective study of aggression in a special secure unit for dangerous patients. *Scandinavian Journal of Psychology, 40*, 57–65.

Bjørkly, S. (2001). *Aggresjonens psykologi—psykologiske perspektiv på aggresjon (Theories of aggression—psychological perspectives on aggression)*. Oslo, Norway: Universitetsforlaget.

Blair, T. (1991). Assaultive behavior: Does provocation begin in the front office? *Journal of Psychosocial Nursing and Mental Health Services, 29*, 21–26.

Bornstein, R. F. (2001). Clinical utility of the Rorschach inkblot method: Reframing the debate. *Journal of Personality Assessment, 77*, 39–47.

Bowlby, J. (1989). *A secure base: Parent-child attachment and healthy human development*. New York: Basic Books.

Brenner, C. (1971). The psychoanalytic concept of aggression. *The International Journal of Psychoanalysis, 52*, 137–144.

Buss, A. H. (1961). *The Psychology of aggression*. New York: Wiley.

Buss, A. H. (1963). Physical aggression in relation to different frustrations. *Journal of Abnormal and Social Psychology, 67*, 1–7.

Dollard, J., Doob, L., Miller, N., Mowrer, O. H., & Sears, R. R. (1939). *Frustration and aggression*. New Haven, Conn: Yale University Press.

Dubin, W. R. (1989). The role of fantasies, countertransference, and psychological defenses in patient violence. *Hospital and Community Psychiatry, 40*, 1280–1283.

Feshbach, S. (1970). Aggression. In: P. H. Mussen (Ed.), *Carmichael's manual of child Psychology.* (Vol. 2). New York: Wiley.

Finnema, E. J., Dassen, T., & Halfens, R. (1994). Aggression in psychiatry: A qualitative study focusing on the characterization and perception of patient aggression by nurses working on psychiatric wards. *Journal of Advanced Nursing, 19,* 1088–1095.

Flannery, R. B., Hanson, M. A., Penk, W. E., & Flannery, G. J. (1996). Violence and the lax milieu? Preliminary data. *The Psychiatric Quarterly, 67,* 47–50.

Fonagy, P. (2003). Towards a developmental understanding of violence. *The British Journal of Psychiatry: The Journal of Mental Science, 183,* 190–192.

Freud, S. (1920). *Beyond the pleasure principle. Standard Edition, (Vol. 18).* London: Hogarth Press.

Friis, S., & Helldin, L. (1994). The contribution made by the clinical setting to violence among psychiatric patients. *Criminal behaviour and mental health : CBMH, 4,* 341–352.

Gacono, C. B., Meloy, J. R., & Bridges, M. (2000). A Rorschach comparison of psychopaths, sexual homicide perpetrators, and non-violent pedophiles: Where angels fear to tread. *Journal of Clinical Psychology, 56,* 757–777.

Howells, K., Watt, B., Hall, G., & Baldwin, S. (1997). Developing programs for violent offenders. *Legal and Criminological Psychology, 2,* 117–128.

Kalogjera, I. J., Bedi, A., Watson, W. N., & Meyer, A. D. (1989). Impact of therapeutic management on use of seclusion and restraint with disruptive adolescent inpatients. *Hospital and Community Psychiatry, 40,* 280–285.

Katz, P., & Kirkland, F. R. (1990). Violence and social structure on mental hospital wards. *Psychiatry, 53,* 262–277.

Linaker, O. M., & Busch-Iversen, H. (1995). Predictors of imminent violence in psychiatric inpatients. *Acta Psychiatrica Scandinavica, 92,* 250–254.

Linehan, M. M. (1993). *Cognitive-behavioral treatment of borderline personality disorder.* New York: Guilford Press.

Lion, J.R., & Pasternak, A. (1973). Countertransference reactions to violent patients. *The American Journal of Psychiatry, 130,* 207–209.

Nestor, P. G. (2002). Mental disorder and violence: Personality dimensions and clinical features. *The American Journal of Psychiatry, 159,* 1973–1978.

Nijman, H. L. I., Merkelbach, H. L. G. J., Allert, W. F. F., & aCampo, J. M. L. G. (1997). Prevention of aggressive incidents on a closed psychiatric ward. *Psychiatric Services, 48,* 694–698.

Nilson, K., Palmstierna, T., & Wistedt, B. (1988). Aggressive behavior in hospitalized psychogeriatric patients. *Acta Psychiatrica Scandinavica, 78,* 172–175.

Okey, J. L. (1992). Human aggression: The etiology of individual differences. *Journal of Humanistic Psychology, 32,* 51–64.

Owen, C., Tarantello, C., Jones, M., & Tenant, C. (1998). Violence and aggression in psychiatric units. *Psychiatric Services, 49,* 1452–1457.

Parke, R. D., & Slaby, R. G. (1983). The development of aggression. In P. H. Mussen (Ed.), *Handbook of child psychology (Vol. 4),* (pp. 547–561), New York: Academic Press.

Pastore, N. (1952). The role of arbitrariness in the frustration–aggression hypothesis. *Journal of Abnormal and Social Psychology, 47,* 728–731.

Pedder, J. (1992). Psychoanalytic views of aggression: Some theoretical problems. *The British Journal of Medical Psychology, 65,* 95–106.

Pepitone, A. (1974). Aggression—A matter of stimulus and reinforcement control. *Contemporary Psychology 19,* 769–771.

Perregaard, R. N., & Bartels, U. (1992). Violence against staff in a mental hospital. Abstract. *First European symposium on aggression in clinical psychiatric practise,* (pp. 22–23). Stockholm: The Psychiatric Institution, Karolinska Institute, Danderyd Hospital.

Powell, G., Caan, W., & Crowe, M. (1994). What events precede violent incidents in psychiatric hospitals. *The British Journal of Psychiatry, 165,* 107–112.

Rice, M. E., Harris, G. T., Varney, G. W., & Quinsey, V. L. (1989). *Violence in institutions: Understanding, prevention and control.* Toronto: Hogrefe and Huber.

Shah, A. K., Fineberg, N. A., & James, D. V. (1991). Violence among psychiatric inpatients. *Acta Psychiatrica Scandinavica, 84,* 305–309.

Tardiff, K. (1989). *Assessment and management of violent patients.* Washington, DC: American Psychiatric Press.

Tedeschi, J. T. (1983). Social influence theory and aggression. In: R. G. Geen & E. I. Donnerstein (Eds.), *Aggression—Theoretical and methodological reviews (Vol. 1).* New York: Academic Press.

Tedeschi, J. T., & Felson, R. B. (1994). *Violence, aggression and coercive actions.* Washington, DC: APA.

Whittington, R., & Wykes, T. (1996). "Going in strong": Confrontive coping by staff. *Journal of Forensic Psychiatry 5,* 609–614.

Zillmann, D. (1979). *Hostility and aggression.* Hillsdale, NJ: Lawrence Erlbaum Associates.

3

From the Individual to the Interpersonal: Environment and Interaction in the Escalation of Violence in Mental Health Settings[1]

RICHARD WHITTINGTON AND DIRK RICHTER

1   THE INDIVIDUAL AND THE INTERPERSONAL AS EXPLANATIONS FOR VIOLENCE

After several decades of controversial scientific research and debate, there is currently no doubt that mental disorders are sometimes associated with a certain elevated risk of violence and aggression (Link & Stueve, 1995). Although people with mental disorders contribute only a very small part to societal violence rates, an illness such as schizophrenia is associated with higher relative risks for affected people to become aggressive and even violent (Angermeyer, 2000; Walsh, Buchanan, & Fahy, 2002). Moreover, there is an overwhelming evidence for moderate to high rates of violence in all kinds of mental health settings (see chapter 1). In order to be able to develop prevention measures against violence in mental health settings, we need to understand which factors contribute to the emergence of this problem. This would not only help to protect staff from physical and psychological injury but

[1]Parts of this chapter have been previously published: Whittington, R., & Richter, D. (2005). Interactional aspects of violent behavior on acute psychiatric wards. *Psychology, Crime and Law, 11*, 1–12.

would also reduce the need for compulsory and coercive measures and, in the end, could contribute to more therapeutic work and treatment environments.

However, a major obstacle to achieving this goal is that there is little agreement among researchers and clinicians on the main causes of aggression and violence in mental health settings. While most commentators recognize the complexity of aggressive behavior and the likely role of multiple causative factors, much of the evidence-based debate has drawn on an epidemiological approach examining associations between demographic, clinical, and aggression variables "within" the patient to develop actuarial models of risk. Reviews of studies on the prediction of violent behavior of psychiatric patients on the basis of their symptoms and appearance have revealed a high rate of false positives even in the short term (Bjørkly, 1995; Steinert, 2002). Thus, even the presence of agitated and/or aggressive behavior is not a perfect predictor of becoming violent in the end.

It should be clear then that we need more sophisticated explanations of aggression and violence in mental health settings on which to base more effective interventions. Henk Nijman has already set up one such model from which we can launch our thinking (Nijman, 2002; Nijman et al., 1999). This model includes patient variables, ward variables, and staff variables which interact with each other and lead to the emergence of violence and aggression. However, the interaction between staff and patients itself remains a black box and it is the aim of this chapter to shine some light into this box. A large number of psychological ideas on stress, arousal, and aggressive behavior as well as sociological theories on the interaction between conflicting parties can be considered for their applicability to this problem. By considering psychiatric aggression where possible, like aggression by people without a diagnosed mental disorder, this behavior—which is usually viewed as purely "abnormal," i.e., due primarily to psychopathology or neuropathology—will be partially "normalized." At the moment, we only have half the picture in this area, drawn from the medical and epidemiological approaches. Once we have the full picture, one in which both pathological and everyday processes are considered, it will be easier to construct interventions which actually work in reducing the scale of the problem.

There is no attempt here to rule out entirely either neurobiological or psychopathological factors in an aggression. On the contrary we are, like many others, aware that a truly comprehensive approach will be multifactorial. We offer here a provisional integration of psychological and sociological approaches to the emergence of violence in psychiatric settings, but it is an integration which is based where possible on biological knowledge. The challenge will be to draw a sharp line between biological factors on the one hand and psychosocial factors on the other because aggressive traits and states are unquestionably influenced by human neurobiology.

The need to reconsider the interpersonal aspects of aggression is obvious when work on aggression in other settings is evaluated. Modern criminology highlights the importance of reciprocal interaction as the main trigger for homicides and other violent crimes. A recent large study of the structure and processes of US-homicides postulates that:

> "Violent crimes are distinct from property crimes in the sense that they consist
> of interactions between at least two parties, which are frequently characterized
> by dynamic exchanges of actions and words." (Miethe & Regoeczi, 2004:1f)

With a similar orientation toward aggressive interactions, an approach from organizational psychology to the general prevention of violence at work is based on the following assumption:

> "Human aggression is typically the product of interpersonal interactions wherein
> two or more persons become involved in a sequence of escalating moves
> and counter moves, each of which successively modifies the probability of
> subsequent aggression." (Cox & Leather, 1994:222)

The same point has been made with reference to violent incidents in prisons. Edgar, O'Donnell, and Martin (2003), describe their analysis of the dynamic interaction which precedes such incidents using the "escalator" tool (Alternatives to Violence Project, AVP, 1996). When asking the participants in a violent incident to describe the steps which lead up to actual violence, a sequence of moves and countermoves is almost always reported with the acts of violence usually described as legitimate responses to provocations by the other prisoner.

Obviously such events take place prior to psychiatric violence as well, but in this setting the pathologizing and medicalizing approach is so dominant that the simple question of what steps led up to the incident is rarely asked. Actually, a patient's individual neurobiology and psychopathology are just additional features that probably only shape the speed and the extent of the patient's reaction. They are facilitators and inhibitors of aggression rather than originators. As will be outlined below, the mental state of the patient and other psychological factors interact with cues from the environment in which this situation occurs. This approach echoes the context-dependent view put forward by social epidemiologists Bruce Link and Ann Stueve who stated more than ten years ago:

> "Rates of violence tend to be somewhat higher for people with mental illness
> than for the general population and for their demographic counterparts.
> Moreover, the association appears to be causal. Several alternative explana-
> tions—methodological and substantive—have been investigated, but none
> receives consistent support. It is possible, however, that mental illness only leads
> to violent behavior under certain conditions." (Link & Stueve, 1995:179)

A very recent Finnish study analyzed the circumstances of homicides by mentally ill offenders (Häkänen & Laajasalo, 2006). In the majority of cases where mentally ill patients were offenders, forensic experts found arguments preceding the homicidal incident, quite similar to the "healthy" control offenders. In the homicides of schizophrenic offenders, however, arguments before the incident were less reported. The situational "trigger" argument was further supported by the finding that only in a minority of cases were weapons taken to the crime scene. In other words, the elevated risk presented by people with a mental disorder is rarely, if ever, due to mental illness alone but occurs when there is a combination of environmental, biological, psychological, and social factors operating together. While consideration of all the possible variables is beyond the scope of this chapter, evidence linking a number of factors in each of these areas to the problem of violence in psychiatric settings will be reviewed.

2   THE LIMITATIONS OF CURRENT INTERVENTIONS

Our focus here is on the role of interpersonal factors and only with regard to one specific variant of psychiatric violence, reactive ("hot," emotional) aggression on wards, and our aim is to examine how theory can help to improve practice and targeted interventions with this behavior. In the search for effective interventions with this problem there are already at least two examples which must be mentioned. Firstly, people with long-standing anger and violence problems, many of whom may spend some time on wards, are often referred for some form of cognitive-behavioral intervention. These interventions are based on robust theoretical constructs, e.g., appraisal, and some of these are considered below. However, there is a limit to the applicability of these structured interventions in the seething group milieu of the psychiatric ward. Traditional anger management and stress inoculation training for people with aggression problems may only be effective when therapists are able to work systematically on core beliefs and behavior in the relative peace of the therapy room. However the risk to staff on, for instance, acute admission wards, is predominantly presented by newly admitted patients in the first day of their admission. At this time, staff will have no information on the patient's core beliefs, etc., and the patient's mental disorder will be at its most severe so the patient's suitability and capacity to engage in traditional treatments is very low. The challenge becomes therefore to see whether the models which have been successful in generating long-term therapeutic interventions can be used to improve deescalation in emergency situations.

Secondly, on the other hand, there are many deescalation training programs for mental health staff that aim at the behavioral modification of nurses and doctors in order to improve their assessment of danger and to prevent violent incidents in the hospital. Although the empirical evidence on the effectiveness of these programs shows mixed results, the approaches seem to work quite well with regard to staff confidence and knowledge about patient violence (see chapter 11). In many of these programs, deescalation is combined with other approaches to aggression management, particularly physical interventions (Calabro et al., 2002; Martin, 1995) as it is widely acknowledged that psychiatric hospital staff need both psychological and physical skills to prevent severe incidents. The main focus of deescalation efforts are obviously to influence the interaction between patients and staff so that risky situations do not result in physical violence and, as the names of the programs indicate, they try to teach skills that help to prevent escalation (see further details in chapter 11). Unfortunately, however, there is no valid elaborated model of escalation or interaction in mental health settings to be found in the literature nor are there sound empirical data that these training programs could be based upon. Therefore, we will outline some theoretical features of interaction and escalation as we go along which could form the basis for a model of deescalation.

3 THE PROVOKING ENVIRONMENT: AVERSIVE STIMULATION

Many aspects of the environment in which the ward-based patient finds him or herself are unpleasant and much of the behavior of the patient in this setting is an understandable response to the aversive experience of being on the ward. The environment can be seen as a source of aversive stimulation (Berkowitz, 1993) and the starting point for many of the problems which follow. Aversive stimulation can be defined as any event which increases emotional and/or physiological arousal and which is experienced as unpleasant by the person. If we look at the average psychiatric ward it is clear that there are many potential sources of aversive stimulation for the patient in terms of both the physical and the human environment. Other patients and staff are of course a potent source, either wittingly or unwittingly, with their tendency to engage in unsolicited touch, to move in too close, to use certain irritating types of nonverbal behavior, e.g., gestures, to use offensive words or tone of voice, even by smelling, or simply by their appearance. Negative arousal quickly becomes anger through rapid transfer of excitation through networks of associations. The general psychological assumption that the experience of injustice and disrespect is one of the most common sources of anger which may then lead to aggression and violence is obviously true for mental health settings, too. Many patients feel they are being treated with disrespect and injustice just by virtue of their involuntary admission into the psychiatric hospital and the ward regime.

How common is aversive stimulation as a factor in violence? Several studies in the early 1990s began an examination of the role of aversive stimulation in the generation of psychiatric aggression (Cooper & Medonca, 1991; Sheridan et al., 1990). Some subsequent studies are comparable to each other because they all use the Staff Observation Aggression Scale (SOAS) developed by Palmstierna and Wistedt (Palmstierna & Wistedt, 1987; see also Chapter 1 this volume). These studies were conducted in Australia, the Netherlands, and Italy (Cheung et al., 1996; Grassi et al., 2001; Nijman et al., 1997) and it can be seen in Figure 1 that there is some parity across the three studies in terms of the proportion of assaults occurring without apparent aversive stimulation (about 40%). It should be pointed out that this does not mean no provocation occurred simply that none was observed or none was considered appropriate for reporting. However, aversive stimulation by staff was reported frequently in the Netherlands relative to Australia and Italy, and provocation by another patient relatively infrequently. In a more detailed examination of aversive stimulation, Whittington and Wykes (1996) used postincident interviews with staff and patients to examine the frequency of aversive stimulation prior to incidents. They defined three types of aversive stimulation (frustration,

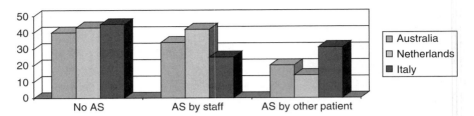

Figure 1. Proportion of patient aggressive incidents preceded by aversive stimulation (AS) in three studies using the SOAS. See text for references.

activity demand, and intrusion) and found that 86% of assaults on nurses were immediately preceded by the assaulted nurse engaging in one or more of these behaviors.

What are the reasons for conflicts in psychiatric settings? Obviously, there are situations that occur again and again where conflicts start. Several studies have found that ward rules and their implementation were frequent causes that led to aggressive situations (Bensley, 1995; Sheridan et al., 1990; see also Chapter 14). Richter (1999) found that everyday interactions such as washing or feeding the patients were more frequent in this respect. Certainly, it depends on the type of setting. In settings with more basic nursing tasks, e.g., in caring for the elderly or people with a learning disability, those situations will trigger more aggressive acts. In general psychiatric settings those triggers are found less. In most cases, staff try to hinder patients from doing something, absconding, violating rules, etc., or try to make patients do something; leave the room, take medication etc.

Very important in this regard is the observation that patients and staff see different reasons for escalating interactions. In a forensic setting, Harris and Varney (1986) asked patients and staff about this topic. Whereas nurses found no explicit reasons for most of the incidents, patients regarded only a small percentage as not being triggered by somebody. Provocations by fellow patients as well as by staff were most frequently identified by the patients. The differences between staff and patients on attributing the causes of aggression and violence have also been confirmed in recent research from other settings. Duxbury (2002) found that staff regarded patient-related internal causes to be mainly responsible for aggressive incidents but, in striking contrast, patients believed that external and situational triggers caused incidents. The same pattern was revealed by an Australian study. Again, Ilkiw-Lavalle and Grenyer (2003) asked patients and nurses for their views of the causes of specific violent incidents in which they had been involved. Although some patients did acknowledge that their mental illness contributed to the incidents, they also highlighted interpersonal and environmental factors that were not mentioned by staff.

It is clear then that the environment, in this case the behavior of other people, plays a role in making violence happen on psychiatric wards. What is not yet clear is the contents of the black box mediating between the environmental stimulus and the aggressive response in this specific setting. Sophisticated models of human aggression have been developed (e.g., Lindsay & Anderson, 2000) which recognize the complexity of factors contributing to "normal" aggression and such complexity needs to be considered with psychiatric violence as well. We will now review some aspects of current knowledge on biological and psychosocial factors which may prove fruitful in developing an understanding of this problem.

4   THE BIOLOGICAL BASIS OF VIOLENCE AND AGGRESSION

In psychiatry (Fonagy, 2003) as well as in nursing studies (Liu & Wuerker, 2005), recent overviews have described the current understanding of the biological under- pinning of violent and aggressive behavior. Current developmental models about this topic reveal that the mechanisms, which for many years have been used to explain how violent behavior is learned or acquired, are wrong. Contrary to previ- ous assumptions, violent predispositions are not acquired through childhood and adolescence but rather "normal" development leads to the unlearning of violent ten- dencies (Fonagy 2003). Aggression is a very early feature of children's behavior and it was assumed thus to be an innate drive which is tamed throughout the early years of life—as Sigmund Freud suggested several decades ago (see Chapter 2, this volume).

The neurobiological mechanisms that are associated with a higher risk for aggressive and violent behavior in adults, meanwhile, are becoming more and more clear (see review by Liu & Wuerker, 2005). Within biological models of aggression, the regulation of emotions plays a central role (Blair & Charney, 2003; Davidson et al., 2000). Current models regard three neural systems of the brain as essential for the emergence of aggression: amygdala, medial frontal cortex, and orbital frontal cortex. However, these systems do not work spontaneously. The neural basis for aggression is a reaction to an external stimulus, e.g., threats, cues, or frustrations. While brain damage, nutritional deficits, and prenatal or birth com- plications are regarded as external organic causes of aggression, several functional deficits can be described on the microlevel of the human brain. Well known and presumed causal mechanisms are related to neurotransmitters such as serotonin, levels of which are found to be lower in aggressive humans. From a neurobiolog- ical perspective "serotonin (5-HT) stands out as the primary modulator of aggres- sion" (Lesch, 2003:34). Another important relation between neurochemicals and aggressive behavior is known from the study of the neuroendocrine stress system (Haller & Kruk, 2003). Environmental challenges here lead to an increase of nora- drenergic neurotransmission, an increase of adrenaline production, and increased glucocorticoid production.

Given the extensive scrutiny that aggression and mental disorder generally receive in the biological sciences, there is surprisingly little research literature on the neurobiological factors underpinning aggression in specific psychiatric disorders (see review by Kohn & Asnis, 2003). For many of the disorders (e.g., Major Depression, Obsessive–Compulsive Disorder, Borderline Personality Disorder, Alzheimer Disease), the above-described dysfunction in the serotonergic system is suggested as an important contributor to aggression. However, for schizophrenia there are currently quite divergent results to be found in the literature and no clear tendency can be extracted from that research. This finding leads to a somewhat cautious statement about the neurobiology of aggression and its practical relevance for prevention. At the beginning of the 21st century and some years after the "decade of the brain," there are a few approaches that might turn out to be of practical relevance, e.g., the control of emotions, but at the moment there are no effective strategies to be seen or even to be expected which could be of any real help. This caution with regard to the practical relevance of biological research is even supported from within the biological research community itself (Niehoff, 1999; Young & Balaban, 2003). On the behavioral level, aggression and violence seem to depend too much on the other mediators mentioned above, so that any research limiting itself to the biological level remains stuck in basic science with little impact on treatment and practice. In order to connect the aggressive response to the aversive stimulus and to improve the management of this response we must go elsewhere inside the black box.

5 PSYCHOPATHOLOGY, PERSONALITY, AND VIOLENCE

Beyond biology, common clinical wisdom usually highlights aspects such as the actual psychopathology or longer lasting personality dispositions of the patient as the main risk factors for becoming violent. As mentioned above, when staff are asked to give reasons for violent incidents, nurses and doctors mainly refer to (assumed) internal mental processes of patients (Duxbury, 2002; Ilkiw-Lavalle & Grenyer, 2003). Perhaps as a result, the possible contribution of internal mental processes has received some attention from psychiatric research in recent decades, especially with schizophrenic patients. The main focus of attention has been on active delusions, hallucinations, and extreme personality traits.

A prominent approach in this regard is that of Bruce Link and colleagues who have found evidence for psychotic delusions as triggers of violent behavior (Link, Andrews, & Cullen, 1992; Link, Monahan, Stueve, & Cullen, 1999; Link & Stueve, 1995). Because the content of such delusions made patients feel threatened by others and/or had the effect of overriding internal controls that worked as shields against violent impulses, this syndrome has been called "threat/control override" (TCO). This theory has received some support from replication studies (Bjørkly & Havik, 2003), but not unanimously (Appelbaum, Robbins, & Monahan, 2000). In a review of studies on delusions and violence, Stal Bjørkly has stated that another possible psychopathological mechanism is emotional distress that might serve as a further mediator between delusions and violent acts (Bjørkly, 2002a). In addition, hallucinations, and especially command hallucinations, have been investigated in connection with their contribution to violence. As with the state of research on delusions, there are some studies that find an association. In another review, Stal Bjørkly has again compiled the findings on this topic (Bjørkly, 2002b) and, according to his results, there is some evidence that voices ordering acts of violence toward others may increase the risk of becoming actually violent. However, this evidence is still tentative (see also Chapter 6 this volume).

A different perspective has been taken in a recent review by Nestor (2002). This review argues for the importance of specific personality dimensions in human aggression and these are, in some cases, connected to positive psychopathological symptoms. The personality dimensions in question are impulse control, affect regulation, threatened egotism or narcissism, and paranoid cognitive style. The first two of these dimensions in particular are impaired in many patients with a wide variety of psychiatric disorders. This review argued that these dimensions operate jointly within the context of specific disorders and associated comorbidities.

The practical relevance of psychopathological and personality factors, however, for dealing with aggressive patients remains unproven. The predictive power of instruments using such dimensions, especially in acute care settings, is no better than good clinical expertise (Steinert, 2002; Steinert et al., 2000; and chapter 6, this volume). In our view, this inaccuracy does not completely compromise the instruments used for prediction, but it does point to the importance of other variables which have been neglected by such research in this area. Once again the individualistic approach, applied at either the neurobiological or the psychopathological levels is found wanting.

6   THE MISSING LINK: INTERACTION

The missing link in understanding, predicting, and managing violence in mental health settings, we would argue, is the idea of interaction. Only when this idea is given its due importance, in first theory and then practice, will it be possible to devise effective interventions. By definition, interpersonal violence between patients and staff requires at least two parties. Our focus is on a specific range of constructs, all of which are concerned with how one person (in this case, the one who becomes the assailant) thinks and draws conclusions about the behavior and motivations of another person (the one who becomes the target of an act of aggression). In the following sections we will argue that the aggressive interaction between patient and staff is shaped by expectations and aversive behavior which will be produced and decoded by each of the people involved. A crucial problem, therefore, is the issue of what and how each party feels and thinks about the other. This problem currently receives a lot of scientific attention in research areas that are not (as yet) closely connected to our topic of psychiatric violence research.

It is worth defining more precisely to what the idea of interaction refers. We are using it to refer to a range of mental and social phenomena all of which are concerned with how the behavior of a person (A) is understood and reacted to by another person (B). These phenomena are psychological and social in that everybody on the ward operates within both their own psychological system and the collective social system of the ward. The ideas thus apply to both patients and staff on the ward. The processes outlined below, unlike the "abnormalities" discussed so far, are applicable to the experience of both parties in the interaction and, to that extent, they are "normal." In other words they can be used to understand aggression in many situations although we would argue that they have particular relevance to understanding the problem here in mental health settings.

To be more specific, the psychological systems operating "within" each individual relating to the behavior of the other during an interaction consists of primary *appraisal* processes in which an incoming stimulus is classified as aversive or non-aversive, and the capacity to judge the intentions of the other person and to see the world from their point of view (*Theory of mind and empathy*). The social system in which both patient and nurse operate when interacting is rooted in these psychological systems but has a life of its own. Here the key processes are the expectations that the person has about the future behavior of the other person in front of them (*double contingency and distrust*) and the sequence of *escalation* (or deescalation). Ultimately, without effective deescalation and enhanced awareness of the importance of interaction among staff, a *stable conflict culture* may emerge. We will now consider each of these in turn.

7   PSYCHOLOGICAL SYSTEM

7.1   Cognitive Appraisal

The importance of the provoking environment and the role of external stimulation in triggering brain systems has been discussed above. But what is the nature of this provocation? How does an incoming stimulus, e.g., touching, become aversive rather than neutral or rewarding? One way of understanding how this happens is set out by Lazarus's cognitive-mediational theory of stress, appraisal, and coping (Lazarus, 1999; Lazarus & Folkman, 1984). This approach places cognitive appraisal and coping at the center of an explanation of how people define, experience and react to stressful events. The theory is not primarily concerned with aggressive behavior *per se* except perhaps as one form of behavior used to cope with stress. However, the appraisal concept has recently been integrated into a model specifically addressing aggressive behavior (Anderson & Bushman, 2002). Two types of stressful primary appraisals are relevant in this context: threat appraisals (if the person anticipates that a physical or psychological loss or harm is imminent) and harm appraisals (if the person has already experienced loss or harm). Coping is seen as a dynamic process whereby the person, having reviewed their coping options, selects an approach which may be cognitive or behavioral, e.g., aggression, and may be directed at dealing with the problem itself, i.e., the source of stressful arousal, in this case the frustrating nurse, or directed at dealing simply with the emotions generated by the source, e.g., changing the way that you think about the frustrating nurse. Among staff, the idea of secondary appraisal is related to the important idea of confidence and self-efficacy which has been the focus of a number of training interventions (see Chapter 11 this volume).

Various aspects of some types of mental disorder can be reformulated in these appraisal and coping terms. Distorted primary appraisal could occur in paranoia and certain cognitive disorders where there is an overinterpretation of the significance of a neutral event for the person's well being. At the next level, coping selection decisions may occur too quickly due to temporary disinhibition as part of a manic phase, or to more stable impulsivity as part of a personality disorder. These decisions may also be restricted due to overreliance on fixed scripts, including aggression, as part of other forms of personality disorder.

Perceived intention and control are two important aspects to evaluate when judging the aversiveness of another person's behavior. When staff aversively stimulate a patient, for example if physically restraining them, it can be with three possible types of intention. It can be done deliberately in order to upset the patient, i.e., punitively; it can be done deliberately but as part of caring for the patient, i.e., therapeutically, e.g., preventing absconding and self-harm; or it can be done accidentally without any intent or awareness of an impact on the patient. With regard to control, some forms of stimulation staff may have control over, e.g., the way they speak, move, or dress, but others they will have no control over, e.g., some aspects of their appearance. Prejudiced patients, for instance, will be aversively stimulated simply by observing a nurse from the relevant disliked group.

It is also important to distinguish the actual and perceived control staff have over their own behavior when aversively stimulating the patient as the patient may perceive a therapeutic or accidental contact as a deliberate attack (cf. hostile attributional bias, Dodge & Coie, 1987). The thing that staff have most control over is their own behavior when interacting with patients. Since, as we have seen, this behavior can be a significant source of negative affect for patients it is also, as we will see below, a significant precedent for violent incidents, and it is appropriate to focus primarily upon this. It is one of the paradoxes of psychiatric care work that good care of some disordered people inevitably involves denying and otherwise controlling their movements and the challenge for all staff who have to do this is how to do it well and generate the least negative affect in their patients. The challenge for organizations is to help benign staff to develop these skills and to identify the small minority of staff who may be using aversive stimulation punitively.

7.2   Theory of Mind and Empathy

Accurate perceptions of intent and control are based on an ability to be aware of the perspective of the other person and, within social cognitive neuroscience, a major research topic at the moment is how we understand others' actions and others' minds. According to the current state of research, the emergence of such skills has an evolutionary basis, because humans had to adjust more and more to a socially complex environment (Brothers, 1997). The neurobiological mechanisms and brain areas associated with these high-level skills have already been detected, e.g., the so-called "mirror neurons" that play an important role in action understanding (Rizzolatto & Craighero, 2004). An in-depth review of social neuroscience is beyond the scope of this chapter and the reader is referred to some recent published overviews (Adolphs, 1999; Blakemore et al., 2004; Frith & Wolpert, 2003). The ideas we present below draw on these reviews but are, of course, preliminary hypotheses, due to the tentative connection currently between social neuroscience and violence research in psychiatry. But the parallels between what we know about social interactions as precursors of violence in mental health settings and the recent findings from social neuroscience are striking.

Understanding other people generally consists of two components. One part is a cognitive process and the other part is an emotional process. While the terminology is still debated within social neuroscience, we will label the cognitive part as the "Theory of Mind" (ToM) and the emotional part as Empathy. ToM is a well-known term in this research area (other labels for the same phenomenon are "mindreading" or "mentalizing") and the concept stems from primatology where originally it was asked whether monkeys have a theory of other monkeys' minds during a social interaction (Frith, 2004). It soon became apparent that this question is applicable to humans as well as to animals and, via autism research, ToM has now also been investigated in schizophrenia (Brüne, 2005; Frith 2004). Patients with schizophrenia often have impaired theories of other people's minds, e.g., intentions, and they also have impaired theories of their own minds (Harrington et al., 2005; Lee et al., 2004).

Empathic abilities have been investigated less often in humans with a schizophrenic disorder. However, some research findings lead to the hypothesis that empathy might also be impaired while suffering from schizophrenia. One reason for this theory is the evidence for an impairment in the recognition of facial expressions which schizophrenic patients show significantly more often than healthy control subjects (Kohler & Brennan, 2004). Another recent experimental study expanded these findings to the recognition of vocal emotions (Kucharska-Pietura, David, Masiak, & Phillips, 2005). Interestingly, echoing recent experimental findings (Kohler et al., 2003), this research has demonstrated that patients with schizophrenia were less able to recognize fear in the facial and vocal expressions of others. This finding, if it could be replicated under real life conditions, has strong implications for the emergence of violence. If one doesn't recognize that the other is fearful, there is no need to alter one's own aggressive behavior.

Only one study so far has directly investigated the connections of ToM, empathy, and violence in schizophrenic patients (Abu-Akel & Abushua'leh, 2004). In this experimental study, violent schizophrenic patients were compared to nonviolent patients with the same disorder. Surprisingly, in this study violence was associated with good ToM-abilities but also with poor empathizing. In this regard, the patients under study were quite similar to patients with an antisocial personality disorder. Possibly the violent patients had an as yet undetected personality disorder, which is not uncommon in violent schizophrenic subjects (Nolan et al., 1999). However, a recent metaanalysis of studies about "cognitive empathy" (i.e., ToM) found a strong association of poor ToM skills with offending (Joliffe & Farrington, 2004). Moreover, this metaanalysis yielded a similarly strong effect for low intelligence and low socioeconomic status. Whether these results are artifacts due to the measuring instruments remains a topic for further research.

While empathic abilities have not been investigated very much in schizophrenic patients, this topic is widely researched in people with the personality disorders just mentioned. For instance, a recent review, entitled "Psychopathy as a disorder of empathy" (Soderstrom, 2003), echoed the findings from the study of Abu-Akel and Abushua'leh (2004). Patients with an antisocial personality disorder generally have good ToM abilities, while many of them are unable to feel empathy with other humans, especially with victims of their crimes. Moreover, the metaanalysis by Joliffe and Farrington (2004) found that the association between affective empathy and offending was only weak but still statistically significant.

This short review of ToM and empathy literature establishes an important issue for psychiatric violence research. Regardless of individual study differences, ToM skills and empathy seem to have effects on the risk of becoming aggressive and violent. The ability to take the perspective of other people is likely to be a protective factor, and vice versa, the inability to make good inferences and to emphasize with the other might probably have negative effects on violence risks. This holds for "healthy" subjects as well as psychiatric patients. As the autism researcher Simon Baron-Cohen has stated, one reason why men become more physically violent than women is that, on average compared to females, men have a reduced capacity for empathy (Baron-Cohen, 2003). Moreover, he suggests a situational effect on empathy which in turn might increase the risk of aggression:

> "Aggression, even in normal quantities, can only occur because of reduced empathizing. You just can't set out to hurt someone if you care about how they feel. [. . .] During aggression you are focused on how you feel, more than how the other person feels." (Baron-Cohen, 2003:37)

What does this mean for the further discussion on psychosocial approaches toward violence in mental health care? Our ability to engage ourselves in an interaction non-violently depends quite a lot on the biologically based skills to get the others' perspective and to get the others' current emotional state. Because this capacity is impaired in many psychiatric patients due to personality traits or due to actual psychopathological states, mental health professionals should be aware of these impairments and adjust their expectations and their own theorizing about the minds of their patients. Many of the situations and conflicts described below seem to emerge from a background of not "getting" the other person's point of view, either cognitively or emotionally. Better awareness and better adjustment of one's theories of minds will surely have a deescalating effect.

8   SOCIAL SYSTEM

8.1   Double Contingency and the Genesis of Distrust

Interaction and escalation are inherently social processes and the psychological systems discussed above obviously operate within a higher-order social system. Sociological theory has a long tradition of trying to understand conflict-loaded interactions and one useful concept that has been proposed is that of double contingency. When looking at social interactions, double contingency refers to the phenomenon where both actors can never be sure about the other's reactions (Parsons & Shils, 1951). In an everyday situation, we find this problem on the street when we encounter somebody and neither of us knows to which side we have to go to make way for the other. The only guide each individual has is the other's anticipated direction and, often enough, we choose the wrong way. Beyond this simple example, double contingency is the basis for the famous dilemmas from game theory, e.g., the prisoners' dilemma, and from this approach we know that the "Tit-for-Tat" strategy (I do what you want me to do, when you do what I want you to do) is the most successful option for all parties involved.

With reference to classical systems theory, Luhmann (1995) has developed this concept much further. In Luhmann's social theory, double contingency is the ground on which an autocatalytic social system emerges. Each actor has only got his/her internal expectations of the other actor's behavior (which are based on a ToM and a capacity for empathy, see above). From here, a circularity about each other's expectations begins. To use the street encounter example again, this means that both of us react not only to our expectations ("single" contingency) but also to our expectations of the other actor's expectations.

When we apply this, admittedly abstract, model to a typical mental hospital ward situation such as a hospital admission, it says that the actors behave according to their expectations. The well-known sociological role theory predicts that, in general, both parties will fulfil their roles: patients will be patient and wait for somebody to care for them and staff will do their complementary caring tasks. What makes it difficult for psychiatric patients as well as for psychiatric staff is that they often cannot behave along these lines. Psychiatric patients, due to their disorders and the circumstances in the mental hospital, are often aroused because of being treated involuntarily. Mental hospital staff, on the other hand, not only have to fulfil caring roles but also other tasks that are closer to those of prison officers when they treat patients against their will to comply with national laws.

As can be easily concluded from this description, both parties often do not comply with their expected roles. The deviation from their roles is in many cases the starting point for distrust of each other, a conclusion which is confirmed by empirical evidence. During and after violent incidents both patients and nurses regard themselves as victims, but, of course, they do so for different reasons. Whereas patients believe themselves to be victims of the behavioral style of the staff and the aversive environment of the hospital, staff believe themselves to be the victim of patient aggression and organizational problems (Duxbury, 2002). Another example is reported by Benson et al. (2003), in which both the patient and staff involved in violent incidents felt that the other party did not conform to their ascribed role in the build-up and thus was to be blamed for its happening. This is exactly what Luhmann predicts as the consequence of double contingency. Trust or distrust in these situations should not be confused with trust as a psychological topic because, viewed sociologically, trust or distrust applies only to the other actor's behavior. When the other party does not fulfil their assumed role (to be patient and to be caring), why should I trust the other? Distrust is likely when role expectations are not met by at least one of the parties.

It can be predicted that distrust might be even stronger because of the status asymmetry between staff and patients which is literally expressed by holding the keys to the entrance door. Ultimately, patients have to follow staff orders. Status asymmetry itself enhances mutual distrust because it triggers another deviation from the standard roles. In the long run, status asymmetry may change the ward's milieu into an overcontrolling and oversanctioning atmosphere. Nursing scientist Eileen Morrison (Morrison, 1990) has described empirically the development that leads to a "tradition of toughness" within psychiatric nurses. Morrison explicitly underlines the distrust some nurses have of patients in general that often is being expressed by—mainly implicit—ward rules about the equal treatment that has to be applied to all patients. Staff have sometimes lost their flexibility to treat patients individually, but individual treatment is required if there is a goal of avoiding aversive stimulation of patients. Similarly, Whittington and Wykes (1994) have shown how some nurses adopt confrontive and/or distancing behavioral strategies toward patients to cope with their fear after being assaulted. It is known from psychological research that extreme excitedness is accompanied by a cognitive deficit (Zillmann, 1994), which results in psychological inflexibility. At the start of the escalating interaction both actors have several options at their disposal (giving in, apologizing, offering different conflict solutions, etc.). The longer the interaction lasts and the more it escalates, the fewer the available options. A very important feature of escalating interactions is the endpoint where one actor only reacts aggressively to the perceived aggression of the other. Both actors are thus subjectively defending themselves against the other.

8.2 Escalation and Conflict

Distrust and the breakdown of ordinary role expectations amplify the arousal and distress caused by the original trigger in a process of rapid escalation. Escalation before aggressive attacks is assumed in some of the textbooks on violence in clinical settings, e.g., Breakwell (1995), but there is still only poor empirical evidence on this important topic because of the methodological problems which plague interaction research. In this respect, again, we have to avoid attributing escalation solely to the patient's behavior. From a sociological perspective, it is the interaction itself that escalates. This assumption is empirically supported by a few studies that have analyzed the order of actions in aggressive interactions (Felson, 1984; Mummendey et al., 1984). Felson, for instance, asked subjects from the general population about the steps that usually happen in conflicts and those identified clearly indicate a worsening escalation: rule violation, orders, reproaches and noncompliance, accounts and insults, threats and physical attacks. Submission and mediation were noted by the respondents as only occurring after physical attacks and the steps to violent attacks were distributed equally between both sides of the conflict. According to Watzlawick et al. (1967) conflicting parties interact in a punctuated manner (see Cox & Leather, 1994; Nolting, 2000), where both sides subjectively only react to the other's reaction.

The same pattern is immediately recognizable when looking at conflict in psychiatric wards (see Figure 2). As we have seen, a typical conflict in a mental health setting starts with a rule violation of a patient observed by a nurse, e.g., teasing fellow patients, smoking in bed. Of course, the rule violation as the first trigger can also be regarded as a reaction to the rules and limits implemented on the wards. The ward rules can be seen as a reaction to expected behavior of mentally ill patients, and so on in an infinite regression. However, the nurse, after the observed rule violation, orders the patient to stop that behavior, which he or she refuses to do, probably while insulting the nurse. A second order by the nurse is followed by increasing arousal in the patient, which could then lead to a threat from the nurse. This threat might be answered with a physical attack by the patient. Usually staff then react to such attacks with physical measures such as restraint/seclusion or compulsory medication. From the patient's perspectives, these measures are experienced as an attack on his/her person and so, very often, violent fights between staff and patient break out in restraint and seclusion situations. Figure 3 illustrates how this analysis works when applied to a specific incident as reported from a patient's perspective to Johnson (1998).

In accordance with some of the literature reviewed above, stimulating patients aversively, e.g., a particular limit-setting style among individual staff seems to be a predictor of becoming a target of patient assaults (Lanza et al., 1991). To put it

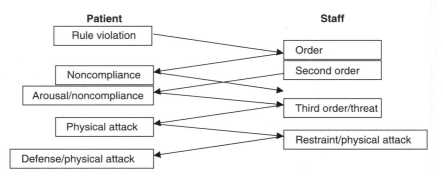

Figure 2. Escalation of a violent incident between staff and patient (after Felson, 1984; Nölting, 2000).

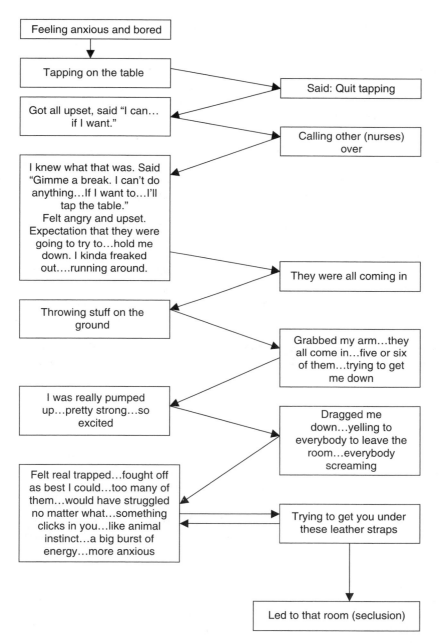

Figure 3. Conflict and escalation in a violent incident, as reported by a patient to Johnson (1998).

sociologically again, conflict is likely when distrust and aversive stimulation leads to a clear, but not necessarily verbal communication of "No!" (Kieserling, 1999; Luhmann, 1995). Luhmann has stressed the point that conflicts may emerge out of minor reasons often not understood even retrospectively. Thus an argument about a trivial problem might lead to a brutal violent attack in the end.

Seen from this perspective, conflicts do not destroy social systems: they are instead the basis of new systems, of conflict systems. In a certain way, conflict systems solve the problem of double contingency in a reversed manner. Within a conflict system both actors expect nothing less than the other actor's aggression: "Tit-for-Tat" with a painful outcome. The social–psychological literature clearly indicates a general tendency toward reciprocity in conflict situations (Patchen, 1993). Both the actor's expectations are now very secure and stable so it is more likely that the conflict will escalate than that it will reduce. Such a stable high-conflict culture can be recognized in many dysfunctional wards and has been observed in detail by Katz and Kirkland (1990).

Of course, conflicts between staff and patients do not always develop into violent attacks. Theoretically, it seems possible that conflicts might be resolved in the early stages of the interaction and this certainly happens in many cases in practice. Unfortunately, to the best knowledge of the authors there is no research investigating successful, i.e., nonviolent, outcomes in aggressive interactions and their predictors. Such research is difficult to conduct because it would have to analyze nonevents, and nonevents are a big challenge in terms of definition and other methodological efforts. But the effort to overcome these obstacles will be rewarded with some vital insights into the problem.

9   CONCLUSION

There is a long tradition in psychiatric research of pathologizing the normal behavior of people with a mental disorder. The professionals' and academics' own theory of the violent mental patient's mind is in this respect as limited and impaired as that of some of the patients to which it is applied. Indisputably some violent behavior has a pathological root but the pendulum has for many years been stuck in one position, that which emphasizes madness and abnormality rather than reason and comprehensibility. We have attempted here to redress the balance a little by examining a number of relatively normal psychological and social processes which need to be added to the equation we are all constructing together to understand and manage this problem. Emphasizing the violent individual alone can quickly lead to repression, therapeutic despair, and the search for silver bullets whereas emphasizing the violent interaction has the potential to positively empower both patients and staff. For the patient, the legitimacy of their perspective and feelings is restored to its rightful prominence. For the staff, an awareness of the importance of their own behavior in generating and maintaining conflict gives an opportunity for change and improved ways of working in this demanding area of psychiatric practice.

REFERENCES

Abu-Akel, A., & Abushua'leh, K. (2004). "Theory of mind" in violent and nonviolent patients with paranoid schizophrenia. *Schizophrenia Research, 69,* 45–53.

Adolphs, R. (1999). Social cognition and the human brain. *Trends in Cognitive Sciences, 3,* 469–479.

Alternatives to Violence Project (1996). *Supplement to the basic and second level manuals.* New York: Alternatives to Violence Education Committee.

Anderson, C., & Bushman, B. (2002). Human aggression. *Annual Review of Psychology, 53,* 27–51.

Angermeyer, M. C. (2000). Schizophrenia and violence. *Acta Psychiatrica Scandinavica, 102*(Suppl. 407), 63–67.

Appelbaum, P. S., Robbins, P. C., & Monahan, J. (2000). Violence and delusions: Data from the MacArthur violence risk assessment study. *The American Journal of Psychiatry, 157,* 566–572.

Baron-Cohen, S. (2003). *The essential difference: Men, women and the extreme male brain.* London: Allen Lane/Penguin.

Bensley, L., Nelson, N., & Kaufman, J. (1995). Patient and staff views of factors influencing assaults on psychiatric hospital employees. *Issues in Mental Health Nursing, 16,* 433–446.

Benson, A., Secker, J., Balfe, E., Lipsedge, M., Robinson, S., & Walker, J. (2003). Discourses of blame: Accounting for aggression and violence on an acute mental health inpatient unit. *Social Science & Medicine, 57,* 917–926.

Berkowitz, L. (1993). *Aggression: Causes, consequences and control.* New York: McGraw Hill.

Bjørkly, S. (1995). Prediction of aggression in psychiatric patients: A review of prospective prediction studies. *Clinical Psychology Review, 15,* 475–502.

Bjørkly, S. (2002a). Psychotic symptoms and violence toward others – a literature review of some preliminary findings, part 1: Delusions. *Aggression and Violent Behavior, 7,* 617–631.

Bjørkly, S. (2002b). Psychotic symptoms and violence toward others – a literature review of some preliminary findings, part 2: Hallucinations. *Aggression and Violent Behavior, 7,* 605–615.

Bjørkly, S., & Havik, O. E. (2003). TCO symptoms as markers of violence in a sample of severely violent psychiatric inpatients. *International Journal of Forensic Mental Health, 2,* 87–97.

Blair, R. J. R., & Charney, D. S. (2003). Emotion regulation: An affective neuroscience approach. In: M. P. Mattson (Ed.), *Neurobiology of aggression: Understanding and preventing violence* (pp. 21–32). Totowa, N. J: Humana Press.

Blakemore, S.-J., Winston, J., & Frith, U. (2004). Social cognitive neuroscience: Where are we heading? *Trends in Cognitve Sciences, 8,* 216–222.

Breakwell, G. (1995). Theories of violence. In: B. Kidd & C. Stark (Eds.), *Management of violence and aggression in health care* (pp. 1–11). London: Gaskell.

Brothers, L. (1997). *Friday's footprints. How society shapes the human mind.* New York/Oxford: Oxford University Press.

Brüne, M. (2005). "Theory of Mind" in schizophrenia: A review of the literature. *Schizophrenia Bulletin, 31,* 21–42.

Calabro, K., Mackey, T., & Williams, S. (2002). Evaluation of training designed to prevent and manage patient violence. *Issues in Mental Health Nursing, 23,* 3–15.

Cheung, P., Schweitzer, I., Tuckwell, V., & Crowley, K. (1996). A prospective study of aggression among psychiatric patients in rehabilitation wards. *The Australian and New Zealand Journal of Psychiatry, 30,* 257–262.

Cooper, A., & Medonca, J. (1991). A prospective study of patient assaults on nurses in a provincial psychiatric hospital in Canada. *Acta Psychiatrica Scandinavica, 84,* 163–166.

Cox, T., & Leather, P. (1994). The prevention of violence at work: Application of a cognitive behavioral theory. *International Review of Industrial and Organizational Psychology, 9,* 213–245.

Davidson, R. J., Putnam, K. M., & Larson, C. L. (2000). Dysfunction in the neural circuitry of emotion regulation—A possible prelude to violence. *Science, 289,* 591–594.

Dodge, K., & Coie, J. (1987). Social-information-processing factors in reactive and proactive aggression in children's peer groups. *Journal of Personality and Social Psychology, 53,* 1146–1158.

Duxbury, J. (2002). An evaluation of staff and patient views of strategies employed to manage inpatient aggression and violence on one mental health unit: A pluralistic design. *Journal of Psychiatric and Mental Health Nursing, 9*, 325–337.

Edgar, K., O'Donnell, I., & Martin, C. (2003). Tracking pathways to violence in prison. In: R. Lee & E. Stanko (Eds.), *Researching violence. Essays on methodology and measurement*. London: Routledge.

Felson, R. (1984). Patterns of social interaction. In: M. Mummendey (Ed.), *Social psychology of aggression: From individual behavior to social interaction* (pp.107–126). Berlin: Springer.

Fonagy, P. (2003). Towards a developmental understanding of violence. *The British Journal of Psychiatry, 183*, 190–192.

Frith, C. C. (2004). Schizophrenia and theory of mind. *Psychological Medicine, 34*, 385–389.

Frith, C. C., & Wolpert, D. (Eds.) (2003). *The neuroscience of social interaction: Decoding, imitating, and influencing the actions of others*. Oxford: Oxford University Press.

Grassi, L., Peron, L., Marangoni, C., Zanchi, P., & Vanni, A. (2001). Characteristics of violent behavior in acute psychiatric inpatients: A five-year Italian study. *Acta Psychiatrica Scandinavica, 104*, 273–279.

Häkänen, H. & Laajasalo, T. (2006). Homicide crime scene behaviors in a Finnish sample of mentally ill offenders. *Homicide Studies, 19*, 33–54.

Haller, J., & Kruk, M. R. (2003). Neuroendocrine stress responses and aggression. In: M. P. Mattson (Ed.), *Neurobiology of aggression: Understanding and preventing violence* (pp. 93–118). Totowa, NJ: Humana Press.

Harrington, L., Siegert, R. J., & McClure, J. (2005). Theory of mind in schizophrenia: A critical review. *Cognitive Neuropsychiatry, 10*, 249–286.

Harris, G., & Varney, G. (1986). A ten-year study of assaults and assaulters on a maximum security psychiatric unit. *Journal of Interpersonal Violence, 1*, 173–191.

Ilkiw-Lavalle, O., & Grenyer, B. (2003). Differences between patient and staff perceptions of aggression in mental health units. *Psychiatric Services, 54*, 389–393.

Johnson, M. (1998). Being restrained: A study of power and powerlessness. *Issues in Mental Health Nursing, 19*, 191–206.

Joliffe, D., & Farrington, D. P. (2004). Empathy and offending: A systematic review and meta-analysis. *Aggression and Violent Behavior, 9*, 441–476.

Katz, P., & Kiskland, F. R. (1990). Violence and Social-structure on Mental-Hospital wards. Psychiatry-Interpersonal and Biological Processes *53*(3), 262–277.

Kieserling, A. (1999). *Kommunikation unter Anwesenden: Studien über Interaktionssysteme*. Frankfurt: Suhrkamp.

Kohler, C. G., & Brennan, A. R. (2004). Recognition of facial emotions in schizophrenia. *Current Opinion in Psychiatry, 17*, 81–86.

Kohler, C. G., Turner, T. H., Bilker, W. B., Brensinger, C. M., Siegel, S. J., Kanes, S. J., et al. (2003). Facial emotion recognition in schizophrenia: Intensity effects and error patterns. *The American Journal of Psychiatry, 160*, 1768–1774.

Kohn, S. R., & Asnis, G. M. (2003). Aggression in psychiatric disorders. In: M. P. Mattson (Ed.), *Neurobiology of aggression: Understanding and preventing violence* (pp.135–149). Totowa, NJ: Humana Press.

Kucharska-Pietura, K., David, A. D., Masiak, M., & Phillips Mary, L. (2005). Perception of facial and vocal affect by people with schizophrenia in early and late stages of illness. *The British Journal of Psychiatry, 187*, 523–528.

Lanza, M., Kayne, H., Hicks, C., & Milner, J. (1991). Nursing staff characteristics related to patient assault. *Issues in Mental Health Nursing, 12*, 253–265.

Lazarus, R. (1999). *Stress and emotion: A new synthesis*. London: Free Association Books.

Lazarus, R., & Folkman, S. (1984). *Stress, appraisal and coping*. New York: Springer.

Lee, K.-H., Farrow, T. F. D., Spence, S. A., & Woodruff, P. W. R. (2004). Social cognition, brain networks and schizophrenia. *Psychological Medicine, 34*, 391–400.

Lesch, K. P. (2003). The serotonergic dimension of aggression and violence. In: M. P. Mattson (Ed.), *Neurobiology of aggression: Understanding and preventing violence* (pp.33–63). Totowa, NJ: Humana Press.

Lindsay, J., & Anderson, C. (2000). From antecedent conditions to violent actions: A general affective aggression model. *Personality and Social Psychology Bulletin, 26,* 533–547.

Link, B. G., Andrews, H. A., & Cullen, F. T. (1992). The violent and illegal behavior of mental patient reconsidered. *American Sociological Review, 57,* 275–292.

Link, B. G., Monahan, J., Stueve, A., & Cullen, F. T. (1999). Real in their consequences: A sociological approach to understanding the association between psychotic symptoms and violence. *American Sociological Review, 64,* 316–332.

Link, B. G., & Stueve, A. (1995). Evidence bearing on mental illness as a possible cause of violent behavior. *Epidemiologic Reviews, 17,* 172–181.

Liu, J., & Wuerker, A. (2005). Biosocial bases of aggressive and violent behavior – implications for nursing studies. *International Journal of Nursing Studies, 42,* 229–241.

Luhmann, N. (1995). *Social systems.* Stanford: Stanford University Press.

Martin, K. (1995). Improving staff safety through an aggression management program. *Archives of Psychiatric Nursing, 9,* 211–215.

Miethe, T., & Regoeczi, W. (2004). *Rethinking homicide: Exploring the structure and process underlying deadly situations.* Cambridge: Cambridge University Press.

Morrison, E. (1990). The tradition of toughness: A study of nonprofessional nursing care in psychiatric settings. *Image-Journal of Nursing Scholarship, 22*(1), 32–38.

Mummendey, A., Linneweber, V., & Löschper, G. (1984). Aggression: From act to interaction. In: M. Mummendey (Ed.), *Social psychology of aggression: From individual behavior to social interaction* (pp.69–106). Berlin: Springer.

Nestor, P. G. (2002). Mental disorder and violence: Personality dimensions and clinical features. *The American Journal of Psychiatry, 159,* 1973–1978.

Niehoff, D. (1999). *The biology of violence: How understanding the brain, behavior, and environment can break the vicious circle of aggression.* New York: Free Press.

Nijman, H. L. I. (2002). A model of aggression in psychiatric hospitals. *Acta Psychiatrica Scandinavica — Supplement, 412,* 142–143.

Nijman, H. L. I., Allertz, W. F. F., Merckelbach, H. L. G. J., à Campo, J. M. L. G., & Ravelli, D. P. (1997). Aggressive behavior on an acute psychiatric admissions ward. *The European Journal of Psychiatry, 11,* 106–114.

Nijman, H. L. I., à Campo, J. M. L. G., Ravelli, D. P., & Merckelbach, H. L. G. J. (1999). A tentative model of aggression on inpatient psychiatric wards. *Psychiatric Services, 50,* 832–834.

Nolan, K. A., Volavka, J., Mohr, P., & Czobor, P. (1999). Psychopathy and violent behavior among patients with schizophrenia and schizoaffective disorder. *Psychiatric Services, 50,* 787–792.

Nolting, A. (2000). *Lernfall Aggression: Wie sie entsteht – wie sie zu vermindern ist.* Reinbek: Rowohlt.

Palmstierna, T., & Wistedt, B. (1987). Staff Observation and Aggression Scale: presentation and evaluation. *Acta Psychiatrica Scandinavica, 76,* 657–673.

Parsons, T., & Shils, E. (1951). *Towards a general theory of action.* Cambridge, MA: Harvard University Press.

Patchen, M. (1993). Reciprocity of coercion and cooperation between individuals and nations. In: R. Felson & J. Tedeschi (Eds.), *Aggression and violence: Social interactionist perspectives* (pp.119–144). Washington, DC: APA.

Richter, D. (1999). *Patientenübergriffe auf Mitarbeiter psychiatrischer Kliniken: Häufigkeit, Folgen, Präventionsmöglichkeiten.* Freiburg: Lambertus.

Rizzolatto, G., & Craighero, L. (2004). The mirror-neuron system. *Annual Review of Neuroscience, 27,* 169–192.

Sheridan, M., Henrion, R., Robinson, L., & Baxter, V. (1990). Precipitants of violence in a psychiatric inpatient setting. *Hospital and Community Psychiatry, 41,* 776–780.

Soderstrom, H. (2003). Psychopathy as a disorder of empathy. *European Child & Adolescent Psychiatry, 12,* 249–253.

Steinert, T. (2002). Prediction of inpatient violence. *Acta Psychiatrica Scandinavica Supplement, 412,* 133–141.

Steinert, T., Woelfle, M., & Gebhardt, R. P. (2000). Aggressive behavior during inpatient treatment. Measurement of violence during inpatient treatment and association with psychopathology. *Acta Psychiatrica Scandinavica, 102,* 107–112.

Walsh, E., Buchanan, A., & Fahy, T. (2002). Violence and schizophrenia: Examining the evidence. *The British Journal of Psychiatry, 180,* 490–495.

Watzlawick, P., Beavin, J., & Jackson, D. (1967). *Pragmatics of human communication: A study of interactional patterns, pathologies, and paradoxes.* New York: W. W. Norton.

Whittington, R., & Wykes, T. (1994). "Going in strong": Confrontive coping by staff. *Journal of Forensic Psychiatry, 5,* 609–614.

Whittington, R., & Wykes, T. (1996). Aversive stimulation by staff and violence by psychiatric patients. *The British Journal of Clinical Psychology, 35,* 11–20.

Young, R. M., & Balaban, E. (2003). Aggression, biology, and context: Dejá-vu all over again? In: M. P. Mattson (Ed.), *Neurobiology of aggression: Understanding and preventing violence* (pp.191–211). Totowa, NJ: Humana Press.

Zillmann, D. (1994). Cognition-excitation interdependencies on the escalation of anger and angry aggression. In: M. Potegal & J. Knutson (Eds.), *The dynamics of aggression: Biological and social processes in dyads and groups* (pp.45–71). Hillsdale, NJ: Erlbaum.

4

Users' Perceptions and Views on Violence and Coercion in Mental Health

CHRISTOPH ABDERHALDEN, SABINE HAHN, YVONNE
D. B. BONNER, AND GIAN MARIA GALEAZZI

1 INTRODUCTION

1.1 The Personal Experience of Coercion

1.1.1 The Personal Experience of Coercion

It is useful to bear in mind, when analyzing user's views on coercion that their opinions stem from their personal experience. Furthermore, it is critical to remember that, for decades, the patients' *experience of illness* was disregarded by the biomedical approach of *disease*. Only through the perseverance of psychoanalysis and its subsequent phenomenological derivatives was the *person and his or her experience of illness* put on the agenda of research. Subsequently, during the 1970s and 1980s, American medical anthropology produced a constructive input pinpointing the conceptual differences between *disease* (objective description of the syndrome), *illness* (subjective narrative of the experience of ailment) and *sickness* (the relational and social dimensions of ill health) (Twaddle, 1981). From then onwards, a symptom can be analyzed as an objective evidence of pathology, or as the outcome of a symbolic and relational transaction between the patient, his complaint and his entourage. The next step in research, under the pressure of the global campaign for Human Rights (United Nations, 1975, 1991, 1993; World Health Organization, WHO, 2002), added new queries to the concern for the quality of *cure* (through evidence-based medicine) and *care* (through the study of the interactions between the sick person's needs and the psychiatric services), i.e., the capacity of the mental health services to protect and promote the human dignity of their patients. Hence, nowadays, when users express their point of view on their experience of illness they tend to underline the impact of the relational characteristics of health personnel on the quality of the treatment they received. That definitely applies to the field of coercive treatment. In fact, the paternalistic model of care in medicine has been challenged during the last decades. Traditionally, professionals in medicine were considered as experts on treatment, and thus felt entitled to treat patients accordingly. Lately however, in most countries, there have been considerable social and legal changes that now stress the autonomy of individuals and their right to self-determination. Medical and social services, as a result, have developed user-centered and consumer-oriented models of care. Nevertheless, the paternalistic model of care still persists in the health sector and, hence, also in psychiatry (Kjellin & Nilstun, 1993).

The slow change observed in psychiatry is connected with the dominant belief of many psychiatrists that their role is to exert power over deviant behavior. Such an approach consequently hinders their ability to adopt a more respectful attitude toward users' feelings and preferences on the treatment goals (Foucault, 1961). This approach is further reinforced by the widely accepted opinion that some patients are a danger to themselves and others. Psychiatric services are hence considered responsible for protecting these patients from themselves. This is the case with patients suffering from acute psychosis or dementias, who show signs of gross behavioral disorganization, confusion, and extreme agitation.

The paternalistic model is also functional (for some professionals) for it circumvents the delicate task of informing, explaining, negotiating, and reaching agreement with a patient who disagrees with the recommended treatment. In addition, it permits the mental health professional to have the last word. The main argument validating this approach is that psychiatric patients' lack insight into their illness. Consequently, coercive measures, such as compulsory admission and forced medication, are considered unavoidable and should not be listed under the heading of violence in psychiatric care.

In most European countries, this intricate situation is regulated by law, authorizing psychiatrists to hospitalize patients (against their will) who are considered a hazard to themselves and others (Dressing & Salize, 2004). Sociological studies have drawn the attention of researchers to the connection between the media's depiction of mental illness (that currently emphasizes the risk of violence) and its impact on the ensuing social policies that support coercive practices (Philo, 1996; Rose, 1998). This shift toward more coercive mental health policies (Priebe et al., 2005), has to do with Governmental:

> "Attempts to pander to inaccurate public perceptions, reactions, and intolerance. Furthermore . . . the public may have been 'whipped up' into this position of intolerance as a result of misleading, inaccurate mass representations of mental illness and mental health issues." (Cutcliffe & Hannigan, 2001).

Furthermore, public concern about the risk of violence, due to the presence of psychiatric patients in the community, has recently pressed some countries to extend the setting of compulsory treatment from hospital to the community (Priebe et al., 2005). Research has recently studied the correlation between media information and hospital admission rates. These studies reveal that political and media information, dealing with crimes committed in the community by psychiatric patients, influence and increase the compulsory admission rates in forensic psychiatric inpatient services (Brophy & McDermott, 2003; Cutcliffe & Hannigan, 2001; Philo, 1996; Rose, 1998). As a result, the responsibility of assessing risks, assigned to psychiatrists despite the lack of reliable predicting tools, is growing. This development, obviously, does not encourage a more flexible approach toward psychiatric patients and confirms the advantages in using the paternalistic model of care.

1.1.2 Coercive Measures in the History of Psychiatry

Coercion, i.e., violent treatment imposed on patients against their will, has always been used and has thus marked the history of psychiatric care. Numerous cases of violent practice have been described in literature, i.e., experimental psychosurgery performed on thousands of patients without their consent (Valenstein, 1986), compulsory sterilization (Roelcke, 2002), systematic extermination of more than 200,000 patients in the T4 Program under the Nazi regime (Tuffs, 2004), and enforced "treatment" against homosexuality (Smith, Bartlett, & King, 2004). Situations of extreme violence, experienced by users, are therefore a reminder to mental health professionals (and society as a whole) of the dangers of psychiatric care. On the other hand, the *desenchaînement* of the inpatients of Bicêtre Hospital (1793), carried out by Pinel and his superintendent nurse Jean-Baptiste Poussin, represents the birth of modern psychiatry as the first symbolic step toward the humanization of care.

1.1.3 Public Response to Coercion

The movements of civil rights and of antipsychiatry have for decades condemned the violent outcomes of coercive psychiatry. They also questioned the legitimacy of authoritarianism in mental health care (Szasz & Alexander, 1968) and, consequently, produced a shift of perspective in psychiatry. Thus laying the foundation for a novel ethical approach, i.e., respect for the individual as a person, and not simply as a patient, with his/her subjective experiences, choices, values, and rights that empowers patients by placing them at the centre of therapy and scientific research.

1.2 Research on Coercion and Users' Views

1.2.1 Research and Users' Role

Historically, the interest for users' perception in health echoes the Quality Assurance approach, developed in trade and industry, which has now expanded to the mental health services. It draws attention to the "user satisfaction criterion" that is an important outcome measure to assess the quality of treatment (Ruggeri et al., 2004). It indicates the necessity to explore the subjective determinants of patient satisfaction, focusing on the whole *process* of care and not solely on psychopathologic outcomes. The shift of perspective in psychiatry emphasizes nowadays the importance of getting psychiatric users involved in their own treatment planning and, as experts, in service planning as well as at all stages of research (Trivedi & Wykes, 2002). See, for example, the debate on the issue of compliance. The Royal Pharmaceutical Society of Great Britain (Mullen, 1997) proposed to replace the term "compliance" with the word "concordance." Such a suggestion reflects the recent role given to users as active collaborators in the outlining of the treatment plan.

This involvement of users in research, i.e., their perceptions and experiences, is considered useful in a number of ways. Paying attention to users' perceptions and experiences of treatment opens new paths for research on violent incidents and coercive measures, i.e., central and conflict-loaded issues in mental health care.

1.2.2 Research on Violent Incidents

Empirical research evidence specifies that violent incidents and their management can be regarded as the product of a complex interaction of variables. These variables comprise:

(a) Patient characteristics, e.g., psychopathology, gender.
(b) Environmental components, e.g., size and crowding of the ward, the general environment.
(c) Interactional factors, e.g., aversive stimulation or provocation.
(d) Staff variables, e.g., attitudes and professional training in aggression management (Daffern & Howells, 2002; Davis, 1991; Nijman, a Campo, Ravelli, & Merckelbach, 1999; Shah, Fineberg, & James, 1991).

Thus situational, interactional, or staff-related variables are now considered possible triggers of aggression and violence.

In 1981, Monahan utilized three standpoints to examine a situation of violence: the victim's point of view, the aggressor's perception, and the situation as a whole (Monahan, 1981). Today most researchers agree with Monahan, and only a few incorporate different perspectives in their surveys. The greater part of research is still based on the psychopathological approach, or a professional bias, that tends to examine only the aggressive characteristics of the patient.

1.2.3 Research on Compulsory Hospitalization

The issue of users' perceptions of coercion related to involuntary hospitalization and treatment (Rose, 1998) has lately received quiet some attention, for the simple reason that compulsory treatments of severe psychiatric cases are difficult to avoid. The shift in research, from the "Thank you theory" to the users' perspective, represents a landmark in the field of mental health, for it can alter old prejudices and allow a broader understanding of the determinants of coercion in psychiatry. The hypothesis of this theory is that users change their ideas on the necessity of a compulsory admission when discharged and, to a certain extent, this happens. Nonetheless, the patients' negative feelings on violence and coercion, attached to compulsory admission, remain (Gardner et al., 1999).

The following paragraphs of this chapter review the available, although scarce, literature of users' views on aggression, violence and coercive practices, and examine its implications on mental health practices and future research.

2   USERS' VIEWS OF VIOLENT INCIDENTS

2.1   Field of Research and Methodology

2.1.1   Field of Research

Research on patients' views of aggression emphasizes the need to analyze this phenomenon in a broader context, making better use of sociological and psycho-sociological concepts, such as "power imbalance," "paternalism," "mutual attribution of blame," "organizational culture," "functional analysis" (Benson et al., 2003; Kumar, Guite, & Thornicroft, 2001). Representatives of the user movement agree with the above statement and thus challenge the use of the one-dimensional biomedical model (O'Hagan, 2004). However, to date only a few empirical surveys include or compare user and staff perspectives, when studying the causes (or precursory signs) of aggressive incidents (Bensley, Nelson, Kaufman, Silverstein, & Shields, 1995; Duxbury & Whittington, 2005; Grewe, Wolpert, & Pflug, 2001; Harris & Varney, 1986; Hinsby & Baker, 2004; Ilkiw-Lavalle & Grenyer, 2003; Lanza & Kayne, 1995; Omerov, Edman, & Wistedt, 2004; Quinsey, 1979). Moreover, these studies focus on users' aggression toward staff (this point has not always been stated) and rarely on users' aggression *vis-à-vis* fellow patients, directed against other users (Crowner, Peric, Stepcic, & Lee, 2005; Crowner, Peric, Stepcic, & Ventura, 1995; Frueh et al., 2005; Love & Hunter, 1999).

2.1.2   Research Methodology

With regard to methods, samples, and focus, the surveys in this field are heterogeneous. For instance, some studies concentrate on users' views on specific incidents (Crowner et al., 1995; Duxbury, 2002; Ilkiw-Lavalle & Grenyer, 2003; Lanza & Kayne, 1995), others on general views. Some research utilizes questionnaires (Duxbury & Whittington, 2005; Gillig, Markert, Barron, & Coleman, 1998), others use individual interviews (Crowner et al., 1995; Fagan-Pryor et al., 2003; Harris & Varney, 1986; Hinsby & Baker, 2004; Johnson, Martin, Guha, & Montgomery, 1997; Lanza & Kayne) or group interviews (Bensley et al., 1995; Kumar et al., 2001). Moreover, these surveys may analyze diverse samples of patients, the latter all having witnessed episodes of aggression during past hospitalization, but coming from different settings (ranging from high security forensic units to psychiatric services).

Most results also concentrate on user experience gathered in one single institution. Finally, several studies compare staff and user perceptions of violence, but at times utilize different methods for collecting data on either users or staff.

Most surveys utilize qualitative methods, i.e., content analysis or the grounded theory approach, to analyze interview data. Yet, only two of these studies (Duxbury, 2002; Duxbury & Whittington, 2005) make use of a standardized, psychometrically tested instrument, designed to examine the patients' attitudes toward aggression and aggression management (The Management of Aggression and Violence Attitude Scale, MAVAS) (Duxbury, 2003).

2.2 Research on Users, Staff, and Informal Carers' Views

2.2.1 Research on Users' Views

Some studies examine participants' perceptions on violent incidents in a broad sense, revealing thus the multiple and complex components of aggression. Benson et al. (2003), for instance, underline that one of the central preoccupations of users concerns the discourse on the mutual attribution of blame. Kumar, Guite, & Thornicroft (2001), using the grounded theory approach, reveals that the imbalance of power observed in the mental health system fosters institutional violence against users.

When users are interviewed on the causes of aggressive behavior, they stress a variety of features, i.e., hospital environment (Johnson et al., 1997; Love & Hunter, 1999), institutional, interpersonal or procedural factors, interpersonal conflicts, and finally personal factors, including illness. However, among all research samples, users consider staff behavior as a central cause of violence, describing it provocative and disrespectful (Bensley et al., 1995; Duxbury, 2002; Duxbury & Whittington, 2005; Fagan-Pryor et al., 2003; Gillig et al., 1998; Harris & Varney, 1986; Ilkiw-Lavalle & Grenyer, 2003; Love & Hunter). For example, Omerov et al. (2004), investigating 41 violent incidents, found that users considered staff provocative, in 75% of the episodes.

2.2.2 Research on Users' and Staff Views

If we now compare research results on users' views (concerning the causes of aggressive behavior) with those of staff, some areas of agreement appear. For instance, users and staff both underline the shortage of resources, i.e., personnel, in igniting aggression. However, most research brings to light substantial differences of opinion between users and staff, whatever the setting or focus of the studies may be: single episodes (e.g., Harris & Varney, 1986), or extensive experiences of the participants (e.g., Duxbury, 2002). For instance, the percentage of episodes in which staff do not identify a cause (or trigger) for violence is generally higher than that of users. Harris and Varney state the following percentages: staff 59%, users 15%. Omerov et al. (2004) present similar percentages: staff do not name a cause in 54% of episodes and users in 10%. As for medication and coercive measures (as perceived triggers of aggression), staff express lower percentages than users

(Bensley et al., 1995; Omerov et al.). Likewise, some circumstances, such as being confined to a room, receiving little information on ward rules (Bensley et al.), or being in conflict with staff or users (Ilkiw-Lavalle & Grenyer, 2003), are rarely reported by staff (as perceived triggers of aggression) and often by users. Furthermore, all surveys underline that provoking and inadequate behavior of staff or lack of helpful communication (as triggers for violence) are rarely mentioned by staff, but highly emphasized by users (Bensley et al.; Duxbury; Lanza & Kayne, 1995; Omerov et al.).

As underlined above, the substantial differences in opinion between users and staff on the perceived causes of violent incidents (e.g., SOAS-forms used by Omerov et al., 2004) allow one to understand, when investigating the grounds of aggressive incidents, that it is advisable to be cautious and thus to rely not only on staff observations.

Another issue investigated is the psychological sequelae caused by experiencing or witnessing violent incidents (Kumar et al., 2001). The negative consequences of assaults, or violence witnessing, are often studied on staff, e.g., Rees and Lehane (1996), but rarely on patients. Yet, as we have seen above, patients frequently report staff behavior as violent (Kumar et al.; Love & Hunter, 1999). Users also underline that the needs of victims of violence in the ward often remain unmet by the care system. To bridge such gaps, programs dealing with aggression are, time and again, organized for users (Kumar et al.).

To sum up the corresponding users' perception, current research now offers evidence that inadequate staff behavior can bring about aggressive incidents (e.g., Shepherd & Lavender, 1999; Whittington & Wykes, 1996).

2.2.3 Research on Informal Carers' Views

If we now take into consideration informal carers (i.e., families, relatives, friends, or other significant persons), we find that, in spite of the prevalence of violence in family settings, only a small number of systematic research surveys investigate the experience of informal carers and their views on aggression, (Steadman et al., 1998; Straznickas, McNiel, & Binder, 1993). The prevalence of violent incidents in a family setting appears similar to that found in samples of health personnel such as nurses. For instance Vaddadi, Gilleard, and Fryer (2002), report that, over a one-year period, in a cross-section of 101 relatives, there is a prevalence of recurrent shouting and swearing (in 42% of the cases), of threatening (22%), of physical violence (24%), and of physical injury (in 4% of the cases). Furthermore, his research group did verify that, six months before admission, a third of relatives had been hit at least once, and over half of them had experienced either verbal abuse, threatening behavior, or temper outbursts (Vaddadi et al., 2002; Vaddadi, Soosai, Gilleard, & Adlard, 1997). Aggressive, agitated, threatening, or unpredictable behavior is commonly associated with psychopathological conditions and also considered the major source of stress and burden for families (Salleh, 1994; Saunders, 2003; Schmid, Spiessl, Vukovich, & Cording, 2003; Vaddadi et al., 2002;

Saunders, 2003; Schmid, Spiessl, Vukovich, and Cording, 2003). Yet studies investigating the impact of such behavioral symptoms on caregivers reveal contradictory results (Kjellin & Östman, 2005; Saunders).

In a nutshell, it is striking to discover how much research has been put into studying violence against staff in clinical settings and how little into analyzing violence within the community and family settings.

3 USERS' SUBJECTIVE EXPERIENCE OF COERCIVE PRACTICES

3.1 Users' Subjective Experience of Admission and Involuntary Commitment

3.1.1 From Inpatient to Outpatient Commitment

Forced admission to hospital or deprivation of autonomy through involuntary commitment is an extreme, but commonly used, practice in psychiatry. Recent reports show that compulsory admissions have not decreased during the last decade in western countries (Dressing & Salize, 2004; Priebe et al., 2005).

The widespread conviction, that persons suffering from psychiatric disorders represent a danger to themselves and to the community (owing to a lack of insight into their illness), legitimizes the mental health policy of emergency compulsory hospitalization, utilized as a preventive measure against social disturbances. Laws on this issue vary from country to country, but usually prescribe the provision of impartial information, and of a legal procedure to appeal against compulsory measures. Psychiatric survivors, consumers (or users) of mental health services express contradictory opinions on this issue. Radical opponents of coercive treatment argue that these laws violate basic human rights, i.e., autonomy and freedom of movement, and should simply be withdrawn. Other users agree that involuntary admission may be useful in situations of extreme crisis (as a last resort, and only as long as serious hazards are feared) provided that other options in less restrictive environments have first been tried, and that legal or advocacy support are guaranteed (O'Hagan, 2004). On the other hand, users generally consider compulsory treatment in the community (outpatient commitment), recently introduced in a number of countries, as an unacceptable extension of social control (from emergency situation to everyday life) that ends by depriving a person of their rights and liberties, at any time and wherever they may reside.

3.1.2 Qualitative Research on Users' Subjective Experience

Personal accounts and qualitative studies on their commitment to a psychiatric hospital describe a number of users' negative feelings, i.e., helplessness, passivity caused by deprivation of personal freedom, humiliation and loss of self-esteem, feelings of isolation and solitude, lack of contact with significant persons, difficulties in meeting basic environmental demands and, finally, the persisting effect of trauma due to compulsory admission (Roe & Ronen, 2003). Qualitative studies report the basic perception that involuntary committed users are not respected as human beings. User accounts, for instance, contain sentences such as "not being involved in one's own care," "receiving care perceived as meaningless and not good," or "being an inferior kind of human being" (Olofsson & Jacobsson, 2001; Olofsson & Norberg, 2001). Results of quantitative studies correspond to the users' views on the after-effects of compulsory admission, reporting evidence of an increase in post-traumatic stress symptomatology in patients (McGorry et al., 1991; Meyer, Taiminen, Vuori, Aijala, & Helenius, 1999; Priebe, Broker, & Gunkel, 1998; Shaw, McFarlane, & Bookless, 1997).

3.1.3   Quantitative Research on Users' Subjective Experience

Quantitative research on commitment in psychiatry has grown recently. The first quantitative surveys on patient experiences of coercion studied the impact of the patient's legal status at admission, comparing voluntary and involuntary admission, and reporting that committed patients showed a lower degree of satisfaction (concerning the admission process) than voluntary patients. Yet subsequently, other surveys highlighted that the legal status of a patient at admission constituted a poor research criterion to evaluate the degree of perceived coercion experienced by a patient during hospitalization. Rogers, for instance, discovered that a number of voluntary patients had reported that family members, friends, community, or hospital staff had put strong pressure (and coercion) on them, before they signed the voluntary application form for hospital admission (Rogers, 1993). On the other hand, in the USA, Hoge and colleagues discovered that 35% of the committed patients reported not having been coerced (Hoge et al., 1997). Furthermore, another study revealed that patients can enter hospital on a voluntary basis, but the moment they ask to be discharged, they receive compulsory commitment status (Poulsen, 1999). Finally, Tuohimaki and colleagues have underlined that a certain number of inpatients (voluntarily and involuntary) seem to be unaware of their legal status anyway, either at admission, or during their hospitalization (Tuohimaki et al., 2001). The results of these different research projects show that comparing results, based on the legal status of patients at hospital admission, remains questionable.

3.1.4   Disregarded Variables of Coercion

The implementation of a reliable research design for observing and recording "objective" coercive acts represents a complex goal for researchers. Moreover, the quantitative approach risks overlooking situations in which users feel subjectively coerced, while "objective" indexes do not reveal coercion. As a matter of fact, a number of studies (that compared objective and subjective measurements) illustrate situations in which users report a high degree of coercion, yet objective evidence of coercion was missing (Kjellin & Westrin, 1998). On the other hand, the disregarded variables of coercion can hide relevant features of pressure or violence that can cause unnecessary suffering to users. Moreover, this situation can impinge negatively on the therapeutic alliance between patient and staff and erode the user's trust in mental health services, therapy, and, overall, in the outcome of care.

3.1.5 The Subjective Dimension of Perceived Coercion

In recent years, the survey predicaments mentioned above have led researchers to privilege the subjective dimension of perceived coercion and thus use this subjective construct for inquiries. This choice, however, has put researchers in the complex situation of having to operationalize a subjective construct (and this process is not simple to carry out, as we have learned with other subjective constructs). As a result, some researchers relied on self-constructed measurement instruments to carry out their survey, while others, such as the MacArthur Research Network on Mental Health and the Law, successfully developed reliable rating instruments to measure systematically the determinants of perceived coercion (Gardner et al., 1993; Lidz et al., 1995).

3.1.6 Instruments to Measure the Determinants of Perceived Coercion

The MacArthur Perceived Coercion Scale (MPCS), a five-item scale that measures perceived coercion at hospital admission (Gardner et al., 1993) was built on the MacArthur Admission Experience Interview (AEI, a semistructured interview) and the MacArthur Admission Experience Survey (AES, a 15 item, paper and pencil derived instrument). Each item of the MPCS comprises a different facet of perceived coercion. The items are: "influence" ("What had more influence on your being admitted: what you wanted, or what other people wanted?"), "control" ("How much control did you have?"), "choice" ("You chose" or "Somebody made you choose"), "freedom" ("How free did you feel to do what you wanted?"), and finally "idea" or "perceived initiative" ("Whose idea was it to come to hospital?"). The MPCS has proved to have a number of psychometric qualities; hence it was adopted by a several teams of researchers, first in North America where it originated, and then in Europe and New Zealand. Moreover, the AEI and the AES also measure other relevant dimensions of coercion in psychiatric treatment, i.e., "coercion-related behavior" (experienced by users during hospital admission) and "procedural justice."

The "coercion-related behavior" is categorized by the MacArthur Collaboration in three clusters: "positive pressure" (persuasion, inducements, and asking for preferences), "negative pressure" (threats, giving orders, deception, and exhibition of force), and "force" (legal and physical forces that impede the patient to refuse what is imposed by staff) (Lidz, 1998).

As for "procedural justice," research highlights that the degree of procedural justice (or process inclusion), perceived by the user, is linked both to their likelihood to be heard, and thus have their opinion taken into account by the decision maker, and to their perception of fairness in the decision making process that concerns them, i.e., up to what point they feel treated with respect and dignity by the decision maker, (Poythress, Petrila, McGaha, & Boothroyd, 2002).

Perceived coercion has also been measured on a visual analogue scale (a Coercion Ladder, ranging from one to ten), producing a global subjective index. This scale was recently introduced as the research instrument in a multicentre study, involving five European Nordic Countries (Hoyer et al., 2002).

A number of studies have been published which have used the MPCS and/or the Coercion Ladder in various countries and psychiatric settings (Bindman et al., 2005; Cascardi & Poythress, 1997; Iversen, Hoyer, Sexton, & Gronli, 2002; Lidz, 1998; Lidz et al., 2000; McKenna, Simpson, & Laidlaw, 1999; Poulsen, 1999; Rain, Steadman, & Morris, 2003; Rain et al., 2003; Sorgaard, 2004; Taborda, Baptista, Gomes, Nogueira, & Chaves, 2004).

3.1.7 Summary

These studies clearly show that the users' perception of coercion is not only related to the patient's legal status at hospital admission (i.e., voluntary versus compulsory) or the use of force and coercion, but also to other sources of pressure. The most consistent findings on this topic reveal an evident relationship between perceived coercion, the use of negative pressure, i.e., threats, exhibition of force, and the absence of procedural justice, i.e., taking no notice of patient opinions during admission.

3.2 Users' Subjective Experience of Coercive Treatment

3.2.1 Research Methodology and Focus

Once again, population samples and research methods differ from study to study, e.g., sometimes surveys use interviews, at other times questionnaires. Nonetheless, research on patients' subjective experience of coercive treatment focuses mainly on four types of coercion: forced medication, physical restraint, mechanical restraint, and seclusion.

3.3 Forced Treatment, The "Closed Door" Policy, and Seclusion

3.3.1 Forced Treatment: Comparing Users' and Staff Perceptions

The professionals' restricted view (generally focused on the harsher methods of coercion mentioned above) stands out against the users' more extensive approach. This disparity becomes evident when surveys compare user and staff perceptions on certain ward activities, such as forced treatment or compulsive nursing, activities that users consider coercive, but professionals do not. Staff do not seem to be aware of these discrepancies and underestimate their faculty of generating negative feelings within patients who then bring them to either judge mental health personnel as untrustworthy, incompetent, neglecting, and mistreating, or else to refuse treatment (Martinez, Grimm, & Adamson, 1999; Olofsson & Norberg, 2001).

3.3.2   Closed Doors as a Form of Restraint

The divergence in perceptions of coercion between users and staff can relate not only to compulsory measures, but also to common ward activities or organization. For instance, the "closed door" policy (based on the proscription to leave the ward or to go out without permission) is applied to compulsory patients, but often to voluntary patients as well. Hence, this policy limits the right to free movement of some patients. Staff consider this restraint as one of the least restrictive practices in a range of coercive measures, yet many patients bluntly judge it compulsory (Poulsen & Engberg, 2001). In fact, Eriksson and Westrin reveal, through their study, that the most common, and first mentioned, method of restraint is "being locked in a room" (Eriksson & Westrin, 1995).

3.3.3   Seclusion

Another type of coercion experienced by users is seclusion. Patients describe this experience as particularly distressing (Hoekstra, Lendemeijer, & Jansen, 2004). "Isolation," they report, sets off critical feelings of "going mad" or "losing control" over reality (Meehan, Vermeer, & Windsor, 2000). Actually, we know that isolation induces a state of oversensitivity to external stimuli, hallucinations, and delusions. However, Kennedy et al. (1994), studying hallucinations in psychiatric patients, found no statistically significant differences in the state of hallucination of users, before or during seclusion.

Wards usually use specific rooms for seclusion. Research investigating this topic reveals that patients often complain about the physical environment of seclusion. The rooms are described as too small, dirty, cold, and smelly, "too quiet" or "too noisy," with dull or dark colored walls, dim or dazzling lights, and uncomfortable beds. Users also disapprove of the routine of withdrawing patients' personal belongings (that may provide them with a little comfort) and the lack of privacy or intimacy in toilets and bathrooms due to staff supervision (Hoekstra et al., 2004; Kennedy, Williams, & Pesut, 1994; Martinez et al., 1999; Norris & Kennedy, 1992; Tooke & Brown, 1992).

3.4   Information on Coercion and Professional Competences of Staff

3.4.1   Information on Coercion

Users describe different factors that can contribute to the negative perception of coercive treatment: the link between information and coercion is one. Information can either flow from staff to patients, or vice versa. In the first case, if staff give little or no information to patients on their reasons for choosing coercive treatment, or on the patients' rights and legal options for appeal, the negative perception of coercive treatments grows in the patient. Conversely, if users do not disclose their feelings and submit to coercive treatment (for fear of the consequences of refusal), negative emotions also arise. We now have evidence that the greater the disagreement between patient and staff, the higher the risk of coercive treatment, and the more intense the patients' disappointment (Meehan et al., 2000; Olofsson & Norberg, 2001).

3.4.2 Professional Competences of Staff

Kumar et al. (2001) emphasize that the professional competence of staff also plays an important role in arousing negative feelings toward treatment. This fact is critical, as we know that, by and large, patients attach great importance to professional competence. Therefore, if mental health personnel lack education or specific training in dispensing coercive measures, patients' negative feelings toward treatment increase swiftly (Kumar et al.).

3.4.3 In Brief

Generally speaking, users perceive coercive practices (used "too often" or "too long") as punitive and as a source of unnecessary violence causing physical injury or long-lasting psychological trauma. These perceptions blemish the professional image of staff, who are repeatedly portrayed as rude, neglecting, avoiding, or aggressive. Only a minority of users express positive opinions about staff and describe personnel (when handling situations of conflict, or applying coercive measures) as friendly, helpful (Hammill, McEvoy, Koral, & Schneider, 1989; Kumar et al., 2001; Martinez et al., 1999; Meehan et al., 2000), or capable of conveying a feeling of protection, safety, and control (Martinez et al.; Meehan et al.; Tooke & Brown, 1992).

3.5 Psychological Repercussions of Coercive Treatment

3.5.1 Loss of Control

Coercive treatment, or the negative behavior of the professionals providing the treatment, impacts profoundly on the core dimensions of the patients' psyche, injuring their sense of integrity, and violating their feelings as persons (Bonner, Lowe, Rawcliffe, & Wellman, 2002; Eriksson & Westrin, 1995). Patients report that the lack of interest and respect for their opinions by staff affects their self-perception and generates feelings of chaos, loss of control, rights, and dignity. In short, they report sensations of helplessness, powerlessness, and failure, and develop the conviction that they have become an inferior kind of human being, with reduced rights and unworthy of help (Greenberg, Moore-Duncan, & Herron, 1996; Haglund, Von Knorring, & Von Essen, 2003; Hoekstra et al., 2004). Studies reveal that patients not only suffer from the impression of being "nothing or nobody," but they also have the impression of being treated like dangerous criminals, adding a feeling of guilt to their sense of inferiority (Olofsson & Jacobsson, 2001; Olofsson & Norberg, 2001; Tooke & Brown, 1992).

3.5.2 Anxiety and Fear

Research also highlights users' other feelings, i.e., anxiety and fear, which happen to be those most reported. The prevalent anxieties mentioned are fear of the side effects of medication, enforced injections, and narrow seclusion rooms. In some cases these feelings are so strong that they engender in certain patients an acute sense of agony (Greenberg et al., 1996; Haglund et al., 2003; Martinez et al., 1999; Meehan et al., 2000; Naber, Kircher, & Hessel, 1996; Norris & Kennedy, 1992; Sequeira & Halstead, 2002a).

3.5.3 Desire to Take Revenge

Other studies reveal that coercive treatment can foster, inpatients, a desire to take revenge and fight back. Users that do not have the opportunity to discuss coercive measures can perceive treatment as mistreatment, with this feeling being aggravated by the impression of having no possibility to defend themselves. Such a clinical experience builds up their feelings of anger and frustration, and can engender a grim, vicious circle of coercion and patient aggression, with an ever-increasing use of coercive measures (Sequeira & Halstead, 2002a).

In contrast, anger can produce reverse feelings of powerlessness, anxiety, loneliness, and depression (Bonner et al., 2002; Hammill et al., 1989; Hoekstra et al., 2004; Kumar et al., 2001; Martinez et al., 1999; Naber et al., 1996; Sheridan, Henrion, Robinson, & Baxter, 1990; Tooke & Brown, 1992).

3.5.4 Concealing Anger and Frustration

Patients also describe another complex, emotional process. A situation in which their fear of the consequences of the decision on treatment drives them to conceal their negative feelings, for they apprehend that their emotions will be interpreted by staff as straightforward symptoms and, thus, bring personnel to use harsher coercive measures. To cut a long story short, they have the choice to either repress their emotions and exhibit an outer image of a "quiet," "passive," "resigned," or "inhibited" person, or to express their anger and frustration and thus risk further coercion (Ilkiw-Lavalle & Grenyer, 2003). As mentioned by Norris and Kennedy, this psychological paradox is yet another burden patients have to carry on their shoulders (Norris & Kennedy, 1992; Olofsson & Norberg, 2001).

3.5.5 Humiliation and Disempowerment

Meehan and colleagues illustrated a problematic, gender-based situation, where female patients were stripped of their clothes and left naked in front of male staff, and then had to report the humiliating and disempowering experience they were forced to live through (Meehan et al., 2000). These situations, or other measures of restraint, can trigger flashbacks of the women's previous traumata, such as sexual abuse (Bonner et al., 2002; Sequeira & Halstead, 1997).

4   RESEARCH RESULTS AND SUGGESTIONS

4.1   Research Results and Suggestions for Practice

4.1.1   Research Results

The results of research emphasize, on one hand the discrepancies of opinion between users and staff on violence and coercion, and on the other, the impact of violence on patients and personnel. Research also underlines the need for further studies on violent incidents with a more efficient involvement of patients and informal carers and better use of their opinions.

The following paragraphs briefly present results based on scientific evidence.

4.1.2   Discrepancies of Opinion Between Users and Staff. The Paternalistic Model

In a nutshell, current research on coercion and aggressive incidents highlights the discrepancies of opinion between users and staff, i.e., users, on the whole, report higher levels of provocative behavior and coercion (experienced during treatment), than staff. These results draw attention to some divergences that are both overlooked and underlie institutional violence (Bowers, Simpson, & Alexander, 2003). Therefore, in present-day psychiatric practice it is wise to handle, with circumspection, the paternalistic model of care (described in the first paragraph of this chapter) and its assumptions that coercive measures are utilized for "the benefit" only of patients that have lost control over their behavior and their capacity to choose adequate treatment. This, controversial approach can now encourage personnel, as in the "zero tolerance" policy (Whittington & Higgins, 2002), to hold in contempt the patient, their subjective experience, and their knowledge. In clinical practice, professional condescension, like neglect and abuse, can hamper reciprocal understanding, conflict solving, and therapeutic alliance building, thus generating a never-ending vicious circle of "aggression and coercion."

4.1.3   Long-Lasting Sequelae

Mental health professionals now know that patients, victims of violent psychiatric incidents, can suffer from long-lasting sequelae that, in common with other victims of violence and abuse, require specific support in order to work through the trauma.

4.1.4   Burnout Syndrome

Staff disregard for users' experience and trauma of institutional violence might be derived not only from a professional attitude (present, for instance, in the paternalistic model), but might be a warning signal of the burnout syndrome. One of the core symptoms of this syndrome is "depersonalization." Once professionals reach this psychological phase, they become incapable of sustaining the emotional burden of care and, in the main, refer to patients as objects. Here again, a vicious circle can build up. The aggressive behavior of patients can feed the burnout syndrome, staff thus become more and more incompetent in handling violent incidents, which, in turn, stimulates the violent counteractions of patients, etc. (Jackson, Clare, & Mannix, 2002).

4.1.5 Defense Mechanism: Denial

Both staff disinterest in users' views and their difficulty to put up with patient hostility against coercive measures can also be an indicator of a defense mechanism: denial. Patients' negative description of care can collide with the staff need to preserve a positive self-perception of being a receptive and caring professional.

4.1.6 Avoidance

Furthermore, professionals exploring users' perceptions of coercion can become aware that they, like the patient, are at risk of being pressured or coerced by hidden social and institutional requests to exert, by and large, more social control (O'Hagan, 2004), thus causing, in them, a growing feeling of uneasiness that they may try to avoid.

4.1.7 Research Methodology

The above-mentioned issues and methodological problems explain, to some extent, why research has had many difficulties in meeting the requirements of systematic data-collecting when studying the accounts of users on coercive measures. Further scientific research is certainly needed to attain a more sensitive and powerful recognition of the user point of view, undoubtedly an important ethical goal.

4.2 Suggestions for Practice

Studies have highlighted a number of useful suggestions to improve clinical practice when dealing with violence and coercion that we shall now summarize in a few words.

4.2.1 Apply Interactional Approaches

Train mental health professionals to analyze, with an interactionalistic approach, violent incidents or aggressive behavior (to avoid the building of destructive vicious circles), use communication skills and management competences to counter interpersonal violence. It is also advisable to involve patients in the planning and implementation of these educational programs for staff.

4.2.2 Build Procedures to Facilitate Direct Contact

After a violent incident or coercive treatment, set up procedures to facilitate direct contact between staff and patients, i.e., fix a timetable and a sheltered setting where the patients can disclose their emotions without fear of being judged (Gillig et al., 1998), or suffer reprisal. Moreover, if an user has been assaulted by a fellow patient or has witnessed violence on the ward, it is advisable that professionals assess whether the patient is suffering from posttraumatic stress symptoms and whether remedial treatment is needed.

4.2.3   Read Conflict-Related Behavior not only in Terms of Pathology

Keep in check the professionals' tendency to read conflict-related behavior exclusively in terms of "pathology" and question the consequent habits of staff who avoid sharing ideas and responsibilities related to violent incidents.

4.2.4   Coach Staff in Mediation Competencies

Coach staff to build up mediation competencies and develop flexible attitudes. Both abilities are strong assets that grow through experience and become crucial instruments for dealing with aggressive incidents and reinforcing collaboration on commonly agreed goals (Fagan-Pryor et al., 2003). Also teach personnel to take into account, seriously, the users' personal options and preferences.

4.2.5   Make Use of Psychiatric Advance Directives or Crisis Cards

These directives comprise the patients' preferences, written statements put on paper autonomously or with the mental health team, in terms of treatment decisions, in case of a major psychiatric crisis that may hinder their cognitive or relational competencies and increase the probability they will be committed to a psychiatric hospital or given a community treatment order (Atkinson, Garner, & Gilmour, 2004; La Fond & Srebnik, 2002; Thomas & Cahill, 2004). In certain states of the USA, psychiatric advance directives are regulated by specific laws and are legally binding, provided the user agrees to use such an instrument and has not endured overt external pressure when transcribing the directives. These crisis cards may be of assistance in reducing perceived coercion (Srebnik et al., 2005).

4.2.6   Protect Patient Integrity

Protecting and defending patient integrity is another fundamental objective to convey to staff. In this respect, it is advisable to train personnel to respect procedural justice, giving users timely, transparent, and accessible information on ward rules and habits, on patient rights and procedures to appeal against forced treatment, and finally, on how to receive advocacy support. Such a work method is of paramount importance to maximize procedural justice on the ward.

4.2.7   Monitor the Gender Issue

Prepare staff to closely follow the gender issue, particularly with regard to coercive measures or in overcrowded wards that lack privacy. These circumstances can encourage abuse or violent behavior from male staff toward female patients (Sequeira & Halstead, 2002b).

4.2.8   Promote the Prevention of Violence

Finally, provide training programs on how to prevent violence on wards, and offer personnel long-term monitoring through supervision.

4.3   Research Results and Suggestions for Further Research

4.3.1   Research Results

The results in research are promising even if, to date, they are few and contradictory. Yet they do represent an unwavering attempt by researchers to help reduce coercive and violent practice.

4.3.2   Coercion as a Dependent Variable

In the late 1990s, Lidz (1998), reviewed the studies on coercion in psychiatry and highlighted the substantial advancement of research, during the last decades, when coercion was analyzed as a dependent variable (in connection with perceived coercion and procedural justice). However, he also brought to light that, due to complex methodological problems, much less was known about coercion as a predictor of other outcomes as independent variables.

4.3.3   Ward Practices Still Rely More on Professional Values Than on Evidence

Lately, research has begun to address the above-mentioned issues, studying for instance, the influence of perceived coercion on patient satisfaction or treatment adherence, or examining more objective aspects, such as coercion and rates of rehospitalization. These studies show encouraging, but not unanimous, results (Bindman et al., 2005; Day et al., 2005; Rain, Steadman, & Robbins, 2003; Rain, Williams et al., 2003; Sorgaard, 2004). Hence, ward practices still have to rely more on professional values and judgments than on evidence from research.

4.4   Suggestions for Further Research

4.4.1   Involve Users and Carers in Research

Nowadays, to foster new understandings on coercion, it is clearly judicious to involve, at all stages of research, users and informal carers to study their interweaving perspectives. Hopefully, such a research effort should bring about a more circumspect use by staff of "objective" coercion and reduce patient experiences of "perceived" coercion. In other words, the goal of utilizing a participatory research method constitutes a relevant ethical target that entails a close collaboration and common endeavor, of staff, patients, and informal carers, to humanize psychiatric care.

4.4.2 Develop Comparative Studies

Scientific acknowledgment of the role played by culture and law in psychiatric coercion underlines the need to develop comparative studies on an international basis, and action-research projects on a local level. The latter represent a valuable tool to implement monitoring and auditing procedures that deal with critical incidents.

Furthermore, local level projects can help to single-out research topics, and thus increase staff knowledge of, and competency during, violent incidents. On this topic, the issues that merit closer scrutiny are: the psychological consequences of aggression and coercion among users, as victims or witnesses; strategies to limit the harmful after-effects of violent incidents; the determinants of aggression in the community directed against family members or informal carers; strategies to prevent aggression in nonclinical settings and to help relatives and informal carers to cope.

4.4.3 Conclusion

This chapter describes the results of research in psychiatry on user perceptions of coercion and violence. This field of research questions the past conviction that aggressive behavior by the patient can only be a symptom, requiring coercion as a response. Preventive violence (that of coercion) is aggression, whatever one declares, and aggression remains the antinomy of cure and support. Therefore the authors of this chapter call for a shift in the agenda of research and practice. They suggest moving from the biomedical, paternalistic model of care, implicit in mono-disciplinary medically oriented research, to a multidisciplinary approach comprising sociological and psycho-sociological analyses, and thus including in the research design the views of patients and informal carers.

REFERENCES

Atkinson, J. M., Garner, H. C., & Gilmour, W. H. (2004). Models of advance directives in mental health care. *Social Psychiatry and Psychiatric Epidemiology, 39*(8), 673–680.

Bensley, L., Nelson, N., Kaufman, J., Silverstein, B., & Shields, J. W. (1995). Patient and staff views of factors influencing assaults on psychiatric hospital employees. *Issues in Mental Health Nursing, 16*(5), 433–446.

Benson, A., Secker, J., Balfe, E., Lipsedge, M., Robinson, S., & Walker, J. (2003). Discourses of blame: Accounting for aggression and violence on an acute mental health inpatient unit. *Social Science & Medicine, 57*(5), 917–926.

Bindman, J., Reid, Y., Szmukler, G., Tiller, J., Thornicroft, G., & Leese, M. (2005). Perceived coercion at admission to psychiatric hospital and engagement with follow-up. A cohort study. *Social Psychiatry and Psychiatric Epidemiology, 40*(2), 160–166.

Bonner, G., Lowe, T., Rawcliffe, D., & Wellman, N. (2002). Trauma for all: A pilot study of the subjective experience of physical restraint for mental health inpatients and staff in the UK. *Journal of Psychiatric and Mental Health Nursing, 9*, 465–473.

Bowers, L., Simpson, A., & Alexander, J. (2003). Patient-staff conflict: Results of a survey on acute psychiatric wards. *Social Psychiatry and Psychiatric Epidemiology, 38*(7), 402–408.

Brophy, L., & McDermott, F. (2003). What's driving involuntary treatment in the community? The social, policy, legal, and ethical context. *Australasian Psychiatry, 11*(Suppl 1), s84–s88.

Cascardi, M., & Poythress, N. G. (1997). Correlates of perceived coercion during psychiatric hospital admission. *International Journal of Law & Psychiatry, 20*(4), 445–458.

Crowner, M. L., Peric, G., Stepcic, F., & Lee, S. (2005). Assailant and victim behaviors immediately preceding inpatient assault. *The Psychiatric Quarterly, 76*(3), 243–256.

Crowner, M., Peric, G., Stepcic, F., & Ventura, F. (1995). Psychiatric patients' explanations for assaults. *Psychiatric Services, 46*(6), 614–615.

Cutcliffe, J. R., & Hannigan, B. (2001). Mass media, "monsters" and mental health clients: The need for increased lobbying. *Journal of Psychiatric and Mental Health Nursing, 8*(4), 315–321.

Daffern, M., & Howells, K. (2002). Psychiatric inpatient aggression: A review of structural and functional assessment approaches. *Aggression and Violent Behavior, 7,* 477–497.

Davis, S. (1991). Violence by psychiatric inpatients: A review. *Hospital and Community Psychiatry, 2*(6), 585–590.

Day, J. C., Bentall, R. P., Roberts, C., Randall, F., Rogers, A., Cattell, D., et al. (2005). Attitudes toward antipsychotic medication: The impact of clinical variables and relationships with health professionals. *Archives of General Psychiatry, 62*(7), 717–724.

Dressing, H., & Salize, H. J. (2004). Compulsory admission of mentally ill patients in European Union member states. *Social Psychiatry and Psychiatric Epidemiology, 39*(10), 797–803.

Duxbury, J. (2002). An evaluation of staff and patient views of and strategies employed to manage inpatient aggression and violence on one mental health unit: A pluralistic design. *Journal of Psychiatric and Mental Health Nursing, 9*(3), 325–337.

Duxbury, J. (2003). Testing a new tool: The Management of Aggression and Violence Attitude Scale (MAVAS). *Nurse Researcher, 10*(4), 39–52.

Duxbury, J., & Whittington, R. (2005). Causes and management of patient aggression and violence: Staff and patient perspectives. *Journal of Advanced Nursing, 50*(5), 469–478.

Eriksson, K. I., & Westrin, C. G. (1995). Coercive measures in psychiatric care. Reports and reactions of patients and other people involved. *Acta Psychiatrica Scandinavica, 92*(3), 225–230.

Fagan-Pryor, E. C., Haber, L. C., Dunlap, D., Nall, J. L., Stanley, G., & Wolpert, R. (2003). Patients' views of causes of aggression by patients and effective interventions. *Psychiatric Services, 54*(4), 549–553.

Foucault, M. (1961). *Histoire de la folie à l'âge classique*. Paris: Plon.

Frueh, B. C., Knapp, R. G., Cusack, K. J., Grubaugh, A. L., Sauvageot, J. A., Cousins, V. C., et al. (2005). Patients' reports of traumatic or harmful experiences within the psychiatric setting. *Psychiatric Services, 56*(9), 1123–1133.

Gardner, W., Hoge, S. K., Bennett, N., Roth, L. H., Lidz, C. W., Monahan, J., et al. (1993). Two scales for measuring patients' perceptions for coercion during mental hospital admission. *Behavioral Sciences and The Law, 11*(3), 307–321.

Gardner, W., Lidz, C. W., Hoge, S. K., Monahan, J., Eisenberg, M. M., Bennett, N. S., et al. (1999). Patients' revisions of their beliefs about the need for hospitalization. *The American Journal of Psychiatry, 156*(9), 1385–1391.

Gillig, P. M., Markert, R., Barron, J., & Coleman, F. (1998). A comparison of staff and patient perceptions of the causes and cures of physical aggression on a psychiatric unit. *The Psychiatric Quarterly, 69*(1), 45–60.

Greenberg, W. M., Moore-Duncan, L., & Herron, R. (1996). Patients' attitudes toward having been forcibly medicated. *The Bulletin of the American Academy of Psychiatry and The Law, 24*(4), 513–524.

Grewe, C., Wolpert, E., & Pflug, B. (2001). Untersuchung zum aggressiven Verhalten stationär psychisch Kranker. In: P. Harttwich & S. Haas (Eds.), *Aggressive Störungen psychiatrisch Kranker* (pp.75–87). Sternenfeld: Verlag Wissenschaft und Praxis.

Haglund, K., Von Knorring, L., & Von Essen, L. (2003). Forced medication in psychiatric care: Patient experiences and nurse perceptions. *Journal of Psychiatric and Mental Health Nursing, 10*(1), 65–72.

Hammill, K., McEvoy, J. P., Koral, H., & Schneider, N. (1989). Hospitalized schizophrenic patient views about seclusion. *The Journal of Clinical Psychiatry, 50*(5), 174–177.

Harris, C., & Varney, G. (1986). A ten-year study of assaults and assaulters on a maximum security psychiatric unit. *Journal of Interpersonal Violence, 1,* 173–191.

Hinsby, K., & Baker, M. (2004). Patient and nurse accounts of violent incidents in a medium secure unit. *Journal of Psychiatric and Mental Health Nursing, 11*(3), 341–347.

Hoekstra, T., Lendemeijer, H. H., & Jansen, M. G. (2004). Seclusion: The inside story. *Journal of Psychiatric and Mental Health Nursing, 11*(3), 276–283.

Hoge, S. K., Lidz, C. W., Eisenberg, M., Gardner, W., Monahan, J., Mulvey, E., et al. (1997). Perceptions of coercion in the admission of voluntary and involuntary psychiatric patients. *International Journal of Law and Psychiatry, 20*(2), 167–181.

Hoyer, G., Kjellin, L., Engberg, M., Kaltiala Heino, R., Nilstun, T., Sigurjonsdottir, M., et al. (2002). Paternalism and autonomy: A presentation of a Nordic study on the use of coercion in the mental health care system. *International Journal of Law and Psychiatry, 25*(2), 93–108.

Ilkiw-Lavalle, O., & Grenyer, B. F. (2003). Differences between patient and staff perceptions of aggression in mental health units. *Psychiatric Services, 54*(3), 389–393.

Iversen, K. I., Hoyer, G., Sexton, H., & Gronli, O. K. (2002). Perceived coercion among patients admitted to acute wards in Norway. *Nordic Journal of Psychiatry, 56*(6), 433–439.

Jackson, D., Clare, J., & Mannix, J. (2002). Who would want to be a nurse? Violence in the workplace – a factor in recruitment and retention. *Journal of Nursing Management, 10*(1), 13–20.

Johnson, B., Martin, M. L., Guha, M., & Montgomery, P. (1997). The experience of thought-disordered individuals preceding an aggressive incident. *Journal of Psychiatric and Mental Health Nursing, 4*(3), 213–220.

Kennedy, B. R., Williams, C. A., & Pesut, D. J. (1994). Hallucinatory experiences of psychiatric patients in seclusion. *Archives of Psychiatric Nursing, 8*(3), 169–176.

Kjellin, L., & Nilstun, T. (1993). Medical and social paternalism. Regulation of and attitudes towards compulsory psychiatric care. *Acta Psychiatrica Scandinavica, 88*(6), 415–419.

Kjellin, L., & Östman, M. (2005). Relatives of psychiatric inpatients—do physical violence and suicide attempts of patients influence family burden and participation in care? *Nordic Journal of Psychiatry, 59*(1), 7–11.

Kjellin, L., & Westrin, C. G. (1998). Involuntary admissions and coercive measures in psychiatric care: Registered and reported. *International Journal of Law and Psychiatry, 21*(1), 31–42.

Kumar, S., Guite, H., & Thornicroft, G. (2001). Service users' experience of violence within a mental health system: A study using grounded theory approach. *Journal of Mental Health, 10*(6), 597–611.

La Fond, J. Q., & Srebnik, D. (2002). The impact of mental health advance directives on patient perceptions of coercion in civil commitment and treatment decisions. *International Journal of Law and Psychiatry, 25*(6), 537–555.

Lanza, M. L., & Kayne, H. L. (1995). Patient assault: A comparison of patient and staff perceptions. *Issues in Mental Health Nursing 16*(2), 129–141.

Lidz, C. W. (1998). Coercion in psychiatric care: What have we learned from research? *Journal of the American Academy of Psychiatry and the Law, 26*(4), 631–637.

Lidz, C., Hoge, S., Gardner, W., Bennett, N., Monahan, J., Mulvey, E., et al. (1995). Perceived coercion in mental hospital admission: Pressures and process. *Archives of General Psychiatry, 52,* 1034–1039.

Lidz, C. W., Mulvey, E. P., Hoge, S. K., Kirsch, B. L., Monahan, J., Bennett, N. S., et al. (2000). Sources of coercive behaviors in psychiatric admissions. *Acta Psychiatrica Scandinavica, 101*(1), 73–79.

Love, C. C., & Hunter, M. (1999). The Atascadero State Hospital experience. Engaging patients in violence prevention. *Journal of Psychosocial Nursing and Mental Health Services, 37*(9), 32–36.

Martinez, R. J., Grimm, M., & Adamson, M. (1999). From the other side of the door: Patient views of seclusion. *Journal of Psychosocial Nursing and Mental Health Services, 37*(3), 13–22.

McGorry, P. D., Chanen, A., McCarthy, E., Van Riel, R., McKenzie, D., & Singh, B. S. (1991). Posttraumatic stress disorder following recent-onset psychosis. An unrecognized postpsychotic syndrome. *The Journal of Nervous and Mental Disease, 179*(5), 253–258.

McKenna, B. G., Simpson, A. I. F., & Laidlaw, T. M. (1999). Patient perception of coercion on admission to acute psychiatric services: The New Zealand experience. *International Journal of Law and Psychiatry, 22*(2), 143–153.

Meehan, T., Vermeer, C., & Windsor, C. (2000). Patients' perceptions of seclusion: A qualitative investigation. *Journal of Advanced Nursing, 31*(2), 370–377.

Meyer, H., Taiminen, T., Vuori, T., Aijala, A., & Helenius, H. (1999). Posttraumatic stress disorder symptoms related to psychosis and acute involuntary hospitalization in schizophrenic and delusional patients. *The Journal of Nervous and Mental Disease, 187*(6), 343–352.

Monahan, J. (1981). *Predicting violent behavior: An assessment of clinical techniques.* Beverly Hills: Sage.

Mullen, P. D. (1997). Compliance becomes concordance. *British Medical Journal, 314*(7082), 691.

Naber, D., Kircher, T., & Hessel, K. (1996). Schizophrenic patients' retrospective attitudes regarding involuntary psychopharmacological treatment and restraint. *European psychiatry : The Journal of the Association of European Psychiatrists, 11*(1), 7–11.

Nijman, H., a Campo, J., Ravelli, D., & Merckelbach, H. (1999). A tentative model of aggression on inpatient psychiatric wards. *Psychiatric Services, 60*(6), 832–834.

Norris, M. K., & Kennedy, C. W. (1992). The view from within: How patients perceive the seclusion process. *Journal of Psychosocial Nursing and Mental Health Services, 30*(3):7–13.

O'Hagan, M. (2004). Force in mental health services: International user and survivor perspectives. *Mental Health Practice, 7*(5), 12–17.

Olofsson, B., & Jacobsson, L. (2001). A plea for respect: Involuntarily hospitalized psychiatric patients' narratives about being subjected to coercion. *Journal of Psychiatric and Mental Health Nursing, 8*(4), 357–366.

Olofsson, B., & Norberg, A. (2001). Experiences of coercion in psychiatric care as narrated by patients, nurses and physicians. *Journal of Advanced Nursing, 33*(1), 89–97.

Omerov, M., Edman, G., & Wistedt, B. (2004). Violence and threats of violence within psychiatric care. A comparison of staff and patient experience of the same incident. *Nordic Journal of Psychiatry, 58*(5), 363–369.

Philo, G. (Ed.). (1996). *Media and Mental Distress.* London: Longman.

Poulsen, H. D. (1999). Perceived coercion among committed, detained, and voluntary patients. *International Journal of Law and Psychiatry, 22*(2), 167–175.

Poulsen, H. D., & Engberg, M. (2001). Validation of psychiatric patients' statements on coercive measures. *Acta Psychiatrica Scandinavica, 103*(1), 60–65.

Poythress, N. G., Petrila, J., McGaha, A., & Boothroyd, R. (2002). Perceived coercion and procedural justice in the Broward mental health court. *International Journal of Law and Psychiatry, 25*(5), 517–533.

Priebe, S., Badesconyi, A., Fioritti, A., Hansson, L., Kilian, R., Torres-Gonzales, F., et al. (2005). Re-institutionalization in mental health care: Comparison of data on service provision from six European countries. *British Medical Journal, 330*(7483), 123–126.

Priebe, S., Broker, M., & Gunkel, S. (1998). Involuntary admission and posttraumatic stress disorder symptoms in schizophrenia patients. *Comprehensive Psychiatry, 39*(4), 220–224.

Quinsey, V. L. (1979). Assessments of the dangerousness of mental patients held in maximum security. *International Journal of Law and Psychiatry, 2*(3), 389–406.

Rain, S. D., Steadman, H. J., & Robbins, P. C. (2003). Perceived coercion and treatment adherence in an outpatient commitment program. *Psychiatric Services, 54*(3), 399–401.

Rain, S. D., Williams, V. F., Robbins, P. C., Monahan, J., Steadman, H. J., & Vesselinov, R. (2003). Perceived coercion at hospital admission and adherence to mental health treatment after discharge. *Psychiatric Services, 54*(1), 103–105.

Rees, C., & Lehane, M. (1996). Witnessing violence to staff: A study of nurses' experiences. *Nursing Standard, 11*(13–15), 45–47.

Roe, D., & Ronen, Y. (2003). Hospitalization as experienced by the psychiatric patient: A therapeutic jurisprudence perspective. *International Journal of Law and Psychiatry, 26*(3), 317–332.

Roelcke, V. (2002). Zeitgeist und Erbgesundheitgesetzgebung im Europa der 1930er Jahre. Eugenik, Genetik und Politik im historischen Kontext. *Der Nervenarzt, 73*(11), 1019–1030.

Rogers, A. (1993). Coercion and voluntary admission: An examination of psychiatric patient views. *Behavioral Sciences and the Law, 11*, 259–267.

Rose, D. (1998). Television, madness and community care. *Journal of Community and Applied Social Psychology, 8*(3), 213–228.

Ruggeri, M., Lasalvia, A., Tansella, M., Bonetto, C., Abate, M., Thornicroft, G., et al. (2004). Heterogeneity of outcomes in schizophrenia: Three-year follow-up of treated prevalent cases. *The British Journal of Psychiatry, 184*(1), 48–57.

Salleh, M. R. (1994). The burden of care of schizophrenia in Malay families. *Acta Psychiatrica Scandinavica, 89*(3), 180–185.

Saunders, J. C. (2003). Families living with severe mental illness: A literature review. *Issues in Mental Health Nursing, 24*(2), 175–198.

Schmid, R., Spiessl, H., Vukovich, A., & Cording, C. (2003). Burden of relatives and their expectations towards psychiatric institutions. A review of the literature and own results. *Fortschritte der Neurologie-Psychiatrie, 71*(3), 118–128.

Sequeira, H., & Halstead, S. (1997). Use of seclusion, restraint and emergency medication. *The British Journal of Psychiatry, 171*, 288–289.

Sequeira, H., & Halstead, S. (2002a). Control and restraint in the UK: Service users' perspectives. *British Journal of Forensic Practice, 4*(1), 9–19.

Sequeira, H., & Halstead, S. (2002b). Restraint and seclusion: Service user views. *The Journal of Adult Protection, 4*(1), 15–24.

Shah, A., Fineberg, N., & James, D. (1991). Violence among psychiatric inpatients. *Acta Psychiatrica Scandinavica, 91*, 305–309.

Shaw, K., McFarlane, A., & Bookless, C. (1997). The phenomenology of traumatic reactions to psychotic illness. *The Journal of Nervous and Mental Disease, 185*(7), 434–441.

Shepherd, M., & Lavender, T. (1999). Putting aggression into context: An investigation into contextual factors influencing the rate of aggressive incidents in a psychiatric hospital. *Journal of Mental Health, 8*(2), 159–170.

Sheridan, M., Henrion, R., Robinson, L., & Baxter, V. (1990). Precipitants of violence in a psychiatric inpatient setting. *Hospital and Community Psychiatry, 41*(7), 776–780.

Smith, G., Bartlett, A., & King, M. (2004). Treatments of homosexuality in Britain since the 1950s. An oral history: The experience of patients. *British Medical Journal, 328*(7437), 427.

Sorgaard, K. W. (2004). Patients' perception of coercion in acute psychiatric wards. An intervention study. *Nordic Journal of Psychiatry, 58*(4), 299–304.

Srebnik, D. S., Rutherford, L. T., Peto, T., Russo, J., Zick, E., Jaffe, C., et al. (2005). The content and clinical utility of psychiatric advance directives. *Psychiatric Services, 56*(5), 592–598.

Steadman, H. J., Mulvey, E. P., Monahan, J., Robbins, P. C., Appelbaum, P. S., Grisso, T., et al. (1998). Violence by people discharged from acute psychiatric inpatient facilities and by others in the same neighborhoods. *Archives of General Psychiatry, 55*(5), 393–401.

Straznickas, K. A., McNiel, D. E., & Binder, R. L. (1993). Violence toward family caregivers by mentally ill relatives. *Hospital and Community Psychiatry, 44*(4), 385–387.

Szasz, T. S., & Alexander, G. J. (1968). Mental illness as an excuse for civil wrongs. *The Journal of Nervous and Mental Disease, 147*(2), 113–123.

Taborda, J. G. V., Baptista, J. P., Gomes, D. A. R., Nogueira, L., & Chaves, M. L. F. (2004). Perception of coercion in psychiatric and non-psychiatric (medical and surgical) inpatients. *International Journal of Law and Psychiatry, 27*(2), 179–192.

Thomas, P., & Cahill, A. B. (2004). Compulsion and psychiatry. The role of advance statements. *British Medical Journal, 329*(7458), 122–123.

Tooke, S. K., & Brown, J. S. (1992). Perceptions of seclusion: Comparing patient and staff reactions. *Journal of Psychosocial Nursing and Mental Health Services, 30*(8), 23–26.

Trivedi, P., & Wykes, T. (2002). From passive subjects to equal partners: Qualitative review of user involvement in research. *The British Journal of Psychiatry, 181*, 468–472.

Tuffs, A. (2004). Doctors' group publishes archive of doctors registered in Nazi era. *British Medical Journal, 329*(7459), 191.

Tuohimaki, C., Kaltiala-Heino, R., Korkeila, J., Protshenko, J., Lehtinen, V., & Joukamaa, M. (2001). Psychiatric inpatients' views on self-determination. *International Journal of Law and Psychiatry, 24*(1), 61–69.

Twaddle, A. C. (1981). Sickness and sickness career—some implications. In: L. Eisenberg & A. Kleinman (Eds.), *The relevance of social science for medicine* (pp.111–134). Dordrecht: Reidel Publishing Co.

United Nations. (1975). *Declaration on the rights of the disabled person*. New York: United Nations.

United Nations. (1991). *Principles for the protection of persons with mental illness and the improvement of mental health care*. New York: United Nations Commissioner for Human Rights.

United Nations. (1993). *Vienna declaration and program of action. World conference on human rights, Vienna 14–25 June 1993*. New York: United Nations.

Vaddadi, K. S., Gilleard, C., & Fryer, H. (2002). Abuse of carers by relatives with severe mental illness. *The International Journal of Social Psychiatry, 48*(2), 149–155.

Vaddadi, K. S., Soosai, E., Gilleard, C. J., & Adlard, S. (1997). Mental illness, physical abuse and burden of care on relatives: A study of acute psychiatric admission patients. *Acta Psychiatrica Scandinavica, 95*(4), 313–317.

Valenstein, E. (1986). *Great and desperate cures: The rise and decline of psychosurgery and other radical treatments for mental illness*. New York: Basic Books.

Whittington, R., & Higgins, L. (2002). More than zero tolerance? Burnout and tolerance for patient aggression amongst mental health nurses in China and the UK. *Acta Psychiatrica Scandinavica Supplement*, (412), 37–40.

Whittington, R., & Wykes, T. (1996). Aversive stimulation by staff and violence by psychiatric patients. *The British Journal of Clinical Psychology, 35*(1), 11–20.

World Health Organization WHO. (2002). *25 questions and answers on health and human rights (Health and human rights publication series, issue 1, July 2002)*. Geneva: World Health Organization.

III

PREDICTION AND MANAGEMENT

5

Diversity and Consistency in the Legal Management of Involuntary Admission and Treatment Across Europe

TROND HATLING, ATHANASSIOS DOUZENIS, AND JIM MAGUIRE

1 INTRODUCTION

Since the 1950s, changes in mental health care and the activities of human rights movements have changed the focus of treatment from a prescriptive type to one that takes into consideration the patients' views and the rights of the mentally ill individual. With this change, the legal framework for involuntary admission and treatment of the mentally ill has been reformed in many European countries (Salize, Dreβing, & Peitz, 2002). It is undisputed that treating the mentally ill without paying attention to their views has led to serious abuses that tarnished the status of psychiatry. Various asylum scandals that took place in western European countries made it evident that safeguards, for the people admitted and treated against their wishes, needed to be firmly in place (Blom-Cooper, 1992). The abuses of psychiatry and the application of various treatments that were directed against individuals opposed to the state, and the fact that in Eastern Europe political dissidents could be branded mentally ill and kept in asylums against their wishes, further underlined the need for respect of the basic human rights of people as well as the need for firm safeguards and a standard procedure that allows for appeal and a second opinion.

The concepts of involuntary admission and treatment are highly politicized concepts and attract the attention of not only psychiatrists and lawyers but of politicians and ministers alike (Symonds, 1998). While there is general agreement that coercion is sometimes justifiable, the disagreement concerns those situations that justify coercion (Høyer, 2000). The criteria of danger either to the patient or to others is accepted by most bodies, while the need of treatment criteria is disputed.

Harmonization of legislation about these issues in Europe has started, but the difficulties that stem from differences in service funding and priorities, as well as local politics, public concerns, and attitudes about the danger of the mentally ill, make this process a slow and laborious one. In concluding their survey on EU legislation and practice, Salize et al. (2002, p. 148) stated:

> "Thus, the main conclusion of this study is that national legal traditions, structures, and standards of quality with regard to the provision of general health care, as well as national approaches or philosophies regarding mental health care, most strongly determine the legal framework, or the practice of involuntary placement, or treatment of mentally ill patients."

The topic of this chapter is the legal aspects of coercion. This is, at best, a crude measure of the patients' perception of coercion, and a number of authors have argued for collecting information about the patient's actual experience (Kjellin et al., 1993; Lidz, 1998; Westrin & Nilstun, 2000). Monahan et al. (1999), used the MacArthur Perceived Coercion Scale, and found that one in ten of the voluntarily admitted feel coerced, and that nearly 40% of those voluntarily admitted claimed they would have been compulsory admitted, had they not accepted admission. Moreover, the legal aspects do not cover to what extent patients, or other agents, regard coercion as justified. So far, studies of patient experiences of compulsory admissions are contradictory (Monahan et al., 1995). Gardner et al. (1999) found they are mainly negative. Edelsohn and Hiday (1990) found that the majority of patients reported positive experiences, while patients interviewed by Luckstedt and Coursey (1995) and Westrin and Nilstun (2000) had mixed opinions. The systematic over-focusing of the media on violence committed by mental patients (Blumenthal & Lavender, 2001), contributes to the public's perception of the mentally ill patient as dangerous. The public is, in general, positive to compulsory admission (Lauber, Nordt, Falcato, & Rössler, 2002), and far more willing to use coercive measures if the person is considered dangerous to themselves or to others (Pescosolido, Monahan, Link, Stueve, & Kikuzawa, 1999). In the future, studies of coercion should thus be expanded to include different bodies, particularly patients; the perception of coercion, and the justification for such measures.

It is erroneous to use the term "involuntary admission" interchangeably with the term "involuntary detention," as the latter, in some countries, includes occasions where the status of a patient is changed from voluntary to involuntary subsequent to admission. In the remainder of this chapter, *involuntary admission* is thus defined as the process leading into the services, while *involuntary detention* is defined as the process preventing patients from leaving the services. Involuntary placement is used as the overall concept, covering both involuntary admission and detention. Indeed, most guidelines and legislative documents distinguish between involuntary placement and involuntary treatment. In these situations, placement may be used solely for assessment/observation purposes. In Belgium, it is known as *hospitalization for observation* and is permissible initially for 40 days, while in Norway the maximum time for such observation is 10 days. It is thus necessary to separate involuntary placement from involuntary treatment, and in the rest of this chapter involuntary treatment is defined as treatment other than involuntary placement, like medication or other kinds of therapeutic activity.

1.1   Method

In writing this chapter the authors examined practices in about 20 European countries through contacts with colleagues in the EViPRG network. In establishing current legislative arrangements, the scientific literature was searched (Medline, Psych Info) using the words: Involuntary, forced, admission, treatment, legal, and Europe, in various combinations. As a next step, the same key words were used in the Google search engine. All entries were browsed. Additionally, one author of this chapter (Douzenis), contacted the Greek members of the study Eunomia (whose contribution is gratefully acknowledged), who were able to suggest some literature about mental health legislation that was in English or French. The information available was categorized using the definitions provided in this chapter.

2   COMPULSORY ADMISSIONS

2.1   Definitional Issues

Admitting or detaining a person with a mental disorder, against his or her wishes, within a mental health inpatient facility or within a community mental health service occurs within mental health services in all European countries. For example, Belgian mental health legislation (1990), allows for compulsory admission within a family setting, although it rarely happens. Various terms are used to describe this practice, often interchangeably in the same country: involuntary or compulsory detention, placement, admission, or hospitalization; certification, being made "temporary" or being deemed to be a "person of unsound mind" (Ireland), being "sectioned" (UK) or formal admission (UK and Greece). Involuntary placement has been defined by the Council of Europe (2000) as:

> "The admission and detention for treatment of a person suffering from mental disorder in a hospital, other medical establishment, or appropriate place, it being understood that the person in question is capable of consent and does not consent to the placement, or the person in question is incapable of consent, and refuses placement."

Table 1 shows the criteria or conditions for persons to be compulsory admitted in a number of European countries, and is an expanded version of Dressing and Salize (2004).

Table 1. Criteria or Conditions of Persons to Be Compulsory Admitted as Specified by Statutes, Law, or Acts

Mental illness and danger criterion	Austria, Belgium, France, Germany, Luxemburg, Netherlands
Mental illness and danger criterion *or* Mental illness and need for treatment criterion	Denmark, Finland, Greece, Ireland, United Kingdom, Portugal, Norway
Mental illness and need for treatment criterion	Italy, Spain, Sweden

The legislation in all countries specifies the danger criterion as a prerequisite for involuntary admissions. In addition, many countries permit involuntary admissions based on the criterion of need for treatment (Dressing & Salize, 2004). In practice, involuntary admission occurs for a range of reasons such as dangerousness, severe mental disorder, severe distress, absence of insight, crisis management, or simply for humane reasons.

Involuntary placement can also take place outside a psychiatric facility—in international literature usually termed "involuntary outpatient treatment" (Bindman, 2004), or "involuntary outpatient commitment" (Swartz & Monahan, 2001). This type of placement is heavily debated, partly empirically based, but also with strong elements of ideology (Szmukler & Holloway, 2000). Most of the studies on this type of involuntary placement have taken place in the United States (e.g., Allen & Smith, 2001; Miller, 1999; Steadman et al., 2001; Torrey & Zdanowitz, 2001). Swartz and Monahan (2001, p. 323), in their introduction to a series of articles on the subject, claimed that:

> "Proposed as a less restrictive alternative to involuntary inpatient commitment, outpatient commitment has amassed a host of supporters and critics, despite a relative paucity of empirical evidence about its risks and benefits."

They end their introduction with:

> "We doubt that supporters or opponents of outpatient commitment will come away from this collection in consensus."

This treatment may consist of taking prescribed medication, reporting to an outpatient clinic or day hospital which monitors the person's condition, or participating in individual, or group, therapy. Hospital release may be conditional on treatment compliance in an outpatient setting.

2.2   Epidemiology of Involuntary Placement in European Countries

The author, in preparing this section, examined practices in 21 European countries with regard to involuntary admission, commitment, or detention of persons with mental illness. An unknown degree of the variations between countries in relation to involuntary admissions is due to definitional issues, reporting mechanisms and practices, and data collection procedures. Some countries base their figures on purely involuntary admission rates, while others include applications for involuntary admission, even if no such admission subsequently occurred. Episodes where a patient's legal status changed from voluntary to involuntary, subsequent to admission, may or may not be included in the data.

Data from the Report on compulsory admission and involuntary detention of mentally ill patients (Salize et al., 2002) are a case in point. The figures, which are from the, then, 15 European Union member states, show wide variability and indicate a strong need for more detailed examination of reporting mechanisms and practices within the member states. Portugal, at 3.2%, has the lowest reported percentage of all inpatient admissions that are involuntary (year 2000) with Sweden officially reporting a quota of 30% (year 1997). Nationwide data is not available in Greece. However, data from the County of Athens (Attica) for 1997 indicates an involuntary admission rate of 75.6% (Douzenis, Michalopoulou, & Christodoulou, 2002).

An even greater variation is seen in the involuntary admission rates, per 100,000 population, in these countries. Portugal, again the lowest, reports a rate of six per 100,000, while Austria reports 175, and Finland tops the table at 218 per 100,000 for the year 2000. Rates of involuntary placements per 100,000 do not correlate with percentages of all inpatient episodes, indicating varying procedures for psychiatric admissions and/or very different levels of access for mentally ill persons to inpatient treatment. These observed differences are in line with other studies (Hansson et al., 1999; Riecher-Rössler & Rössler, 1993; Zinkler & Priebe, 2002). A number of hypotheses have been put forward to explain the differences in involuntary admission rates and quotas between, and within, countries: differences in legislation, and in interpretation of the legislation, availability of beds, degree of urbanization, degree of mental illness in the population, patient characteristics such as diagnosis, gender, and sociodemographic factors, personnel characteristics as well as level of education, ethics, and attitudes, institutional and ward characteristics like hospital responsibility, ward atmosphere, and staffing level, and characteristics of community services like educational and staffing level. So far, no firm conclusions have been made regarding the importance of each of these factors.

2.3 European Regulation of Involuntary Placement

At a European level much attention has been given to the rights of people with mental disorders. In 1950, the European Convention for the Protection of Human Rights and Fundamental Freedoms stated that:

> "Everyone who is deprived of his liberty by arrest or detention shall be entitled to take proceedings by which the lawfulness of his detention shall be decided speedily by a court and his release ordered if the detention is not lawful." (Article 5, paragraph 4).

Subsequent recommendations from groups such as the Committee of Ministers of the Council of Europe (1983), and the Parliamentary Assembly of the Council of Europe (1994), have formulated guidelines for legislators and practitioners alike.

The 1994 recommendation was timely, as several member states were reviewing or drafting new mental health legislation. It led to the creation of a Working Party on Psychiatry and Human Rights (2000). This, in turn, led to the formulation of a White Paper on the protection of human rights and the dignity of people suffering from mental disorder, especially those placed as involuntary patients in a psychiatric establishment (Council of Europe, 2000). The eighth general report of the European Committee for the Prevention of Torture and Inhuman or Degrading Treatment or Punishment or CPT (1998), was devoted to involuntary placement in psychiatric establishments. Then, in 2004, recommendation 10 from the Committee of Ministers of the Council of Europe provided a template for legislators and practitioners alike addressing, among many other issues, criteria for routine and emergency involuntary placement and treatment (Articles 17–28). It remains to be seen to what extent these guidelines will change the present substantial differences in legal regulations and clinical practice throughout Europe.

It is within this context of increased protection of the rights of the mentally ill that much of the legislation governing involuntary placement of persons with mental disorder was drafted. However, it is worth noting that, in many European countries, measures to protect the rights of mentally ill persons who are involuntarily admitted pre-existed initiatives on these matters by overarching European bodies.

Interestingly, the aforementioned guidelines and recommendations on involuntary placement may not be sufficient to ensure standardized practices, as it is by no means clear what legislative approaches should be taken to lower involuntary placement rates. Salize et al. (2002), report paradoxical effects on commitment rates immediately after the implementation of new laws in Belgium and Austria. England experienced a dramatic increase in formal (compulsory) admissions from 1984 to 1996. This followed the enactment of new mental health legislation in 1983. Hotopf, Wall, Buchanan, Wessley, and Churchill (2000) suggest this rise is due to changes in the psychiatric services, a reduction in psychiatric beds in particular, and changing societal pressures on psychiatrists away from libertarianism and toward coercion.

In many countries, the written application to have someone involuntarily admitted can be, and often is, initiated by a relative or other concerned person. The certificate must be completed (with a second, or more, opinion obtained) within a defined period of time, or the document becomes legally invalid and the procedure must begin again. The Irish Mental Treatment Act of 1945 may have been unique in requiring the signatures of two general practitioners (GP) for involuntary detentions to private psychiatric facilities, while requiring only one for public hospital detentions. The higher standard of having a second GP opinion was extended in practice to all involuntary detentions, public or private, in the 1980s and 1990s, an example of standards in practice being pitched higher than the minimum requirements in law. Another example of standards in practice exceeding those required in law is seen in some Italian regions. The governing mental health legislation (law 833 of 1978) allows a nonpsychiatrist physician to complete the involuntary detention documentation, even for the second (known as *sustaining*) stage of the process. Several regions have imposed the higher standard of requiring a psychiatrist's opinion for the second stage.

In most cases, European countries have enacted legislation specifically in relation to mental health. Currently, several nations have more than one mental health act in operation. Where there is a specific mental health legislation, involuntary placement is always addressed.

In countries where there is no specific mental health legislation, mental health service users have recourse to the law under general legislation, covering the rights of all users of health services. Proponents of nonspecialized regulation argue that the approach serves to de-stigmatize mental illness. This contention has yet to be tested empirically.

Of the 21 countries considered in this section all, except Italy and some German states, have updated their governing laws, acts, or regulations in the last 30 years. Ireland has enacted a new Mental Health Act (2001) but, while awaiting its full implementation, technically still operates under the Mental Treatment Act (1945) and subsequent regulations. In practice, the higher standards of the 2001 Act are being observed.

In some countries the governing statutes, regulations or acts have countrywide applicability, while in others the legislation changes from one region to another. Germany, being a federation of states (Bundesländer), is an obvious example of the latter with its 16 separate laws governing mental health care (Salize et al., 2002).

2.4 Emergency Involuntary Placement

In most countries, involuntary placement can be either normal/routine or an emergency procedure. Varying legislative approaches also exist in relation to emergency situations, where involuntary placement is deemed necessary. Emergency procedures are particularly necessary in countries where the normal application, and approval, procedure is rigorous and therefore time consuming. The Belgian system, which requires the approval of a Judge of Peace, a lawyer, and possibly an independent psychiatrist, is a good example. The presence of the criterion of "imminent danger" is grounds for an emergency procedure under French law. In most countries, a physician who is not qualified in psychiatry may initiate, in writing, an emergency involuntary admission. Indeed, several nations permit this approach to initiation of the procedure, even in nonemergency situations. All countries require that the decision is reviewed or endorsed by one or more psychiatrists, or in some countries clinical psychologists, very soon after the original decision. An independent review is also required in all countries except Belgium, Greece, and Spain.

Any comparison of mental health legislation is confounded by the extensive degree of detail found within the various acts. To illustrate this point, one might consider how multi-faceted the involuntary placement process can be. Under the law it is usually stipulated who may initiate a detention certificate. However, some acts are not specific about the identity of the initial applicant, leaving considerable room for interpretation of who this may be. Then there are varying requirements for who else is required to sign the paperwork. The legislation may necessitate the involvement of a general practitioner, or other physician, alone or as well as one or more psychiatrists.

Next, there are various time-bound elements to be complied with, such as the maximum period of time from the initial application to secondary, and subsequent, opinions, or the period of time from assessment to compulsory detention and, where permissible at all, the maximum allowable time from involuntary detention to completion of the certificate. The clock is running once again, once detention has commenced, counting out a legally required period, at the end of which the detention order expires, if not reapproved.

2.5   Involuntary Detention Subsequent to Voluntary Admission

The reasons given for changing a patient's legal status from voluntary to involuntary are similar to those given for initial involuntary admission. In many cases, it occurs because the patient refuses voluntary treatment that the mental health team believes is necessary. The legal procedural requirements for changing a person's status in this way are no different to those for initial detention in all the European countries reviewed in this study, with minor differences in Sweden and Finland. Another reason why subsequent involuntary detentions occur arises from the legal requirement in all European countries to reapprove the initial involuntary detention within a stated period of time. In all countries, two or more reapprovals of the original decision are allowed and the time periods are stipulated. Some countries, like Norway, do not permit a change from voluntary to involuntary while the patient is hospitalized. The patient must be discharged, and then involuntarily admitted through an ordinary procedure.

2.6   Rights of Patients Placed Involuntarily

A characteristic of modern mental health legislation is the mention of the rights of involuntary patients. The wording in the various acts differs little and most enshrine rights, such as the right to appeal the placement, the right to have a visit from a lawyer, personal physician, or inspectorate, ombudsman, patient counselor, the right to respect (Belgium), the right to privacy of personal mail, the right to vote (France), and the right to have a visit from a lawyer, personal physician, or inspectorate, ombudsman, patient counselor (Denmark), control commission (Germany), or mental health commissioner (Ireland). Sometimes these rights are legislated for in a separate act (Finland) (Salize et al., 2002).

Advocacy is another entitlement incorporated into several of the mental health acts. Patient counselors are provided for in the Danish Act (1989), and Austria has its *patientenanwalt* service, with offices based in the hospitals. In other countries, such as the Netherlands and Ireland, the inspector/commissioner is invested with the advocacy function along with all their other responsibilities. This seems less satisfactory than have specially appointed personnel for this role. Of course, in many countries, lawyers or other persons must be appointed as patient advocates if the patient is appealing the placement to the control commission (Norway) or in the courts.

2.7   Conclusion

There are many factors influencing involuntary admission rates and quotas, and probably legislation plays only a minor role (Bagby & Atkinson, 1988; Hatling, Krogen, & Ulleberg, 2002). Variables such as standards of care, service location (Madianos & Economou, 1999), availability of inpatient beds (Hotopf et al., 2000; Kokkonen, 1993), interpretation of the legislation (Humphreys & Ryman, 1996), and intuitive decision-making (Appelbaum, 1997; Rogers, 1999), probably bring a strong influence to bear on local practices. So far, the complexity of these mechanisms is poorly understood, and there is an urgent need for cross-national studies including legal perspectives, service characteristics and user, provider, and public perspectives.

Psychiatry has, for a long time, accepted the responsibility for the duty of care (medical paternalism), and the duty of protecting other people from the risk of being harmed by a mentally ill person (social paternalism) (Westrin, 1997). Different legal actions by policymakers have, over the decades, attempted to restrict this responsibility, moving more of the deciding power to the legal system. The strengthening of the user perspective implicit in these actions has, at the same time, been questioned by the public, fearing for their own health and safety. The many high-profile criminal cases in different European countries involving psychiatric patients implies that reducing the use of compulsory placement in psychiatric facilities cannot be restricted to the services themselves, but must include efforts to increase the public's feeling of safety.

3   INVOLUNTARY TREATMENT IN EUROPE

3.1   Introduction

As with involuntary placement, the practice on involuntary treatment has been criticized by the civil rights movement, and both the EU court of Civil Rights and United Nations Declarations has emphasized the patient's competence to decide on treatment, even if placed involuntary (Høyer, 2000; Salize et al., 2002).

3.2   Definitional Issues

There is no clear distinction between involuntary placement and involuntary treatment, nor between involuntary treatment and forced medication, as a kind of coercive measure. An example of the latter is Kaltiala-Heino et al. (2000), who use compulsory medication, involuntary medication, and forced medication interchangeably when writing about the same empirical phenomenon, but from the article it is not possible to identify if this is a treatment or a coercive measure.

According to Salize et al. (2002), a number of treatments or interventions can, potentially, be applied compulsorily across Europe. This includes pharmaceutical intervention, electroconvulsive therapy (ECT), psychotherapy, psychosurgery, treatment of somatic comorbidity, and forced feeding. While some of these interventions are explicitly permitted in some countries, in other countries the same interventions can be permitted only with defined conditions, and are explicitly prohibited in others. ECT is the only intervention where they found countries in all three categories. They could find no common patterns regarding how the 15 countries in their study regulated coercive application of interventions (Salize et al. 2002, p. 30).

Even if there are distinctions in the law between involuntary placement and involuntary treatment, the distinction is often less clear in clinical practice. According to Steinert and Smith (2004), involuntary treatment is defined by whether or not the patient is touched, or held, during the administration of medication. In instances when the staff told the patient that he would be physically forced to take the medication, without being touched, it was not defined as involuntary treatment. In other countries, such as Norway, this would clearly be defined as involuntary treatment.

3.3 Epidemiology of Involuntary Treatment in European Countries

Due, possibly, to the lack of distinction between involuntary placement and treatment presented in the introduction to this chapter, few studies are published regarding the epidemiology of involuntary treatment. In Denmark, according to Sundhedsstyrelsen (2003), involuntary treatment was used against 523 persons in 2002, out of a total of 25,000 inpatients, a quota of about 2%. ECT was used against 76 persons. If the variety of concepts used in Kaltiala-Heino et al. (2000), could be interpreted as involuntary treatment only, 8.4% of a population of about 1,500 patients in Finland was involuntary treated. Hatling and Krogen (1998) estimated that approx. 6.6% of about 14,000 inpatients, in Norway in 1994, were treated involuntary with pharmaceuticals.

3.4 European Regulation of Involuntary Treatment

Four legal areas will be presented: is there a legal distinction between involuntary placement and involuntary treatment, is it possible to be involuntary placed without being involuntary treated, what types of treatment can be delivered involuntary, and to what extent is informed consent required?

Table 2. Distinction Between Involuntary Placement and Involuntary Treatment in a Number of European Countries

	Number	Countries
Distinction	8	Austria, Denmark, Germany, Luxemburg, Netherlands, Sweden, UK, Norway.
No distinction	12	Belgium, Finland, France, Greece, Ireland, Italy, Portugal, Spain, Lithuania, Poland, Slovakia, Czech Republic.

In Table 2 we present countries with and without a legal distinction between involuntary placement and involuntary treatment.

Eight European countries define involuntary placement and involuntary treatment as distinct modalities in their legal frameworks, while 12 countries do not have that distinction. A legal distinction, of involuntary placement from involuntary treatment, might increase awareness for safeguarding patients' rights when applying coercive interventions (Salize et al., 2002).

In Table 3, countries are separated according to whether they allow involuntary placement without involuntary treatment.

Table 3. Legal Distinction Allowing Involuntary Placement Without Involuntary Treatment

	Number	Countries
Distinction	10	Austria, Denmark, Germany, Luxemburg, Netherlands, Sweden, UK, Poland, Slovakia, Czech Republic, Norway.
No distinction	10	Denmark, Finland, France, Ireland, Italy, Luxemburg, Portugal, Spain, Sweden, Lithuania.

An equal number of European countries in our study have, and do not have, this distinction. Those who do not make this distinction probably base it on the assumption that the aim of involuntary placement is to deliver the necessary needed treatment. As can be seen from Tables 2 and 3, regardless of distinguishing between involuntary placement and involuntary treatment on a legal level, there are countries where patients must accept treatment whenever being placed involuntarily, as is the case in Sweden, Denmark, or Luxembourg.

Even if involuntary placement, and administration of treatment involuntarily, is not legally distinct, some countries in their legislation allow the placement of a patient in a psychiatric unit against his will but make it plain that the psychiatrist can withhold treatment in order to have a better assessment of the mental health needs of the patient, and in order to reach a more conclusive diagnosis. Bearing in mind that the decision to treat is a medical one (psychiatric), one assumes that the psychiatrists in the states where the law does not specifically allow admission without treatment, will still decide when to start medical treatment and will not be forced to start treatment "upon admission."

In most legislation, treatment means administration of psychiatric medication and nothing more, although some countries make a specific reference to ECT, or other treatments like individual, and group, therapy (Salize et al., 2002). When the application of involuntary or coercive treatment measures is not explicitly defined in law, the civil rights of involuntarily placed persons are usually safeguarded by other means or procedures (Salize et al., 2002).

In Table 4, countries are classified by requiring, or not requiring, informed consent for involuntary treatment.

Table 4. Informed Consent for Involuntary Treatment Required

	Number	Countries
Informed consent required	5	Austria, Germany, Ireland, Netherlands, Sweden
Informed consent not required	15	Belgium, Denmark, Finland, France, Greece, Italy, Luxemburg, Port, Spa, UK, Lithuania, Poland, Slovakia, Czech Republic, Norway

In countries which do not require informed consent, involuntarily placed patients might be treated without consent in cases of emergency, or at times when they lack the mental capacity to consent. From a clinical perspective this can also be seen as a logical interpretation of the law. Patients who refuse treatment for their illness are not doing so because they want to stay ill but because they do not realize they are ill because of a lack of insight into common symptoms of psychotic illnesses. Thus, by admitting someone who is grossly psychotic and disturbed against their will, it is implicit that those persons lack the capacity of consent, regardless of them giving it or not. It can also happen that the patient consents to treatment but they are so obviously disturbed at the time that their consent is not valid, neither is any agreement they enter into. In this respect, it is difficult to understand the law in the states requiring consent. It seems that the term consent has a different legal meaning, or that it suggests a different procedure, in order to safeguard patients' rights.

3.5 Conclusion

As can be observed from this chapter, there are substantial legal differences between European countries regarding involuntary treatment. There are few studies illuminating to what extent involuntary treatment is used and, similarly, on the type of involuntary treatment actually used. Though there is conceptual, and political, as well as scientific, agreement for the need to protect the civil rights of patients, we still have quite a long way to go in order to establish agreement between the legal perspective focusing on protecting patient rights, and the clinical perspective focusing on treating the patient for his or her illness (Szmukler & Holloway, 2000).

REFERENCES

Allen, M., & Smith, V. F. (2001). Opening Pandora's Box: The practical and legal dangers of involuntary outpatient commitment. *Psychiatric Services, 52*(3), 342–346.

Appelbaum, P. S. (1997). Almost a revolution: An international perspective on the law of involuntary commitment. *The Journal of the American Academy of Psychiatry and the Law, 25*(2), 135–147.

Assembly of the Council of Europe (1994). *Recommendation 1235 on psychiatry and human rights.* Strasbourg: Council of Europe.

Bagby, R. M., & Atkinson, L. (1988). The effects of legislative reform on civil commitment admission rates: A critical analysis. *Behavioral Sciences and the Law, 6,* 45–61.

Bindman, J. (2004). Involuntary outpatient treatment in England and Wales. *Current Opinion in Psychiatry, 15,* 595–598.

Blom-Cooper, L. (1992). *Report of the committee of inquiry into complaints about Ashworth Hospital (Cm2028).* London: HMSO.

Blumenthal, S., & Lavender, T. (2001). *Violence and mental disorder. A critical aid to the assessment and management of risk.* London: Jessica Kingsley Publishers Ltd.

Council of Europe (1950). *The European Convention for the Protection of Human Rights and Fundamental Freedoms.* E.T.S. No.5, Rome.

Council of Europe (2000): *White Paper on the protection of the human rights and dignity of people suffering from mental disorder, especially those placed as involuntary patients in a psychiatric establishment.* CM(2000) 23 Addendum, appendix 1. Strasbourg: Council of Europe.

Council of Europe Committee of the Ministers (1983). *Recommendation No R (83)2 to member states on legal protection of persons suffering from mental disorder placed as involuntary patients.* Strasbourg: Council of Europe.

Council of Europe Committee of the Ministers (2004). *Recommendation No. REC(2004)10 concerning the protection of the human rights and dignity of persons with mental disorder.* Strasbourg: Council of Europe.

Douzenis, A., Michalopoulou, P., & Christodoulou, G. N. (2002). Factors influencing formal admission in Athens. In: T. Palmstierna & H. Nyman (Eds.) *Management strategies and guidelines. Prevention and treatment of aggression* (pp.11–17). Sweden: Larserics Digital Pro.

Dressing, H., & Salize, H. J. (2004). Compulsory admissions of mentally ill patients in European Union Member States. *Social Psychiatry and Psychiatric Epidemiology, 39,* 797–803.

Edelsohn, G. A., & Hiday, V. H. (1990). Civil commitment: A range of patient attitudes. *Bulletin of the American Academy of Psychiatry and the Law, 18,* 65–77.

European Committee for the Prevention of Torture and Inhuman or Degrading Treatment or Punishment (1998): *Eighth general report, CPT/Inf (98)12.* Strasbourg: CPT.

Gardner, W., Lidz, C. W., Hoge, S. K., Monahan, J., Eisenberg, M. M., Bennett, N. S., et al. (1999). Patients' revisions of their beliefs about the need for hospitalization. *The American Journal of Psychiatry, 156,* 1385–1391.

Hansson, L., Muus, S., Saarento, O., Vinding, H. R., Göstas, G., Sandlund, M., et al. (1999). The Nordic comparative study on sectorized psychiatry: Rates of compulsory care and use of compulsory admissions during a one-year follow-up. *Social Psychiatry and Psychiatric Epidemiology, 34,* 99–104.

Hatling, T., & Krogen, T. (1998). *Bruk av tvang i norsk psykiatri – en empirisk gjennomgang.* NIS-rapport STF78 F98506. Trondheim.

Hatling, T., Krogen, T., & Ulleberg, P. (2002). Compulsory admissions to psychiatric hospitals in Norway. International comparisons and regional variations. *Journal of Mental Health, 11,* 623–634.

Hotopf, M., Wall, S., Buchanan, A., Wessley, S., & Churchill, R. (2000). Changing patterns in the use of the Mental Health Act 1983 in England, 1984–1996. *The British Journal of Psychiatry, 176,* 479–484.

Høyer, G. (2000). On the justification for civil commitment. *Acta Psychiatrica Scandinavica Supplement, 399*(101), 65–71.

Humphreys, M., & Ryman, A. (1996). Knowledge of emergency compulsory detention procedures among general practitioners in Edinburgh: Sample survey. *British Medical Journal, 312*, 1462–1463.

Kaltiala-Heino, R., Korkeila, J., Touhimäki, C., et al. (2000): Coercion and restrictions in psychiatric treatment, Journal of European psychiatry, *15*, 213–219.

Kjellin, L., Westrin, C. -G., Eriksson, K., Axelsson-Östman, M., Candefjord, I. -L., Ekblom, B., et al. (1993). Coercion in psychiatric care: Problems of medical ethics in a comprehensive empirical study. *Behavioral Sciences and the Law, 11*, 323–334.

Kokkonen, P. (1993). Coercion and legal protection in psychiatric care in Finland. *Medicine and Law, 12*, 113–124.

Lauber, C., Nordt, C., Falcato, L., & Rössler, W. (2002). Public attitude to compulsory admission of mentally ill people. *Acta Psychiatrica Scandinavica, 105*, 385–389.

Lidz, C. W. (1998). Coercion in psychiatric care: What have we learned from research. *The Journal of the American Academy of Psychiatry and the Law, 26*, 631–637.

Luckstedt, A., & Coursey, R. D. (1995). Consumer perceptions of pressure and force in psychiatric treatments. *Psychiatric Services, 46*, 146–152.

Madianos, M. G., & Economou, M. (1999). The impact of a community mental health center on psychiatric hospitalizations in two Athens areas. *Community Mental Health Journal, 35*(4), 313–323.

Mental Health Act Poland August 19 1994 (1994). Warsaw: Acts Register.

Miller, R. D. (1999). Coerced treatment in the community. *Forensic Psychiatry, 22*(1), 183–196.

Monahan, J., Hoge, S. K., Lidz, C., Roth, L. H., Bennett, N., Gardner, W., et al. (1995). Coercion and commitment: Understanding involuntary mental hospital admission. *International Journal of Law and Psychiatry, 18*, 249–263.

Monahan, J., Lidz, C. W., Hoge, S. K., Mulvey, E. P., Eisenberg, M. M., Roth, L. H., et al. (1999). Coercion in the provision of mental health services: The MacArthur Studies. In: J. P. Morrissey & J. Monahan (Eds.) *Research in community and mental health. Coercion in mental health services — International perspectives.* Stamford: JAI Press.

Pescosolido, B. A., Monahan, J., Link, B., Stueve, A., & Kikuzawa, M. S. (1999). The public's view of the competence, dangerousness, and need for legal coercion among persons with mental illness. *American Journal of Public Health, 89*, 1339–1345.

Riecher-Rössler, A., & Rössler, W. (1993). Compulsory admission of psychiatric patients – an international comparison. *Acta Psychiatrica Scandinavica, 87*, 231–236.

Rogers, A. (1999). Broadening the agenda of coercion research: Addressing the sociopolitical context of risk, violence and mental disorder. In: J. M. Morrissey & J. Monahan (Eds.) *Coercion in mental health services – international perspectives. Research in community and mental health. Volume 10.* Stamford: JAI Press.

Salize, H. J., Dreβing, H., & Peitz, M. (2002). *Compulsory admission and involuntary treatment of mentally ill patients — Legislation and practice in EU member states.* Mannheim, Germany: Central Institute of Mental Health.

Steadman, H. J., Gounis, K., Dennis, D., Hopper, K., Roche, B., Swartz, M., et al. (2001). Assessing the New York City involuntary outpatient commitment pilot program. *Psychiatric Services, 52*(3), 330–336.

Steinert, T., & Smith, P. (2004). Effect of voluntariness of participation in treatment on short-term outcome of inpatients with schizophrenia. *Psychiatric Services, 55*(7), 786–791.

Sundhedsstyrelsen. (2003). *Anvendelse af tvang i psykiatrien 2002*, Nye tal fra Sundhedsstyrelsen, 2003:20. København.

Swartz, M. S., & Monahan, J. (2001). Special section on involuntary outpatient commitment: Introduction. *Psychiatric Services, 52*(3), 323–324.

Symonds, B. (1998). The philosophical and sociological context of mental health care legislation. *Journal of Advanced Nursing, 27*(5), 946–954.

Szmukler, G., & Holloway, F. (2000). Reform of the Mental Health Act. Health or safety? The *British Journal of Psychiatry, 177*, 196–200.

Torrey, E. F., & Zdanowicz, M. (2001). Outpatient commitment: What, why and for whom. *Psychiatric Services, 52*(3), 337–341.

Westrin, C. -G. (1997). Compulsory psychiatric care – an arena for conflicts and research. *Nordic Journal of Psychiatry, 51*(Suppl. 39), 57–61.

Westrin, C. -G., & Nilstun, T. (2000). Psychiatric ethics and health services research. Concepts and research strategies. *Acta Psychiatrica Scandinavica, 101,* 47–50.

Working Party on Psychiatry and Human Rights (2000). *White Paper on the protection of the human rights and dignity of people suffering from mental disorder, especially those placed as involuntary patients in a psychiatric establishment.* Strasbourg.

6

Prediction of Violence in Inpatient Settings

TILMAN STEINERT

1 INTRODUCTION

Taking into account the high incidence of violence in psychiatric institutions (see Chapter 3) and the hazards posed thereby to the physical and mental health of staff, there is a need for procedures and instruments for the prediction of violence in clinical routine. This applies not just to safety within institutions but also clinicians who have to deliberate patients' rights and the possible danger to the public before their discharge. In the UK, practice guidelines suggest that best practice should include a documented risk assessment before any patient is discharged to the community (Reed, 1997). However, to develop and evaluate formal instruments is a second step after robust predictors of violence have been determined. At first glance, the conditions seem similar regarding community violence and the risk of violence posed by discharged patients with mental disorders. A large body of research has identified a set of variables which are consistently associated with violent delinquency, among them personality traits, nonspecific and specific historical items, psychiatric diagnoses, and clinical symptoms (Bonta, Law, & Hanson, 1998; Dolan & Doyle, 2000; Harris & Rice, 1997; Hodgins, Mednick, Brennan, Schulsinger, & Engberg, 1996; Swanson, Holzer, Ganju, & Iono, 1990). Thereafter, predictive instruments such as PCL-R (Hare, 2003), the HCR-20 (Douglas, Ogloff, Nicholls, & Grant, 1991), and the ICT (Monahan et al., 2000) have been developed and evaluated within the last decade (Webster, Douglas, Belfrage, & Link, 2000). Repeatedly, it has been shown that static and historical variables make a major contribution to the incidence of violence in the community than clinical variables which can underlie therapeutic influences (Bonta et al.; Buchanan, 1999; Dolan & Doyle; Harris & Rice). Many studies with rather different methodological approaches provide evidence that the risk of violence in the community is increased by a diagnosis of major mental disorder (Eronen, Hakola, & Tiihonen, 1996; Hodgins et al.; Swanson et al., not confirmed, however, by the MacArthur study findings, Steadman et al., 1998), substance abuse (Hodgins et al.; Räsänen et al., 1998; Swanson et al.), ideas of persecution, especially so-called "threat control override" symptoms (Boeker & Haefner, 1973; Link, Stueve, & Phelan, 1998), medication noncompliance (Swartz et al., 1998), "concentrated poverty" in the neighborhood (Silver, Mulvey, & Monahan, 1999), history of violence, male gender, and young age (Bonta et al.; Monahan & Appelbaum, 2000).

In contrast, in inpatient settings only a few predictors of violence have been consistently confirmed, though plenty of research has been carried out in many countries on the subject (Steinert, 2002). Therefore, there has been only modest progress in the development of instruments and research on the accuracy of predictions of violence in inpatient settings. The purpose of this review will be to give an overview of the results of studies in inpatient settings, to suggest hypotheses for the inconsistency of findings, and finally, in a necessarily shorter part, to review findings regarding the accuracy of predictions.

2   STATISTICAL PREDICTORS OF INPATIENT VIOLENCE

Generally, predictions of inpatient violence are short-term predictions (days or weeks), in contrast to predictions in forensic psychiatry, which comprise months or years. Given the continuous decrease in the incidence of violence during inpatient treatment (Steinert, Sippach, & Gebhardt, 2000), the risk of violence by inpatients certainly is rather dynamic and dependent on many variables and cannot be considered as a static property. Variables related to the violent behavior of psychiatric inpatients can be:

(1) Patient-related:
   (i) Historical
   (ii) Demographical
   (iii) Diagnostic
   (iv) Psychopathological
   (v) Behavioral
   (vi) Biological
(2) Environment-related:
   (i) Behavior of staff and fellow patients
   (ii) Ward atmosphere (furniture, rooms, rules, number and character of fellow patients, number, skills and personality of staff)
(3) Interactional

While most research that has been conducted regarding the community violence of mentally ill people is limited to a small set of variables, e.g., diagnosis, gender, criminal records, much more information could be available in inpatient settings.

However, most research has been done with those variables which can be easily obtained—patient variables—and the least with interactional variables, which are difficult to define for research purposes. There is no evidence that environmental and interactional influences are less important in their contribution to the origin of violence. Until now, the relative weight of environmental versus patient-related variables has not yet been determined.

2.1 Patient Variables

Gender. There are a considerable number of studies which found no gender differences in patients engaged in violent acts (Beck, White, & Gage, 1991; Hodgkinson, Mc Ivor, & Phillips, 1985; Miller, Zadolinnyj, & Hafner, 1993; Myers & Dunner, 1984; Tardiff & Sweillam, 1982), others found a higher prevalence in males (Kay, Wolkenfeld, & Murrill, 1988; Pearson, Wilmot, & Padi, 1986; Steinert, Hermer, & Faust, 1996), others a higher prevalence in females (Binder & McNiel, 1990; Kiejna, Janska-Skomorowska, & Baranowski, 1993; Rasmussen & Levander, 1996). A recent study designed with the objective to yield further evidence in this conflicting matter (Krakowski & Czobor, 2004) found positive psychotic symptoms more likely to result in verbal and physical assaults in women during inpatient treatment, where as violence in men was more frequent during subsequent community treatment and was related to substance abuse.

Age. Whereas young age is a well established risk factor for violence in the community, this could be confirmed for inpatient violence in only some studies (Aquilina, 1991; Convit, Isay, Otis, & Volavka, 1990; Hoptman, Yates, Patalinjug, Wack, & Convit, 1999), others did not find such associations (Miller et al., 1993; Rasmussen & Levander, 1996; Steinert, Wiebe, & Gebhardt, 1999).

Diagnosis. There is no consistent pattern of study results, which diagnoses are associated with a higher risk of inpatient violence. Some studies reported higher rates in patients with schizophrenia (Noble & Rodger, 1989; Steinert, Vogel, Beck, & Kehlmann, 1991; Watson, Segal, & Newhill, 1993), others did not (Kay et al., 1988; Miller et al., 1993; Walker & Seifert, 1994). A higher prevalence of aggression among people with nonparanoid schizophrenia was reported (Shader, Jackson, Harmatz, & Appelbaum, 1977; Tardiff & Sweillam, 1982), but also the opposite (Grossman, Haywood, Canavaugh, Davis, & Lewis, 1995). Other studies reported a higher prevalence of chronic patients (Noble, 1997), of patients with substance abuse disorders (Myers & Dunner, 1984), with personality disorders and bipolar disorder (Miller et al.), and with dementia and mental retardation (Cooper & Mendonca, 1991; Spießl, Krischker, & Cording, 1998).

History. Previous violent behavior is the only robust predictor of violent inpatient behavior since many studies confirmed this finding and no contradictory findings have been published (Steinert, 2002). This applies to previous inpatient violent behavior (Arango, Barba, González-Salvador, & Ordónez, 1999; Blomhoff, Seim, & Friis, 1990; McNiel, Binder, & Greenfield, 1988; Steinert et al., 1996), violence prior to admission (Janofsky, Spears, & Neubauer, 1988; Yesavage, 1984), premorbid violent behavior outside of institutions (Krakowski, Convit, Jaeger, Shang, & Volavka, 1989), and violence in family of origin (Blomhoff et al.; Hoptman et al., 1999). Actuarial instruments like HCR-20 and PCL-SV that are highly estimated in the prediction of future violence in forensic patients seem to have only very limited value in civil inpatients on general wards (Nicholls, Ogloff, & Douglas, 2004; Rasmussen & Levander, 1996), particularly in relation to the necessary efforts needed for the application of these complex instruments. The number of previous hospitalizations (Greenfield, McNiel, & Binder, 1989; Rossi et al., 1985) and the total length of hospitalization (Chang & Lee, 2004; Steinert et al., 1999) are further historical variables of which associations with violent behavior have repeatedly been described. A history of suicide attempts was associated with violence in some studies, in which the samples consisted predominantly or exclusively of personality disorders (Hillbrand, 1995; Myers & Dunner, 1984). In patients with psychotic disorders, violent and suicidal behaviors are rather independent (Apter et al., 1991; Krakowski & Czobor, 2004; Steinert et al., 1999).

Psychopathology. Probably the risk of violence generally increases with the severity of psychopathological symptoms, as measured by the Positive and Negative Syndrome Scale (PANSS) total score or the BPRS (Arango et al., 1999; Krakowski, Czobor, & Chou, 1999; Steinert, Woelfle, & Gebhardt, 2000), though contradictory findings with regards to this subject have also to be mentioned (Krakowski, Jaeger, & Volavka, 1988). A strong argument for the role of psychopathology is the finding that most violent behavior occurs in the first few days of inpatient treatment with the proportion of patients involved continuously decreasing in the course of treatment (Steinert, Woelfle, & Gebhardt, 2000). Much less clear is the contribution of specific symptoms. It seems to belong to basic clinical knowledge that symptoms such as delusions and hallucinations, especially command hallucinations, signal an increased risk of violent acts. However, though some studies support this view (Janofsky et al., 1988; McNiel, Eisner, & Binder, 2000; Rogers, Nussbaum, & Gillis, 1988; Taylor et al., 1998), others do not (Arango et al.; Goodwin, Alderson, & Rosenthal, 1971; Kasper, Rogers, Adams, 1996; Steinert, Woelfle, & Gebhardt, 2000). A delusional symptom which actually is associated with abrupt violence outbursts, person misidentification (the so-called Capgras syndrome) (Bourget & Whitehurst, 2004), is too rare to influence statistics. Somewhat contraintuitively, a symptom that has repeatedly been found associated with violence is formal thought disorder (Arango et al.; Hoptman et al., 1999; Steinert, Woelfle, & Gebhardt, 2000). In a psychiatric ward or institution, some social skills and communication skills are required for many of the daily living activities. Formal thought disorder leads to impairment in communication, and when communication fails or may be misleading, the probability of violence increases.

Negative symptoms show no clear association with violent behavior (Steinert, Woelfle, & Gebhardt, 2000), but there is an evidence that sheltered living, a sheltered working situation, low intelligence and poor social situation, all of them indirect indicators of reduced social skills, are associated with an increased risk of violence during inpatient treatment (Spießl et al., 1998).

2.2 Biological Variables

There has been some research on biological variables supposed to be predictors of violent behavior, such as brain damage, neurological soft signs, creatin kinase serum level, and serum cholesterol level (overview in Steinert, 2002). The results are contradictory or solitary and not yet sufficiently confirmed.

2.3 Behavior

An alternative approach to a psychopathological description of patients, certainly more from the nurses' point of view, is the description of patient behavior ante-ceding violent outbursts. Even if such descriptions seem less sophisticated, they have the advantage of a close, timely association to the violent event, whereas psychopathology ratings by doctors and psychologists generally have not been performed just before or after such an event. This aspect is particularly important because it has been shown in several studies (Richter & Berger 2001; Steinert et al., 1991) that inpatient violence in most cases does not succeed as an abrupt outburst but typically as an escalating conflict (thus justifying the use of de-escalation trainings, see Chapter 10). Behaviors observed prior to violent incidents are confusion, irritability, boisterousness, verbal threats, physical threats, and attacks on objects (Woods & Almvik, 2002). There is evidence that only a minor part of aggressive patient behavior is a direct consequence of psychopathological symptoms, whereas a major part can be attributed to similar psychological motives in those not mentally disturbed (Nolan et al., 2003; Steinert, Hermer, & Faust, 1995), with psychopathological symptoms having rather an unspecific disinhibit-ing effect.

2.4 Environment

It is common sense psychiatric knowledge that staff behavior, staff attitudes, and staff personality traits play a major role in provoking or preventing violent conflict escalations, even if from a scientific viewpoint there is not yet much evidence (Palmstierna & Wistedt, 1995; Whittington & Wykes, 1994a, 1994b). This applies similarly to the use of seclusion and restraint, the high variance of which is prob-ably explained by staff attitudes, not different patient characteristics (Fisher, 1994). There is some evidence that lack of experience among staff is associated with higher rates of inpatient violence (James, Fineberg, Shah, & Priest, 1990). Gebhardt and Steinert (1999) demonstrated that a change in hospital policy (dis-tributing "difficult" admitted patients to several wards instead of concentrating them on a single ward) had a high impact on the incidence of aggressive behav-iors, reducing not verbal, but physical aggression. "Crowding" of patients, the con-centration of too many persons with abnormal behaviors in too little space, can be a risk factor for violence, too (Lanza, Kayne, Hicks, & Milner, 1994; Palmstierna, Huitfeld, & Wistedt, 1991).

The impact of staffing levels and the number of beds per ward on the incidence of violence is a frequent issue for discussion, but there is no data available from multivariate or longitudinal studies that would allow clear conclusions. Another aspect of common sense psychiatric knowledge in many countries is the influence of the physical environment, e.g., furniture, food, quality of living and sleeping rooms, private sphere, so-called "hotel standard." Though there is no evidence from scientifically sound studies, clinical experience over decades tells us that a good environment and respect for patient privacy are able to reduce the level of aggression and suicidality. The almost complete lack of research regarding the impact of architecture on patients' behavior and mental state in psychiatric institutions shows that a very important aspect of institutional policy has been neglected by researchers, maybe underestimated as "matter of administration."

2.5   Interaction

Within the last decade, psychiatrists have learnt that most psychiatric disorders are the results of interactions, e.g., of interactions of genetic factors with early and actual environmental factors. Probably the phenomenon of inpatient violence is, similarly, a result of complex interactions between biological and psychological patient properties, victim behavior, and institutional influences. Some models of interactions are described in this book (see Chapter 5), but adequate research designs still need to be developed.

2.6   Limitations

The question seems justified as to why so much research on well-observable incidents in many countries has produced only a rather scant amount of clear facts of clinical value. Several reasons can be identified which should be taken into account before further research in this issue is undertaken:

(1) Restriction to patient variables and neglect of the impact of environment
(2) Poor comparability of results due to different measurements of violence (Steinert, 2002; Steinert & Gebhardt, 1998)
(3) A problem that causes much bias and requires some further explanation: lack of a clearly defined reference population

The reference population in all studies on community violence is quite clear: it is the general population of the same region and its respective rate of offences or violent offences, in some studies paralleled with respect to gender, age, social class, etc. But what is the reference population of studies on inpatient violence? Most published studies were performed on a single admission ward, the reference population being the nonviolent patients of the same ward. Obviously, the results obtained in this way are highly biased by the admissions policy of the respective ward and should not be generalized. It can be shown that the determination of significant risk variables in such relatively small samples is strongly dependent on the sample composition and yields varying results according to the applied inclusion and exclusion criteria (Steinert, 2002). A more reasonable approach that has been rarely applied is the use of the total of all hospital admissions or all admissions with a specific diagnosis within a certain, sufficiently long period, as a reference population in order to obtain comparable results (for example Spießl et al., 1998). However, even results obtained in this way are of limited clinical value for purposes of prediction, if patients with similar risk variables are aggregated on the same ward by hospital policy.

3 ACCURACY OF PREDICTION

There are a limited number of studies that prospectively evaluate the accuracy of prediction of inpatient violence by clinicians. Twenty years ago, research projects on the prediction of inpatient and out-patient violence usually yielded depressing results. Monahan (1981) demonstrated that predictions were not much better than chance and at that time were false twice as often as they were correct. Werner, Rose, & Yesavage (1983) found that 15 psychiatrists and 15 psychologists were not able to predict inpatient violence within a period of only one week. These researchers had made psychiatrists decide whether admitted patients would engage in assaults within the first seven days of their hospitalization. The decisions were based on BPRS ratings and information about violence preceding admission exclusively. No correlation between predictions and subsequent observed violence could be found in this study. Similarly disappointing were the results of Janofsky et al. (1988) who asked psychiatrists to predict assaults and suicidal behavior within the next seven days based on an interview at the patient's admission. Some progress in the quality of studies or of prediction seems to be achieved since then. Lidz, Mulvey, and Gardner (1993) performed a study with nearly 2,000 patients in emergency departments for whom clinical staff predicted violence for the next six months (that means, most of the prediction period referred to community violence). The accuracy of the predictions was significantly better than chance with a sensitivity of 60% and specificity of 58%. However, for women the predictions were no better than chance because the rates of violence among female patients had been significantly underestimated.

A series of studies on the accuracy of clinical predictions were performed by McNiel and Binder. First, in 1988, they studied the relationship between confidence and accuracy in clinical assessments of patients' short-term risk of violence. A total of 78 different physicians estimated the probability of physical attacks in 317 inpatients during the first week of hospitalization and the degree of confidence in their estimates. Only when clinicians had a high degree of confidence were their estimates rather good (McNiel et al., 1988). In 1991 McNiel and Binder reported a study which examined a sample of civil, involuntarily committed patients (n = 149) (McNiel & Binder, 1991). The accuracy of the predictions of physicians and nurses in predicting violence during the first seven days of hospitalization was assessed. The risk of violence was rated as a percentage of probability. The intuitive clinical ratings in this probabilistic approach turned out to be much better than chance. Risk estimates by doctors and nurses were moderately good with a correlation of 0.46 between physician and nurse assessments. In another, similar, study with 226 inpatients, the same authors (McNiel & Binder, 1995) determined a sensitivity of 67% and a specificity of 69% of the clinical predictions for a period of seven days, if the clinicians had rated the probability of violence 27% or greater. The accuracy of prediction was better for psychotic than for nonpsychotic patients, and the authors could demonstrate that overweighting of static variables such as gender led to systematic errors. This is contrary to what has been emphasized for the prediction of community violence where static variables like age, gender, and history were found to be superior to dynamic (clinical and environmental) variables. A similar rate of correct predictions as in the studies described before was found in a study of Hoptman et al. (1999). Haim, Rabinowitz, Lereya, and Fenning (2002) studied physician and nurse ability in predicting violence on the basis of clinical knowledge in 308 consecutively admitted inpatients. The rate of violence was 10.7% in this sample, and physicians and nurses performed equally well. Nonoccurrence of violence was more successfully predicted than violence with a high specificity but low sensitivity. Nijman, Merckelbach, Evers, Palmstierna, and à Campo (2002) used visual analogue scales to determine the accuracy of predictions of clinical staff. With these unaided clinical assessments, 75% of patients could be correctly classified whether they would be aggressive during their inpatient stay or not.

The other way of making predictions is the use of formal instruments for the risk assessment, an approach which suffers somewhat from the poor knowledge of robust risk variables. McNiel and Binder (1994) created a rather simple actuarial screening instrument consisting of five items which had been correlated with violence in previous studies. Categorizing the presence of three or more positive items as high risk, a discrimination between violent and nonviolent patients could be achieved with a sensitivity of 57% and a specificity of 70%. The Brøset-Violence Checklist (Woods & Almvik, 2002) is a short instrument for predictions of inpatient violence within the next 24 hours which has been developed in Norway. Six behavior characteristics: confusion, irritability, boisterousness, verbal threats, physical threats, and attacks against objects, have to be rated as present or absent. The instrument has satisfactory psychometric properties with a high specificity and moderate sensitivity. Abderhalden et al. (2004) developed a German version and found again a sensitivity of 64% and a specificity of 94% in the predictions, consistent with the original Norwegian version. The number of correct classifications was similar to clinical predictions.

Another approach was a self-report questionnaire for a risk of violence which has been developed by Plutchik and van Praag (1990), but it has not stimulated further research and seems not to be in clinical use.

3.1   Limitations

All predictions of violence in psychiatric institutions are compromised by good clinical management. Even if clinical staff are blind to predictions made within the frame of a research project, good psychiatric teams continuously make their own prognoses, based on their experience and all the available knowledge of the patient. If a patient is identified as someone with an increased risk of violence, maybe because of a history of violence, acute psychopathology, and acute anger because of adverse experiences such as involuntary admission, well-educated psychiatric teams will do their best to deescalate the situation with preventative measures such as calming down, keeping contact with the patient, giving medication, or, if necessary, using seclusion. Thus, good clinical management leads to false positive predictions and, vice versa, a 100% correct prediction of violent behavior, either as a clinical assessment or by some formalized instrument, would be an evidence of rather poor clinical management.

4 CONCLUSION

Research on inpatient violence has yielded knowledge on three important aspects which should be considered in education and training: assessing the patient's history with respect to violent behavior, assessing carefully the psychopathological state and its potential effects on behavior, and recognizing actual conflicts and potential motives for violent escalations. Whether the further development and implementation of standardized tools for prediction will be a promising pathway for safer and better management in psychiatric institutions is still an open question. Certainly, such tools can be helpful for less experienced staff, but it has not yet been convincingly demonstrated that they have a better accuracy than predictions based on clinical assessments by experienced professionals. In the author's opinion, after years of research on this issue, a prediction based on a good clinical assessment performed by an experienced team yields a high quality standard which should not be underestimated. Such kinds of multidisciplinary team assessment are like share values. They contain all the available and relevant information, even if it may be difficult or impossible to determine exactly the weight of the single contributing variables.

REFERENCES

Abderhalden, C., Needham, I., Miserez, B., Almvik, R., Dassen, T., Haug, H. J., et al. (2004). Predicting inpatient violence in acute psychiatric wards using the Brøset-Violence-Checklist: A multicentre prospective cohort study. *Journal of Psychiatric and Mental Health Nursing, 11*, 422–427.

Apter, A., Kotler, M., Sevy, S., Plutchik, R., Brown, S. L., Foster, H., et al. (1991). Correlates of risk of suicide in violent and nonviolent psychiatric patients. *The American Journal of Psychiatry, 148*, 883–887.

Aquilina, C. (1991). Violence by psychiatric in-patients. *Medicine, Science, and the Law, 31*, 306–312.

Arango, C., Barba, A. C., González-Salvador, T., & Ordónez, A. C. (1999). Violence in inpatients with schizophrenia: A prospective study. *Schizophrenia Bulletin, 25*, 493–503.

Beck, J. C., White, K. A., & Gage, B. (1991). Emergency psychiatric assessment of violence. *The American Journal of Psychiatry, 148*, 1562–1565.

Binder, R. L., & McNiel, D. E. (1990). The relationship of gender to violent behavior in acutely disturbed psychiatric patients. *The Journal of Clinical Psychiatry, 51*, 110–114.

Blomhoff, S., Seim, S., & Friis, S. (1990). Can prediction of violence among psychiatric inpatients be improved? *Hospital and Community Psychiatry, 41*, 771–775.

Boeker, W., & Haefner, H. (1973). Gewalttaten Geistesgestörter. *Eine psychiatrisch-epidemiologische Untersuchung in der Bundesrepublik Deutschland.* Berlin: Springer.

Bonta, J., Law, M., & Hanson, K. (1988). The prediction of criminal and violent recidivism among mentally disordered offenders: A meta-analysis. *Psychological Bulletin, 123*, 123–142.

Bourget, D., & Whitehurst, L. (2004). Capgras syndrome: A review of the neurophysiological correlates and presenting clinical features in cases involving physical violence. *Canadian Journal of Psychiatry, 49*, 719–725.

Buchanan, A. (1999). Risk and dangerousness. *Psychological Medicine, 29*, 465–473.

Chang, J. C., & Lee, C. S. (2004). Risk factors for aggressive behavior among psychiatric inpatients. *Psychiatric Services, 55*, 1305–1307.

Convit, A., Isay, D., Otis, D., & Volavka, J. (1990). Characteristics of repeatedly assaultive psychiatric inpatients. *Hospital and Community Psychiatry, 41*, 1112–1115.

Cooper, A. J., & Mendonca, J. D. (1991). A prospective study of patient's assaults on nurses in a provincial psychiatric hospital in Canada. *Acta Psychiatrica Scandinavica, 84*, 163–166.

Dolan, M., & Doyle, M. (2000). Violence risk prediction. Clinical and actuarial measures and the role of the psychopathy checklist. *The British Journal of Psychiatry, 177*, 303–311.

Douglas, K. S., Ogloff, R. P., Nicholls, T. L., & Grant, I. (1991). Assessing risk for violence among psychiatric patients: The HCR-20 risk assessment scheme and the psychopathy checklist: Screening version. *Journal of Consulting and Clinical Psychology, 61*, 917–930.

Eronen, M., Hakola, P., & Tiihonen, J. (1996). Mental disorders and homicidal behavior in Finland. *Archives of General Psychiatry, 53*, 497–501.

Fisher, W. A. (1994). Restraint and seclusion: A review of the literature. *The American Journal of Psychiatry, 151*, 1584–1590.

Gebhardt, R. P., & Steinert, T. (1999). Should severely disturbed psychiatric patients be distributed or concentrated in specialized wards? An empirical study on the effects of hospital organization on ward atmosphere, aggressive behavior, and sexual molestation. *European Psychiatry, 14*, 291–297.

Goodwin, D. W., Alderson, P., & Rosenthal, R. (1971). Clinical significance of hallucinations in psychiatric disorders. *Archives of General Psychiatry, 24*, 76–80.

Greenfield, T. K., McNiel, D. E., & Binder, R. L. (1989). Violent behavior and length of psychiatric hospitalization. *Hospital & Community Psychiatry, 40*, 809–814.

Grossman, L. S., Haywood, T. W., Canavaugh, J. L., Davis, J. M., & Lewis, D. A. (1995). State psychiatric hospital patients with past arrests for violent crimes. *Psychiatric Services, 46*, 790–795.

Haim, R., Rabinowitz, J., Lereya, H., & Fenning, S. (2002). Predictions made by psychiatrists and psychiatric nurses of violence by patients. *Psychiatric Services, 53*, 622–624.

Hare R. (2003). *Hare Psychopathy Checklist-Revised (PCL-R)*. Technical manual. Second edition. Toronto: Multihealth Systems.

Harris, G. T., & Rice, M. E. (1997). Risk appraisal and management of violent behavior. *Hospital and Community Psychiatry, 48*, 1168–1176.

Hillbrand, M. (1995). Aggression against self and aggression against others in violent psychiatric patients. *Journal of Consulting and Clinical Psychology, 63*, 668–671.

Hodgins, S., Mednick, S. A., Brennan, P. A., Schulsinger, F., & Engberg, M. (1996). Mental disorder and crime. Evidence from a Danish birth cohort. *Archives of General Psychiatry, 53*, 489–496.

Hodgkinson, P. E., Mc Ivor, L., & Phillips, M. (1985). Patient assaults on staff in a psychiatric hospital. A two-year retrospective study. *Medicine, Science, and the Law, 25*, 288–294.

Hoptman, M. J., Yates, K. F., Patalinjug, M. B., Wack, R. C., & Convit, A. (1999). Clinical prediction of assaultive behaviour among male psychiatric patients at a maximum-security forensic facility. *Psychiatric Services, 50*, 1461–1466.

James, D. V., Fineberg, N. A., Shah, A. K., & Priest, R. G. (1990). An increase in violence on an acute psychiatric ward. A study of associated factors. *The British Journal of Psychiatry, 156*, 846–852.

Janofsky, J. S., Spears, S., & Neubauer, D. N. (1988). Psychiatrists' accuracy in predicting violent behavior on an inpatient unit. *Hospital and Community Psychiatry, 39*, 1090–1094.

Kasper, M. E., Rogers, R., & Adams, P. A. (1996). Dangerousness and command hallucinations: An investigation in psychotic inpatients. *The Bulletin of the American Academy of Psychiatry and the Law, 24,* 219–224.

Kay, S. R., Wolkenfeld, F., & Murrill, L. M. (1988). Profiles of aggression among psychiatric patients. 1. Nature and prevalence. *The Journal of Nervous and Mental Disease, 176,* 539–546.

Kiejna, A., Janska-Skomorowska, M., & Baranowski, P. (1993). Medical procedure with aggressive patients: Experiences of the psychiatric clinic in Wroclaw. *Psychiatria Polska, 27,* 501–513.

Krakowski, M., Convit, A., Jaeger, J., Shang, L., & Volavka, J. (1989). Neurological impairment in violent schizophrenic inpatients. *The American Journal of Psychiatry, 146,* 849–853.

Krakowski, M., & Czobor, P. (2004). Gender differences in violent behavior: Relationship to clinical symptoms and psychosocial factors. *The American Journal of Psychiatry, 161,* 459–465.

Krakowski, M., Czobor, P., & Chou, J. C. (1999). Course of violence in patients with schizophrenia: Relationship to clinical symptoms. *Schizophrenia Bulletin, 25,* 505–517.

Krakowski, M., Jaeger, J., & Volavka, J. (1988). Violence and psychopathology: A longitudinal study. *Comprehensive Psychiatry, 29,* 174–181.

Lanza, M. L., Kayne, H. L., Hicks, C., & Milner, J. (1994). Environmental characteristics related to patient assault. *Issues in Mental Health Nursing, 15,* 319–335.

Lidz, C. W., Mulvey, E. P., & Gardner, W. (1993). The accuracy of predictions of violence to others. *Journal of the American Medical Association, 269,* 1007–1011.

Link, B. G., Stueve, A., & Phelan, J. (1998). Psychotic symptoms and violent behaviors: Probing the components of "threat/control-override" symptoms. *Social psychiatry and psychiatric epidemiology, 1*(Suppl. 33), S55–S60.

McNiel, D. E., & Binder, R. L. (1991). Clinical assessment of the risk of violence among psychiatric inpatients. *The American Journal of Psychiatry, 148,* 1317–1321.

McNiel, D. E., & Binder, R. L. (1994). Screening for risk of inpatient violence: Validation of an actuarial tool. *Law and Human Behavior, 18,* 579–586.

McNiel, D. E., & Binder, R. L. (1995). Correlates of accuracy in the assessment of psychiatric inpatients' risk of violence. *The American Journal of Psychiatry, 152,* 901–906.

McNiel, D. E., Binder, R. L., & Greenfield, T. K. (1988). Predictors of violence in civilly committed acute psychiatric patients. *The American Journal of Psychiatry, 145,* 965–970.

McNiel, D. E., Eisner, J. P., & Binder, R. L. (2000). The relationship between command hallucinations and violence. *Psychiatric Services, 51,* 1288–1292.

Miller, R. J., Zadolinnyj, K., & Hafner, R. J. (1993). Profiles and predictors of assaultiveness for different psychiatric ward populations. *The American Journal of Psychiatry, 150,* 1368–1373.

Monahan, J. (1981). *The clinical prediction of violent behaviour.* Washington, DC: US Government Printing Office.

Monahan, J., & Appelbaum, P. (2000). *Reducing violence risk.* In: S. Hodgins (Ed.) Violence among the mentally ill. Effective treatments and management strategies. Dordrecht: Kluwer Academic Publishers.

Monahan, J., Steadman, H. J., Appelbaum, P. S., Robbins, P. C., Mulvey, E. P., & Silver, E. (2000). Developing a clinically useful actuarial tool for assessing violence risk. *The British Journal of Psychiatry, 176,* 312–319.

Myers, K. M., & Dunner, D. L. (1984). Self and other directed violence on a closed acute care ward. *The Psychiatric Quarterly, 56,* 178–188.

Nicholls, T. L., Ogloff, J. R., & Douglas, K. S. (2004). Assessing risk for violence among male and female civil psychiatric patients: The HCR-20, PCL:SC, and VSC. *Behavioral Sciences and the Law, 22,* 127–158.

Nijman, H., Merckelbach, H., Evers, C., Palmstierna, T., & à Campo J. (2002). Prediction of aggression on a locked psychiatric admission ward. *Acta Psychiatrica Scandinavica, 105,* 390–395.

Noble, P. (1997). Violence in psychiatric in-patients: Review and clinical implications. *International Review of Psychiatry, 9,* 207–216.

Noble, P., & Rodger, S. (1989). Violence by psychiatric in-patients. *The British Journal of Psychiatry, 155,* 384–390.

Nolan, K. A., Czobor, P., Roy, B. B., Platt, M. M., Shope, C. B., Citrome, L. L., et al. (2003). Characteristics of assaultive behavior among psychiatric inpatients. *Psychiatric Services, 54,* 1012–1016.

Palmstierna, T., Huitfeld, B., & Wistedt, B. (1991). The relationship of crowding and aggressive behavior on a psychiatric intensive care unit. *Hospital and Community Psychiatry, 42,* 1237–1240.

Palmstierna, T., & Wistedt, B. (1995). Changes in the pattern of aggressive behaviour among in-patients with changed ward organisation. *Acta Psychiatrica Scandinavica, 91,* 32–35.

Pearson, M., Wilmot, E., & Padi, M. (1986). A study of violent behaviour among in-patients in a psychiatric hospital. *The British Journal of Psychiatry, 149,* 232–235.

Plutchik, R., & van Praag, H. M. (1990). A self-report measure of violence risk. Part II. *Comprehensive Psychiatry, 31,* 450–456.

Räsänen, P., Tiihonen, J., Isohanni, M., Rantakallio, P., Lehtonen, J., & Moring, J. (1998). Schizophrenia, alcohol abuse, and violent behavior: A 26-year follow-up study of an unselected birth cohort. *Schizophrenia Bulletin, 42,* 437–441.

Rasmussen, K., & Levander, S. (1996). Crime and violence among psychiatric patients in a maximum security psychiatric hospital. *Criminal Justice and Behavior, 23,* 455–471.

Reed, J. (1997). Risk assessment and clinical risk management: The lessons from recent enquiries. *The British Journal of Psychiatry, 170*(Suppl. 32), 4–7.

Richter, D., & Berger, K. (2001). Patient assaults of staff. A prospective study of the incidence, circumstances and sequelae. *Der Nervenarzt, 72,* 693–699.

Rogers, R., Nussbaum, D., & Gillis, R. (1988). Command hallucinatons and criminality: A clinical quandary. *The Bulletin of the American Academy of Psychiatry and the Law, 16,* 251–258.

Rossi, M., Jacobs, M., Monteleone, M., Olsen, R., Surber, R. W., Winkler, E. L., et al. (1985). Violent or fear-inducing behavior associated with hospital admission. *Hospital and Community Psychiatry, 36,* 643–647.

Shader, R. I., Jackson, A. H., Harmatz, J. S., & Appelbaum, P. S. (1977). Patterns of violent behavior among schizophrenic inpatients. *Diseases of the Nervous System, 38,* 13–16.

Silver, E., Mulvey, E. P., & Monahan, H. (1999). Assessing violence risk among discharged psychiatric patients: Toward an ecological approach. *Law and Human Behavior, 23,* 237–255.

Spießl, H., Krischker, S., & Cording, C. (1998). Aggressive Handlungen im Psychiatrischen Krankenhaus. *Psychiatrische Praxis, 25,* 227–230.

Steadman, H. J., Mulvey, E. P., Monahan, J., Robbins, P. C., Appelbaum, P. S., & Grisso, T. (1998). Violence by people discharged from acute psychiatric inpatient facilities and by others in the same neighborhoods. *Archives of General Psychiatry, 55,* 393–401.

Steinert, T. (2002). Prediction of inpatient violence. *Acta Psychiatrica Scandinavica, 106,* 133–142.

Steinert, T., & Gebhardt, R. P. (1998). Wer ist gefährlich? Probleme der Validität und Reliabilität bei der Erfassung und Dokumentation von fremdaggressivem Verhalten. *Psychiatrische Praxis, 25,* 221–226.

Steinert, T., Hermer, U., & Faust, V. (1995). Die Motivation aggressiven Patientenverhaltens in der Einschätzung von Ärzten und Pflegepersonal. *Krankenhauspsychiatrie, 6,* 11–16.

Steinert, T., Hermer, K., & Faust, V. (1996). Comparison of aggressive and non-aggressive schizophrenic inpatients matched for age and sex. *European Journal of Psychiatry, 10,* 100–107.

Steinert, T., Sippach, T., & Gebhardt, R. P. (2000). How common is violence in schizophrenia despite neuroleptic treatment? *Pharmacopsychiatry, 33,* 98–102.

Steinert, T., Vogel, W. D., Beck, M., & Kehlmann, S. (1991). Aggressionen psychiatrischer Patienten in der Klinik. Eine 1-Jahres-Studie an 4 psychiatrischen Landeskrankenhäusern. *Psychiatrische Praxis, 18,* 155–161.

Steinert, T., Wiebe, C., & Gebhardt, R. P. (1999). Aggressive behavior against self and others among first-admission patients with schizophrenia. *Psychiatric Services, 50,* 85–90.

Steinert, T., Woelfle, M., & Gebhardt, R. P. (2000). Aggressive behavior during in-patient treatment. Measurement of violence during in-patient treatment and association with psychopathology. *Acta Psychiatrica Scandinavica, 102,* 107–112.

Swanson, J. W., Holzer, C. E., Ganju, V. K., & Iono, R. T. (1990). Violence and psychiatric disorder in the community: Evidence from the epidemiologic catchment area surveys. *Hospital and Community Psychiatry, 41,* 761–770.

Swartz, M. A., Swanson, J. W., Hiday, V. A., Borum, R., Wagner, R., & Burns, B. H. (1998). Taking the wrong drugs: The role of substance abuse and medication non-compliance in violence among severely mentally ill individuals. *Social Psychiatry and Psychiatric Epidemiology, 33,* S75–S80.

Tardiff, K., & Sweillam, A. (1982). Assaultive behavior among chronic inpatients. *The American Journal of Psychiatry, 139,* 212–215.

Taylor, P. J., Leese, M., Williams, D., Butwell, M., Daly, R., & Larkin, E. (1998). Mental disorder and violence. A special (high security) hospital study. *The British Journal of Psychiatry, 172,* 218–226.

Walker, Z., & Seifert, R. (1994). Violent incidents in a psychiatric intensive care unit. *The British Journal of Psychiatry, 164,* 826–828.

Watson, M. A., Segal, S. P., & Newhill, C. E. (1993). Police referral to psychiatric emergency services and its effect on disposition decisions. *Hospital and Community Psychiatry, 44,* 1085–1090.

Webster, C., Douglas, K. S., Belfrage, H., & Link, B. G. (2000). Capturing change. In: S. Hodgins (Ed.) *Violence among the mentally ill. Effective treatments and management strategies* (pp.119–144). Dordrecht: Kluwer Academic Publishers.

Werner, P. D., Rose, T., & Yesavage, J. A. (1983). Reliability, accuracy and decision—making strategy in clinical predictions of imminent dangerousness. *Journal of Consulting and Clinical Psychology, 51,* 815–825.

Whittington, R., & Wykes, T, (1994a). Violence in psychiatric hospitals: Are certain staff prone to being assaulted? *Journal of Advanced Nursing, 19,* 219–225.

Whittington, R., & Wykes, T. (1994b). An observational study of associations between nurse behaviour and violence in psychiatric hospitals. *Journal of Psychiatric and Mental Health Nursing, 1,* 85–92.

Woods, P., & Almvik, R. (2002). The Brøset-Violence Checklist (BVC). *Acta Psychiatrica Scandinavica, 106,* 103–105.

Yesavage, J. A. (1984). Correlates of dangerous behavior by schizophrenics in hospital. *Journal of Psychiatric Research, 18,* 225–231.

7

Nonphysical Conflict Management and Deescalation

DIRK RICHTER

1 INTRODUCTION

For many decades, mental health staff used mainly physical techniques to manage aggressive and violent situations. Mechanical or physical restraint and/or seclusion were the only explicit interventions that staff were used to. When other techniques, e.g., verbal interventions, were used, they happened more implicitly or through the intuition of selected nurses and doctors. The physical part of aggression management was reinforced by distinctive training programs for (more or less violent) self-defense and other interventions that came up in the 1970s (Gertz, 1980; St. Thomas Psychiatric Hospital, 1976).

Until the present, nonphysical techniques are only rarely taught and actively trained. A recent systematic review of the effectiveness of aggression management training programs revealed that most programs which combined physical and non-physical techniques had their origins in self-defense orientations (Richter 2004, 2005; see Chapter 11). This situation is mirrored by the state of research on aggression management techniques in mental health in general. Most published books on this topic contain mainly recommendations about physical techniques, which are illustrated by pictures or drawings (Mason & Chandley, 1999; Richter, Fuchs, & Bergers, 2001). Recommendations for nonphysical behavior are rarely published (but see Harris & Morrison, 1995; Leadbetter & Paterson, 1995; Paterson & Turnbull, 1999).

This situation in practice and research is not very satisfying. It is obvious that nurses, doctors and other mental health workers need adequate options for every stage of the escalation curve. Although not all potential violent situations can be managed solely by nonphysical techniques, at present staff are undertrained and underequipped concerning nonphysical interventions. The following review tries to provide the reader with state-of-the-art information on nonphysical conflict management and interpersonal deescalation.

This chapter draws heavily from the literature outside mental health, due to the lack of genuine psychiatric approaches. Interestingly, the basic assumptions and even some specialist techniques are quite similar among diverse fields. Such fields range from hostage negotiations to international conflicts (Donohue, 2003). As is easily imagined, many other professions have also to face the task of managing aggressive situations. Aggressive situations in mental health care are not categorically different from situations that the police are confronted with (Hücker, 1997) or that are to be found in services for children and adolescents with challenging behavior (Dutschmann, 2003a, 2003b; Omer, 2004). On the whole, however, according to a chapter on deescalation in a recent handbook on violence in general, deescalation techniques are poorly researched and practiced in areas other than mental health (Eckert & Willems, 2002).

2   SITUATIONAL DYNAMICS AND CONFLICT ESCALATION

Many aggression management approaches refer to an escalation curve that illustrates the increasing emotional arousal in the conflict situation. Although the notion of a curve is simplifying the complexity of aggressive situations a little, the curve highlights the empirically well-known fact that most potential violent situations inside and outside of psychiatry grow out of a situational escalation. For mental health care, several studies have shown that violence is preceded by identifiable events and patient behavior (Aiken, 1984; Powell, Cann, & Crowe, 1994; Richter & Berger, 2001; Whittington & Patterson, 1996). In most of these situations, conflict happened between staff and patient or between two or more patients. By using a simple but very intriguing methodology, Nijman, Allertz, Merckelbach, à Campo, and Ravelli (1997) have mapped the locations of violent situations in a closed ward. The ward map revealed that most incidents happened in the staff office, in front of the ward entrance and in the day rooms. In these places interactions between staff, patients, and visitors take place, people get close to each other and conflicts arouse out of "normal" encounters (asking for medication, etc.). It can be estimated that in more than two-thirds of all violent incidents such conflicting interactions can be retrospectively analyzed.

Another well-established fact is that the events and situations that lead to violence in psychiatric institutions are observed quite divergently between staff and patients. Whereas staff attribute aggressive behavior mainly to the mental illness itself, patients are more likely to see situational aspects and staff behavior as precursors (Bensley,

Nelson, Kaufman, Silverstein, & Shields, 1995; Duxbury, 2002; Harris & Varney, 1986; Ilkiw-Lavalle & Grenyer, 2003). Taken together, this research suggests that staff behavior is nearly as important as a precursor to violent incidents as patient behavior. This conclusion is further supported by research findings about explicit staff behavior, limit-settings styles and even open coercion (Lancee, Gallop, McCay, & Toner, 1995; Morrison, 1990, 1992). Of course, in special situations such behavior cannot be avoided at any time. However, such behavior may be one decisive factor in triggering patients' angry, hostile, and potentially violent reactions. Dominance orientation can become dangerous for two reasons. First, because it may shape the ward milieu so that aggression and counteraggression set the tone on the ward. Second, staff that are prone to dominance orientation are likely to react more aggressively and violently toward even minor hostile behavior (Omer, 2004). This is in no way meant to blame staff for aggression and violence with which they are confronted, it just means that staff should be aware of their own reactions and behavior.

What do we know about situations that are likely to escalate? Unfortunately, the research methodology applied to investigate the precursors of aggression and violence is mainly focusing on patient behavior (e.g., Bowers, Simpson, & Alexander, 2003). Although it is important to identify risk factors associated with patient behavior, it is at least as important to know about staff behavior, the whole situation that the interaction is embedded in and to understand the interactional trajectory. As mental health workers who are trained in psychology and psychiatry, we are biased toward an individualistic perspective that looks only to cognitions and emotions. However, communication interactionists who have specialized in the field of conflict management try to see the "relational logic" (Donohue, 2003) that emerges from the interaction of the parties involved. Escalation, in this sense, means that hostile and aggressive behavior has the tendency to be mutually reinforcing, so that each party's reactions lead to greater harm with each new round of actions.

From unpublished research material in a study conducted by the author (Richter, 1999; Richter & Berger, 2001) it was possible to identify typical situations retrospectively that, via escalation, have led to violent assaults on staff:

- Patient is aroused, staff intervene (tries to calm patient down, reprimands, etc.)
- Staff asks patient for some action (to take medicine, to take off clothes, etc.), patient denies
- Staff try to avert patient actions (absconding, annoying fellow patients, etc.)
- Patient asks staff for something (PRN medication, cigarettes, etc.), staff deny
- Staff try to settle conflicts between patients
- Patient is in a delusional state, misjudges staff

The escalation from interaction to violence might take several hours, but it also might only take several seconds. This is the reason why an escalation curve is misleading when you try to apply it to "real" situations. The escalation curve suggests an ideal type of interaction with a steady increase of tensions, which usually is not the case.

However, the escalating conflict that follows the basic situations above are mainly triggered by the diverging goals and intentions of the two parties. Whereas staff try to fulfill their therapeutic and safety roles, patients often try to aim at short-term goals that support their subjective quality of life and, most importantly, their subjective needs and identity. Striving for needs and identity are generally the main causes that trigger violence, regardless of the social context and institution. John Burton, a leading violence theorist has stated, after reviewing the general literature on violence causation:

> "The conclusion to which we are coming is that seemingly different and separate social problems, from street violence to industrial frictions, to ethnic and international conflicts, are symptoms of the same cause: institutional denial of needs of recognition and identity and the sense of security when they are satisfied, despite losses through violent conflict." (Burton, 1997:38)

This is also true for interpersonal conflicts in mental health care. When the incompatibility of staff and patient intentions becomes clearer to both sides, the escalation is fueled by emotions (e.g., anger) and cognitions (e.g., prior experiences). In general, expectations shape our role behavior as well as the observation of the other party involved. Therefore, the incompatibility of the two parties' expectations can be regarded as the key factor for conflict escalation (Messmer, 2003). As a nurse, I expect a patient to comply with my orders, and as a patient I expect a nurse to show a caring (and not security) behavior (see the qualitative data provided by Benson et al., 2003). When these or other expectations are violated it is very likely that distrust emerges. Distrust is one of the most important cognitions that lead to further increasing aggression. Both sides, staff and patient, feel being aversively stimulated by the other's behavior (Whittington & Richter, 2005; Whittington & Wykes, 1996; see Chapter 3).

The feeling of being provoked by the other party will, in many cases, lead to assertive reactions which will stimulate the opponent in return. Distrust and aversive stimulation can lead both parties into the above-mentioned relational logic of escalation, where inflammatory language is only the overt signal of underlying cognitions and emotions. Being trapped in this logic of escalation will, then, lead to more or less fixed expectations about the other party's behavior: This nurse wants to harm me and I have to defend myself. As indicated by this example, cognitive processes will turn to narrowness and rigidity the more the interaction escalates (Omer, 2004). Questioning participating staff and patients after a violent incident, Benson and colleagues (2003) found discourses of blame on both sides. In conflict theory, this "paranoid" expectation and its connected rigidity is regarded to be one of the most powerful cognitive frames that makes conflict solution so difficult. Breaking this logic and its expectation frame is, therefore, a key task for nonviolent conflict resolution.

At this point it is important to stress the role of the patient's psychopathology. The symptoms of the actual mental disorder surely shape the patient's observational and appraisal abilities. Further, the control of impulsivity and of conflict solving skills are impaired by the disorder. Experimental psychological research has shown that subjects who score highly on trait hostility will also express higher levels of state hostility (Lindsay & Anderson, 2000). However, the basic conflict situation is still based on an interaction. Without a triggering event from the social environment of the patient, which has been regarded as an aversive stimulus, the escalation would not have begun. Thus so far, violence by psychiatric patients is not totally different from violence committed by healthy subjects. For a common sense approach to research on interpersonal violence in general, the risk factors can be divided into the following categories: predisposing factors and processes, situational elements, and triggering events (Reiss & Roth, 1993). To prevent a violent escalation, staff have only minimal chances to affect the predisposing psychopathology in the short term. Even the situation of the often involuntarily admission cannot be changed easily. What staff can do is try to avoid the stimulus that may trigger the patient's aggression.

3   STRESS MANAGEMENT AND ANGER MANAGEMENT

The concepts of interactive escalation and aversive stimulation again stress the importance that staff behavior takes. Therefore, staff behavior is the crucial point where the prevention of violence is initiated. If patients feel aversively stimulated by staff, this usually does not happen by the staff's intention, rather it will happen unintentionally. Many mental health workers who currently work in psychiatric institutions have to face a huge work-load and organizational pressure and, thus, feel highly distressed (Siegrist, Rödel, & Siegrist, 2003). Obviously, actual working condition will surely impact on the encounters between staff and patients. Staff who suffer from distress will not be able to react as calmly and therapeutically as they probably intend to do.

Current working conditions in mental health care and the stressful situations that are associated with aggression itself make it necessary that staff are able to cope with their own distress and anger in order behave in a way that aggression and violence can be avoided. Therefore, stress management and anger management are the basis for applying deescalation skills effectively. The key step to managing your personal emotions is self-awareness (Nay, 2004). As mental health workers, we have to know our personal signs that indicate stress and arousal. These indicators might be physical signs (e.g., sweating, elevated heart frequency) or psychological signs (e.g., polarized thinking, labeling). Because such indicators are highly individualistic, anger therapists recommend setting up a personal anger scale that includes the whole range of reactions in connection with experienced anger (Nay:84ff).

The following stress management skills have successfully been converted from a police training program (Hücker, 1997) into training for mental health staff:

- *Management of personal emotions*: Mental health staff have to cope with high levels of frustration and need to be very tolerant. To achieve emotional stability in distressing situations it is appropriate to avoid negative stances that will lead to self-fulfilling prophecies (e.g., to find a patient's behavior or appearance "unbearable," to think of a patient's behavior as "unacceptable," to feel "indignant" at a patient's argument).

- *Role distance*: Mental health staff must be able to know and eventually to dissociate themselves from the expectations and norms that are connected to psychiatry and psychiatric nursing. In some situations it is more appropriate not to follow the professional rules (e.g., enforcing personal hygiene on the patient in any case).
- *Empathy/Role-taking*: Although professional norms already highlight staff empathy while being in a therapeutic encounter, empathy is difficult to maintain in distressing or even aggressive situations. However, trying to find out what the patient is currently feeling and thinking is of its own worth especially in aggressive interactions. It might be that the patient's behavior is fully justified.
- *Ambiguity tolerance*: Interpersonal conflict is, by definition, associated with opinions and intentions that diverge from the staff's point of view. In many situations, staff need to tolerate and accept different perspectives and to cope with the distance between patients and themselves. This is another skill in not reacting too emotionally toward hostile behavior.

Another practical method is the use of instructions by self-talk. Based on psychological research on anger, Nay (2004:136ff) recommends the use of specific instructions that are adjusted to different stages of anger. These include:

- Preparing for provocation: "This may upset me, but I know how to deal with it."
- Impact and confrontation: "What difference will this make in a week or a month?"
- Coping with arousal of anger: "My muscles are getting tight. That's my signal for a relaxation breath."
- After the confrontation: "I could have used a calming phrase. Let me rethink how I could have handled it better."

Further, each mental health worker has to find out the best way to cope individually with distressing situations. Different personal temperaments make it impossible to adopt all stress management rules alike. After several years of practiced deescalation and stress management, a personal style of conflict management will surely emerge.

4   BASIC RULES OF CONFLICT MANAGEMENT

Obviously, deescalation is not an option for all aggressive and potentially violent incidents. In some situations physical techniques against aggressive patients are unavoidable. Which option to choose depends on several context factors: the current situation on the ward, the patient's psychiatric symptoms, the patient's conflict solving skills and impulsivity control, staff experience of conflict management, and, of course, the intensity of conflict. The type of aggression or violence is also highly relevant. Instrumental violence (acts that are related to specific goals) have to be handled differently than emotional violence (behavior that emerges from interpersonal tension) (Dutschmann, 2003a, 2003b). For instrumental violence, general cognitive behavioral interventions are more appropriate than specific body language or rhetoric skills which are better applied to situations with high arousal.

Generally, verbal interventions are possible for patients who are not highly delusional or disorganized (e.g., patients with dementia) (Alpert & Spillmann, 1997). Quite common, but difficult to master, are triggered displaced aggressions. Patients sometimes feel more provoked by fellow patients, relatives or other mental health workers than the one who becomes assaulted in the end. Triggered displaced aggressions are a combination of two aversive stimulations by different people where a minor stimulus can lead to an excessive violent outburst (Miller, Pedersen, Earlywine, & Pollock, 2003).

Because the conflicts they are to handle are so diverse and specific, it is generally recommended to first consider and learn several basic rules rather than to stick to highly ambitious skills or techniques which may only be appropriate in special situations (which doesn't mean that the mastery of such skills may not be advantageous, details of specific skills are provided below). The following recommendations are mainly about general attitudes toward conflicts, about staff involvement into such conflicts, and about the adequate timing of interventions (for a similar list of principles, see Leadbetter & Paterson, 1995; Paterson & Turnbull, 1999; Stevenson, 1991). Of course, there are further possibilities to prevent violence and aggression. Although scientifically widely neglected, mental health workers with job experience usually acknowledge the influence of factors like ward architecture (Gulak, 1991; Kumar & Ng, 2001; Welter, 1997) and, more importantly, ward milieu (Johnson & Morrison, 1993; Katz & Kirkland, 1990; see Chapter 14). There is, for instance, some empirical evidence that the concentration of "difficult" patients on separate wards does affect the ward milieu negatively (Gebhardt & Steinert, 1999). However, because of problems in operationalizing the specific causes, the impact of these factors is very difficult to assess and to use in organizational change processes. There is probably some indirect positive effect from dedicated training programs. Staff from wards who have implemented training for effective nonviolent conflict management report that the milieu has changed positively with the training. This impression seems plausible because nonviolent conflict management is very likely to change the communication style of staff. Another option is given for staff who work with chronic aggressive patients. For this group, several behavioral treatments (e.g., skills training, anger management, token interventions) have been established and empirically tested (Alpert & Spillmann, 1997; Goldstein, Nensén, Daleflod, & Kalt, 2004; Wong, Woolsey, Innocent, & Liberman, 1988). For people with learning disabilities, cognitive behavioral approaches have proved to be effective (Ball, Bull, & Emerson, 2004).

Before going into details of conflict management and deescalation, two important warnings have to be given. First, the reader has to be aware that the following recommendations must not be used in a cook-book manner. It is possible that the same intervention applied to the same patient works successfully in one situation but not in another. The remarks about role distance earlier also have their importance here: Don't stick to the rules too tightly. A well-known example from experience for many psychiatric nurses is that the appearance of an authoritarian doctor can, in some situations, change an aggressive patient into a calm and compliant one. Sometimes it is possible to enforce a conflict resolution, namely when the force is associated with capability, legitimacy, and credibility (Schellenberg, 1996). This example should make clear that conflict management means, in the first place, to decide pragmatically and adequately for the special situation. Second, and this warning is related to the first, the reader has to be aware that he or she is not able to apply effective deescalation techniques from reading this or other printed matter on the topic. Deescalation does not work without in-depth training. Experience from several training programs has further shown that it is appropriate to train personnel from one ward together, so that every staff member receives the same knowledge and each one can rely on his or her colleague.

The first basic rule stresses the general attitude toward the patient and his or her aggression. The attitude should be empathy, concern, respect, sincerity, and fairness. This attitude should be accompanied by a caring and therapeutic intention. Staff have to be aware that, apart from patients with specific personality disorders, human beings and, therefore, patients, are usually not voluntarily aggressive or even violent. In general, aggression and violence are triggered by the subjective notion that one has to defend oneself against another's intimidations, provocations or unjust behavior (Anderson & Bushman, 2002; Miethe & Regoeczi, 2004; Miller, 2001), however, justified these accusations might be from a different point of view. Likewise, there is ample evidence that low self-esteem is related to aggression and delinquency (Donnellan, Trzesniewski, Robins, Moffitt, & Caspi, 2005). Further research results stress the point that insults to personal honor will increase the risk of aggressive reactions (Beersma, Harinck, & Gerts, 2003).

These findings have received support from experimental social psychology. With reference to the specific problem in which cases mentally healthy subjects do escalate a social conflict, results of experiments revealed that escalation did occur in cases of feeling highly offended and judging the opponent's behavior as inappropriate (Mummendey, Löschper, Linneweber, & Bornewasser, 1984). The same is true even for mentally ill offenders who are treated in forensic hospitals (Gilligan, 1996) and also applies to most acts of instrumental violent. Patients who violently try to abscond from the ward, understandably, see their quality of life severely reduced by the closed door. Thus, aggressive and potentially violent patients subjectively face a serious problem that they cannot cope with in any other way. The attitude of empathy and respect may in many cases help to find out which problem it is that triggers the patient's aggression and, at the same time, is the basis for interpersonal conflict resolution in so far as the patient can feel more accepted and understood by staff.

The second rule of conflict management is to assess the risks that are associated with each available option. Most important are the realistic expectations. Can this situation really be mastered without physical options? Because of the situation's acuity the answer to this question has, in many cases, to be given by intuition. If staff don't feel safe enough to manage this situation by nonphysical options alone, they should switch over to plan B, i.e., the preparation of physical interventions. Several studies have shown that younger and less experienced staff face greater risks of being assaulted (e.g., Richter, 1999; Richter & Berger, 2001). One reason for this is unrealistic confidence in personal skills.

Third, the next basic rule is not to control the patient, but to control the situation. Conflict management within an interaction has the goal of getting the best out of the situation for both parties, a win–win situation as it is commonly termed in game theory (Davidson & Wood, 2004). The goal to avoid violence depends on both parties' reactions. However, it is impossible to predict the outcome of an interaction in advance. If the patient has the impression that staff are trying to control or even coerce him or her into specific behavior, hostile reactions are very likely to emerge. Therefore, staff behavior should not be too intrusive or provocative. Theoretically, the explicit use of power in the early stage of an escalating interaction is justified only in cases where the power relation between both parties is very clear and where it is obvious that the use of power will not shape the way into an intractable conflict (Bonoma & Tedeschi, 1974). But there are therapeutic and practical reasons against the use of power and coercion, which are related to each other. Staff and patients have to work together after the crisis incident. Patients rarely forget who was using too much power and coercion. Staff have also to work therapeutically with patients. The use of power usually contradicts a therapeutic relationship.

Fourth, in cases where this is possible, risk assessment, decision making, responsibilities, and actions should be shared with fellow colleagues. Several reasons make this rule obligatory. Conflict situations are associated with high emotional tension, and staff decisions might be biased by their own emotional involvement. Although deescalation works better within a one-to-one interaction, fellow staff should know about the plan, should try to calm down other patients and should be aware of possible crisis interventions to save the participants from injuries.

Fifth, deescalation works more successfully when it is done as an early intervention (Leadbetter & Paterson, 1995). This is again illustrated by the escalation curve. The more both parties' behavior and tensions are similar to "normal" dimensions, the better they are able to plan a nonviolent intervention and to react to it. In other words, deescalation is usually inappropriate in situations that are accompanied by high risks and tensions.

Sixth, one of the main subgoals in deescalation is to gain time. Very often, aggressive interpersonal communication, e.g., accusations and shouting, proceeds quickly. Emotional arousal makes quick responses very likely, and participants feel subjectively under pressure to respond so that the opponent will not get the impression that one has given in. Experimental psychological research has, however, shown that time pressure leads to less thorough information processing and, consequently, to inadequate decisions (De Dreu, 2003; Van Cleef, De Dreu, & Manstead, 2004). A gain in time may not only lead to better decisions, but will also reduce the interpersonal tension. A simple, but very successful technique is to look the other way, e.g., out of a window for some seconds, when you feel under pressure to respond.

Seventh, spatial considerations are equally important and distance keeping between staff and patient has several advantages. Anxious arousal can be induced by getting to close to each other, which in turn, may lead to defensive actions (Smith & Cantrell, 1988). Another advantage concerns personal safety: sufficient space will safeguard against immediate hits or blows.

Eighth, deescalation interventions have to be applied with apparent self-confidence and certainty, without being provocative. Like several other principles and techniques in this regard, this rule asks for a balanced procedure. If staff show too much complacency, it may be regarded as arrogant and provocative. No, or too little, self-confidence may give the impression that staff are not able to codetermine the outcome of difficult situations. This problem is known from research on aggressive children, where parents who permanently give in are known to increase the demands and aggressive actions of their children. Omer (2001, 2004) has coined the term "complementary escalation" for this kind of escalation which stands in contrast to the well-known type of reciprocal escalation.

Ninth, power plays between staff and patients have to be avoided. Quite often, major conflicts grow out of minor disputes or misunderstandings. The question of whose perspective is right or whose is wrong leads to mutual argument. Conflicts are fueled by each party's notion that one cannot give in, because this might show weakness. Apparently unimportant differences become issues of personal identity and honor. For experienced and self-confident staff, this kind of conflict should not be necessary in many cases. Although the patient may be totally wrong from a staff's point of view, prevention of violence should be reason enough to give in cases where this would not cause serious consequences (Maier, 1996). Of course, staff cannot make promises or concessions that will lead to conflict in later situations.

Tenth, staff should be aware of general safety issues. Aggressive situations often occur in ward environments where there are several other people. The safety of fellow patients or inexperienced staff should always be kept in mind. As one does not know the outcome of a deescalation attempt from the start, the place of such an intervention should be carefully considered. Where possible, an open way to flee should be in reach and potentially dangerous objects should be removed.

There are several common misunderstandings and self-induced pitfalls related to the management of conflict situations. Although mentioned earlier, it cannot be overstated that the outcome of the situation does not depend solely on patient behavior. As said above, staff are very likely to mainly attribute aggression and violence to the mental disorder and to underestimate contextual and personal factors that may contribute to the outcome.

Related to this problem are two further common misunderstandings. Many interpersonal conflicts are based on different notions about what has been said or done. Current sociological and communication research stresses the point that communication is not just a message from A to B, as many readers may have learned in recent decades. Communicative messages are coconstructed by both sender and receiver (Luhmann, 1995; Stewart & Logan, 1997). This means that a message is encoded by A and has to be decoded by B. Encoding as well as decoding are highly individualistic and idiosyncratic processes which are influenced by the personality, current mental state and, very importantly, by biographical experiences. This is the reason why A and B may fall into the trap of self-fulfilling prophecies. When I, as a mental health worker, have had experience with specific patients who are not able to comply with nonviolent interventions, I won't apply them next time. The opposite is also true: When I, as a patient, have had only bad or even victimizing experiences during my last admission, I will expect that the next nurse I encounter will also behave like that, regardless of how he or she actually behaves. Friendly or therapeutically encoded messages will, then, probably be decoded as a "trick" to convince me to comply.

Another common notion is that communication is just a verbal message, and that the spoken word is in charge of the interaction. This is not, in fact, the case. Associated with encoding or decoding are nonverbal cues such as body language, facial expression, gestures, loudness, and tone. This is especially true when emotional arousal can be "felt" as it usually happens in interpersonal conflicts (Turner, 2002). The "feeling" of emotions points to the fact that the spoken word alone is not enough to get the big picture of the scene. Therefore, the total personal appearance presented to the patient is highly important. Details about nonverbal communications are given in Section 5.

In conclusion, the impact of both verbal and nonverbal communication cannot be assessed by the sender of the message alone. Similar, or even more important than the sender's intentions, is the receiver's observation of the sender and his or her message. Although it is difficult to apply to aggressive encounters, the person who wants to deescalate the tension has to see the whole situation through the patient's eyes. Deescalation is closely connected to the question of how my behavior will be regarded by my opponent. As already stated, this is a difficult task even in conflicts without mentally ill participants. This gets even more difficult if mental disorder shapes the observation. As a mental health worker, you can never be sure which kind of film is currently being seen by the patient, especially in the case of paranoia or other schizophrenic symptoms. However, precise knowledge about specific mental disorders and their symptoms, and, most importantly, a greater experience in working with mentally ill patients will allow staff to further empathize with the patient.

5   NONVERBAL COMMUNICATION: BODY LANGUAGE, FACIAL EXPRESSIONS, AND GESTURES

The mastering of body language and related physical features is one of the most important and at the same time one of the most difficult tasks when learning nonviolent conflict management. As already mentioned, verbal communication is usually overemphasized in deescalation. This emphasis on verbal communication is in stark contrast to research findings which stem from the 1960s where, in general, nonverbal communication was found to be more important for sending emotional signals (Mehrabian & Ferris, 1967; Mehrabian & Wiener, 1967). Related to the overemphasis of words in interactions is the common notion that humans are rational beings who calculate their decisions and actions thoroughly in order to make the best out of each situation. This anthropological misunderstanding may be one reason why we, as modern individuals, have many problems in understanding and coping with aggression. Aggression and other negative emotional states, so it seems to us, are deviant features that often enough do surprise us.

Recent theories of language evolution, however, have stressed the point that early humans and their predecessors used "emotional languages" that relied mainly on the sense modality of vision (Ekman, 1999a; Turner, 2000, 2002). Long before auditory languages emerged, the theory goes, humans had to solve the task of reading the body language of their fellows to reaffirm their support and solidarity silently in difficult situations and, thus, to be aware of the other's emotional state. It seems that body language and especially facial expressions make up the basic language which is very important for "reading" emotions. Current psychology of emotion has stressed the notion that there are some basic emotions universal in all human beings (and, probably, in nonhuman primates, too) (Ekman, 1993, 1999a). Among the list of basic emotions are topics like anger, fear, disgust, embarrassment, or shame. These emotions are basic features in several regards. What is important here, is that basic emotions mainly emerge automatically and unconsciously. A much discussed topic within the psychology of emotion is the question whether there are distinctive facial expressions that are related to basic emotions. While it is clear that a facial expression is not exactly the appearance of an internal state and that humans can, to a certain extent, artificially choose their facial expressions freely, the relation of mimics to unconscious emotions cannot be questioned any longer (Ekman, 1999b).

As mental health workers who try to deescalate interpersonal tensions, we have, therefore, to be aware that our facial expressions are made up automatically. In a way, our mimicking and other body language features reveal our "true" basic emotions, regardless of what we are trying to express verbally. Facial expression and body language that can be observed by others make it impossible not to communicate, as Paul Watzlawick's 1960s meta-communication axiom has already stated (Watzlawick, Beavin, & Jackson, 1967). Therefore, the most important task in this regard is to know what we look like when we are distressed by an interpersonal conflict. As we normally do not walk in front of a mirror while having a dispute with our partner, most of us do not know what kind of body language we present to others. Role plays recorded on video may give the first impression of what our body reveals to others, much surprise is guaranteed. While trying to master our own body language, the next task is to avoid incongruent impressions toward the other party of the conflict (Stevenson, 1991). Our body language should give the same message as our verbal communication. If verbal and nonverbal channels do contradict, an observer will most likely regard the nonverbal expression as "true" and the verbal signals as faked. Nevertheless, although emotions and facial expressions come up automatically, it is not impossible to suppress or to alter expressions to the way we want (Ekman, 1997).

The goal of physical expression in deescalation is to give the distressed opponent a feeling of comfort and safety. Details of nonverbal communication surely depend on the (multi-)cultural settings and the ethnic origins of all the people involved. Staff have to be aware that some aspects of nonverbal communication are culture bound. It is likely that nonverbal behavior can lead to misunderstandings on both sides. Thus, the following recommendations which have proved to be effective on the European continent in general, have to be considered carefully when translated into local mental health settings. In line with our verbal communication, our body language should minimize threats and give a clear signal of openness with regard to the patient's concerns. The gestures of our arms are a powerful vehicle to provide these signals. Lowered, uncrossed arms with open hands show that we are not aggressive. A relaxed appearance is also given by the posture of the head and the gaze of the eyes. An upright position of the head, combined with subtle tilts to the left and right may induce the observation that one is interested in the other person and actively listening. Active or empathic listening (see next section) is further supported by head nodding and maintaining eye contact without staring. All gestures should be slow and gentle. Sudden movements toward another person may be regarded as an attack and should be avoided. Sufficient spatial distance should also be provided. Psychotic patients sometimes have a need for larger distances during an encounter. Children and retarded patients with learning disabilities may, on the other hand, benefit from closer body contact.

Aggressive body language, in contrast, tries to make the body appear larger. When putting hands on hips, the elbows go wide to impress the opponent. This posture is usually underlined by a very upright position and the chin higher than usual. Facial expression is of high importance when the body "speaks" aggressively. Eyes become smaller and staring, disapproving frowns may be observed. These signals may be accompanied by insulting gestures. Thrusting arms, pointed up fingers, etc. may show readiness for battle. Directing or ordering gestures underline the asymmetry of the encounter and signal who wants to be the boss. A defensive body language, in contrast, will make the body smaller to minimize the surface. Vital organs might be covered; the chin covers the neck to protect it. When defending, arms are usually held across the chest or face. Facial expression will show the common signs of fear, e.g., wide open eyes or submission.

Without explicitly being verbal, several vocal features are relevant, too. The tone of the voice may be aggressive, e.g., loud and deep or ironic. In distressing situations, nervousness or anger often cannot be hidden. For instance, women's voices reveal distress when the tone becomes high or even shrill. While trying to deescalate an aggressive situation, the mental health worker should try to maintain a normal level of volume and tone. To keep the intonation at a normal level will also help to manage your own stress and emotions.

In conclusion, body language and nonverbal expression of emotional states play an important role for the management of interpersonal conflicts in mental health care. Having said this, the mastering of these features is not an easy task. To know the personal appearance does not automatically lead to the adequate use of nonverbal communication techniques. It takes several hours of training and experience to be able to use such techniques in a professional manner. A caveat has also to be mentioned: Artificial manipulations of, say, facial expressions, may end up sending mixed messages. Because basic emotions and associated expressions have so much power, they cannot easily be ruled out by volitional acts. Professional stage actors can surely talk about this problem. However, as a few mainly experimental studies from nonmental health care have shown, body language may be one factor in preventing assaults, for it does affect perceptions of vulnerability or nonvulnerability and of submissiveness (Grayson & Stein, 1981; Murzinsky & Degelman, 1996). More successful than just manipulating one's expression is to change the thinking about conflicts and their solutions. Thus, technique alone doesn't make a good conflict management worker, stress management, and basic conflict management rules are at least similarly important (see above).

6   VERBAL DEESCALATION TECHNIQUES

In Section 2, the escalation of interpersonal conflicts was characterized by cognitions and expectations of distrust and "paranoia." These cognitions are usually accompanied by emotional distress, anger, or fear. A basic goal of verbal deescalation is to regain the trust of the distressed patient. This can only happen when the emotional tension has run down, which in this regard is another basic goal. One skill for achieving these goals is active and empathic listening. Active/empathic listening is likely to improve mutual trust and understanding, while handling the emotions. Active listening contains the following techniques (Beyondintractability.org, 2003; Changingminds.org, 2005; Conflict Resolution Network, 2005):

Enhance the patient's self-esteem and confidence through a nonjudgmental and noncritical manner.

- Listen for both content and meaning
- Respond to the emotional message
- Respond honestly
- Paraphrase the patient's message to indicate your understanding
- Do not interrupt while the patient is talking
- Do not give advice
- Do not discount the patient's feelings
- Indicate a clear interest in the patient's opinion and acknowledge his/her position ("I see what you mean"; "I'd like to hear more about it")

In case of complaints or verbal attacks the goal should be to defuse the strong emotions attached to the verbal claims (Conflict Resolution Network, 2005):

- Do not defend or justify yourself at this point
- Try to deal with the patient's emotions (shouting occurs because the patient does not think he/she is being heard): "I can see how upset you are," etc.
- Acknowledge the patient's position (which does not mean accept it)

Although it is sometimes hard to do, in special situations it is appropriate to totally agree with the patient's complaints or arguments (Maier, 1996). The patient may not be right in stating that this or that symptom is a side effect of their medication, but in a heated dispute there is no real chance to convince him or her of the psychiatrist's view. Rather, a better way is to wait for an emotional cool-down and then try to discuss this issue at another time.

When the emotional tension is no longer overwhelmingly in charge of the situation, several rhetorical techniques are possible to restabilize the interaction (Hücker, 1997):

- Lead the talk back to the initial issue. In cases of personalizing arguments and minor verbal abuse, staff should try to take the emotion out of the scene: "Could we talk about . . . again?"
- Overhear accusations. Without devaluating gestures (e.g., whole arm from up to down) or facial expressions staff should reissue the former topic of discussion: "We should talk about . . ."
- Admit time for responses. After difficult questions or decisions, staff should allow enough time for answers: "Take your time." "Think carefully . . ."
- Sophisticated giving in: "You're right, one can see it from this point of view, but we should talk about . . ."

Conflict theorists generally recommend the use of I-messages in difficult situations. I-messages help to personalize yourself and stress one's own point of view: "I feel . . ." You-messages, in contrast, often lead to blaming the patient: "You did this or that, you didn't comply to the order (etc.)." Such accusations will certainly fuel lengthy arguments about what and why somebody did or didn't do something. Obviously, the use of I-messages has to be chosen carefully. I-messages are not appropriate in every situation or every style. Phrases like "I know exactly that . . ." or "I have no time for that . . ." are not really helpful (Hücker, 1997). Further, the verbalized relation of a patient's behavior to a staff member's internal emotional state is surely an attempt to blame the patient.

Theoretically, one of the simplest techniques in nonviolent conflict management is simply to not use special styles of communication or verbal interventions. Again, this is easier said than done, because emotional arousal helps us to forget about this rule. However, the following responses have been described as roadblocks to communication (Davidson & Wood, 2004) or as communication killers (Dutschmann, 2003a):

- Ordering
- Warning
- Moralizing
- Arguing

- Blaming
- Shaming
- Judging
- Name-calling
- Analyzing
- Probing
- Irony/sarcasm
- Praising
- Belittling

Another intervention that is not useful is the "Why-question." Why-questions ("Why do you always behave like this?"; "Why did you do this again?") are often regarded as reprimanding statements. They may fuel the patient's anger because why-questions in this way make clear that the mental health worker can't empathize with the patient. Further, the patient feels under pressure to justify his or her behavior which will not be difficult and will lead to generalized statements about other persons or situations.

Similarly, open-ended questions are more suitable than closed questions, where the answering options are only "yes" or "no." Closed questions likely lead to the impression that someone will be pressed into a rigid position. Open-ended questions ("What did you feel in this moment?"; "How would you describe your position?"; "How could we get out of this situation together?") are statements that try to keep the conversation going. They may also help to let the patients personalize themselves, so that a better understanding will be possible (Dutschmann, 2003a). Additional advantages of open-ended questions are the chance to gain time, because the patient is not forced to give a quick answer, and to involve the patient in the decision-making process.

Altogether, these techniques offer several options to mental health workers for solving interpersonal conflicts by verbal means. Again, even seemingly simple verbal interventions need training and experience to be applied successfully. Reasons for this are the emotional arousal which is felt by staff in aggressive situations and the indispensable "fit" of the intervention to the respective situation.

7   CONCLUSIONS

Nonviolent conflict strategies and skills have only recently reached a certain popularity within the mental health workers' community. Still, published (and, it seems, practiced) genuine psychiatric approaches are very rare and, up to now, not very sophisticated. This review should have made clear that mental health care can greatly profit from experiences in other fields. As mentioned earlier, aggressive conflicts in psychiatry are not totally different from those in other areas. However, it is necessary to identify the specific psychiatric demands and problems to enhance solutions that fit into current mental health care.

The author is convinced that thoroughly applied deescalation skills will be an important tool for many mental health workers who stand between two dangers: to use too much force or to do nothing when faced with violent behavior. Good deescalation skills help staff to cope actively with difficult situations without using physical force. Nonviolent conflict management is a way out of passivity, and at the same time avoids provoking violent counter-reactions (Omer, 2004).

REFERENCES

Aiken, G. J. M. (1984). Assaults on staff in a locked ward: Prediction and consequences. *Medicine, Science, and the Law*, 24, 199–207.

Alpert, J. E., & Spillmann, M. K. (1997). Psychotherapeutic approaches to aggressive and violent patients. *The Psychiatric Clinics of North America*, 20, 453–472.

Anderson, C. A., & Bushman, B. J. (2002). Human Aggression. *Annual Review of Psychology*, 53, 27–51.

Ball, T., Bush, A., & Emerson, E. (2004). Challenging Behaviors: Psychological interventions for severely challenging behaviors shown by people with learning disabilities. *Clinical Practice Guidelines*. Leicester: British Psychological Society.

Beersma, B., Harinck, F., & Gerts, M. J. J. (2003). Bound in honor: How honor values and insults affect the experience and management of conflicts. *The International Journal of Conflict Management*, 14, 75–94.

Bensley, L., Nelson, N., Kaufman, J., Silverstein, B., & Shields, J. W. (1995). Patient and staff views of factors influencing assaults on psychiatric hospital employees. *Issues in Mental Health Nursing*, 16, 433–446.

Benson, A., Secker, J., Balfe, E., Lipsedge, M., Robinson, S., & Walker, J. (2003). Discourses of blame: Accounting for aggression and violence on an acute mental health inpatient unit. *Social Science and Medicine*, 57, 917–926.

Beyondintractability.org, Empathic listening (2003). Boulder, Colorado. http://www.beyondintractability.org/m/empathic_listening.jsp

Bonoma, T. V., & Tedeschi, J. T. (1974). The relative efficacies of escalation and de-escalation for compliance-gaining in two-party conflicts. *Social Behavior and Personality*, 2, 212–218.

Bowers, L., Simpson, A., & Alexander, J. (2003). Patient-staff conflict: Results of a survey on acute psychiatric wards. *Social Psychiatry and Psychiatric Epidemiology*, 38, 402–408.

Burton, J. (1997). *Violence explained*. Manchester: Manchester University Press.

Changingminds.org, Listening (2005). http://www.changingminds.org/techniques/listening/listening.htm Accessed 22.02.05.

Conflict Resolution Network, Conflict Resolution Kit (2005). Chatswood (Australia), http://www.crnhq.org/freeskill3.html

Davidson, J., & Wood, C. (2004). A conflict resolution model. *Theory Into Practice*, 43, 6–13.

De Dreu, C. K. W. (2003). Time pressure and the closing of mind in negotiation. *Organizational Behavior and Human Decision Processes*, 91, 280–295.

Donnellan, M. B., Trzesniewski, K. H., Robins, R. W., Moffitt, T. E., & Caspi, A. (2005). Low self-esteem is related to aggression, antisocial behavior and delinquency. *Psychological Science*, 16, 328–335.

Donohue, W. A. (2003). The promise of an interaction-based approach to negotiation. *The International Journal of Conflict Management*, 14, 167–176.

Dutschmann, A. (2003a). *Aggressionen und Konflikte unter emotionaler Erregung: Deeskalation und Problemlösung* (Das Aggressions-Bewältigungs-Programm ABPro). Tübingen: DGVT-Verlag.

Dutschmann, A. (2003b). *Verhaltenssteuerung bei aggressiven Kindern und Jugendlichen: Der Umgang mit gezielten -instrumentellen -Aggressionen* (Das Aggressions-Bewältigungs-Programm ABPro). Tübingen: DGVT-Verlag.

Duxbury, J. (2002). An evaluation of staff and patient views of strategies employed to manage inpatient aggression and violence on a mental health unit: A pluralistic design. *Journal of Psychiatric and Mental Health Nursing, 9,* 325–337.

Eckert, R., & Willems, H. (2002). Eskalation und Deeskalation sozialer Konflikte: Der Weg in die Gewalt. In: Heitmeyer, W., & Hogan, J. (Hrsg.), *Internationales Handbuch der Gewaltforschung* (pp. 1457–1480). Wiesbaden: Westdeutscher Verlag.

Ekman, P. (1993). Facial expression and emotion. *The American Psychologist, 48,* 384–392.

Ekman, P. (1997). Should we call it expression or communication? *Innovations in Social Science Research, 10,* 333–344.

Ekman, P. (1999a). Basic emotions. In: T. Dalgleish & M. Power (Eds.), *Handbook of Cognition and Emotion* (pp. 45–60). Chichester: Wiley.

Ekman, P. (1999b). Facial expressions. In: T. Dalgleish & M. Power (Eds.), *Handbook of Cognition and Emotion* (pp. 301–320). Chichester: Wiley.

Gebhardt, R. -P., & Steinert, T. (1999). Schwierige Patienten konzentrieren oder verteilen? Auswirkungen von innerer Sektorisierung, partieller Stationsöffnung und Geschlechtermischung auf das Behandlungsmilieu. *Psychiatrische Praxis, 26,* 61–66.

Gertz, B. (1980). Training for prevention of assaultive behavior in a psychiatric setting. *Hospital and Community Psychiatry, 31,* 628–630.

Gilligan, J. (1996). *Violence: Reflections on a National Epidemic.* New York: Vintage Books.

Goldstein, A. P., Nensén, R., Daleflod, B., & Kalt, M. (Eds.). (2004). *New Perspectives on Aggression Replacement Training: Practice, Research, and Application.* Chichester: Wiley.

Grayson, B., & Stein, M. I. (1981). Attracting assault: Victims' nonverbal cues. *Journal of Communication, 31,* 68–75.

Gulak, M. B. (1991). Architectural guidelines for state psychiatric hospitals. *Hospital and Community Psychiatry, 42,* 705–707.

Harris, D., & Morrison, E. F. (1995). Managing violence without coercion. *Archives of Psychiatric Nursing, 9,* 203–210.

Harris, G. T., & Varney, G. W. (1986). A ten-year study of assaults and assaulters on a maximum security psychiatric unit. *Journal of Interpersonal Violence, 1,* 173–191.

Hücker, F. (1997). *Rhetorische Deeskalation.* Stuttgart: Boorberg.

Ilkiw-Lavalle, O., & Grenyer, B. F. S. (2003). Differences between patient and staff perceptions of aggression in mental health units. *Psychiatric Services, 54,* 389–393.

Johnson, K., & Morrison, E. F. (1993). Control or negotiation: A health care challenge. *Nursing Administration Quarterly, 17,* 27–33.

Katz, P., & Kirkland, F. R. (1990). Violence and social structure on mental hospital wards. *Psychiatry, 53,* 262–277.

Kumar, S., & Ng, B. (2001). Crowding and violence on psychiatric wards: Explanatory models. *Canadian Journal of Psychiatry, 46,* 433–437.

Lancee, W. J., Gallop, R., McCay, E., & Toner, B. (1995). The relationship between nurses' limit-setting styles and anger in psychiatric inpatients. *Psychiatric Services, 46,* 609–613.

Leadbetter, D. & Paterson, B. (1995). De-escalating aggressive behavior. In: B. Kidd & C. Stark (Eds.), *Management of Violence and Aggression in Health Care* (pp. 49–84). London: Gaskell.

Lindsay, J. J., & Anderson, C. A. (2000). From antecedent conditions to violent actions: The General Affective Aggression Model. *Personality and Social Psychology Bulletin, 26,* 533–547.

Luhmann, N. (1995). *Social Systems.* Stanford: Stanford University Press.

Maier, G. J. (1996). Managing threatening behavior: The role of talk down and talk up. *Journal of Psychosocial Nursing and Mental Health Services, 34,* 25–30.

Mason, T., & Chandley, M. (1999). *Managing violence and aggression: A manual for nurses and health care workers.* Edinburgh: Churchill Livingstone.

Mehrabian, A., & Ferris, S. R. (1967). Inference of Attitudes from Nonverbal Communication in Two Channels. *Journal of Consulting Psychology, 31,* 248–258.

Mehrabian, A., & Wiener, M. (1967). Decoding of Inconsistent Communications. *Journal of Personality and Social Psychology, 6,* 109–114.

Messmer, H. (2003). Konflikt und Konfliktepisode: Prozesse, Strukturen und Funktionen einer sozialen Form. *Zeitschrift für Soziologie, 32,* 98–122.

Miethe, T. D., & Regoeczi, W. C. (2004). *Rethinking Homicide: Exploring the Structure and Process Underlying Deadly Situations.* Cambridge: Cambridge University Press.

Miller, D. T. (2001). Disrespect and the experience of injustice. *Annual Review of Psychology, 52,* 527–553.

Miller, N., Pedersen, W., Earlywine, M., & Pollock, V. E. (2003). A theoretical model of triggered displaced aggression. *Personality and Social Psychology Review, 7,* 75–97.

Morrison, E. F. (1990). The tradition of toughness: A study of nonprofessional nursing care in psychiatric settings. *Image: Journal of Nursing Scholarship, 22,* 32–38.

Morrison, E. F. (1992). A coercive interactional style as an antecedent to aggression in psychiatric patients. *Research in Nursing and Health, 25,* 421–431.

Mummendey, A., Löschper, G., Linneweber, V., & Bornewasser, M. (1984). Social-consensual conceptions concerning the progress of aggressive interactions. *European Journal of Social Psychology, 14,* 379–389.

Murzinsky, J., & Degelman, D. (1996). Body language of women and judgments of vulnerability. *Journal of Applied Social Psychology, 26,* 1617–1626.

Nay, W. R. (2004). *Taking charge of anger: How to resolve conflict, sustain relationships, and express yourself without losing control.* New York: Guilford Press.

Nijman, H. L. I., Allertz, W. F. F., Merckelbach, H. L. G. J., à Campo, J. M. L. G., & Ravelli, D.P. (1997). Aggressive behavior on an acute psychiatric admission ward. *European Psychiatry, 11,* 106–114.

Omer, H. (2001). Helping parents deal with children's acute disciplinary problems without escalation: The principle of nonviolent resistance. *Family Processes, 40,* 53–66.

Omer, H. (2004). *Non-violent resistance: A new approach to violent and self-destructive children.* Cambridge: Cambridge University Press.

Paterson, B., & Turnbull, J. (1999). De-escalation in the management of aggression and violence: Towards evidence-based practice. In: J. Turnbull & B. Paterson (Eds.), *Aggression and Violence: Approaches to Effective Management* (pp. 95–123). Basingstoke: Palgrave Macmillan.

Powell, G., Caan, W., & Crowe, M. (1994). What events precede violent incidents in psychiatric hospitals? *British Journal of Psychiatry, 165,* 107–112.

Reiss, A. J., & Roth, J. A. (Eds.). (1993). *Understanding and preventing violence: Panel on the understanding and control of violent behavior.* Washington, DC: National Academy Press.

Richter, D. (1999). *Patientenübergriffe auf Mitarbeiter psychiatrischer Kliniken. Häufigkeit, Folgen, Präventionsmöglichkeiten.* Freiburg: Lambertus.

Richter, D. (2004). Trainingsmaßnahmen zur Gewaltprävention und zur Anwendung physischer Maßanahmen. In: Ketelsen, R., Schulz, M., & Zechert, C. (Hrsg.), *Seelische Krise und Aggressivität: Der Umgang mit Deeskalation und Zwang* (pp. 127–137). Psychiatrie-Verlag: Bonn.

Richter, D. (2005). *Effekte von Trainingsprogrammen zum Aggressionsmanagement in Gesundheitswesen und Behindertenhilfe: Systematische Literaturübersicht.* Münster: Westfälische Klinik Münster.

Richter, D., & Berger, K. (2001). Patientenübergriffe auf Mitarbeiter -Eine prospektive Untersuchung der Häufigkeit, Situationen und Folgen. *Nervenarzt, 72,* 693–699.

Richter, D., Fuchs, J. M., & Bergers, K. -H. (2001). *Konfliktmanagement in psychiatrischen Einrichtungen.* Gemeindeunfallversicherungsverband Westfalen-Lippe, Rheinischer Gemeindeunfallversicherungsverband. Münster/Düsseldorf: Landesunfallkasse Nordrhein-Westfalen.

Schellenberg, J. A. (1996). *Conflict Resolution: Theory, Research, and Practice.* Albany: State University of New York Press.

Siegrist, K., Rödel, A., & Siegrist, J. (2003). Theoriegeleitete Mitarbeiterbefragung im Krankenhaus als Instrument betrieblicher Gesundheitsförderung. *Das Gesundheitswesen, 65,* 612–619.

Smith, B. J., & Cantrell, P. J. (1988). Distance in nurse-patient encounters. *Journal of Psychosocial Nursing and Mental Health Services, 26,* 22–26.

St. Thomas Psychiatric Hospital (1976). A program for the prevention and management of disturbed behavior. *Hospital and Community Psychiatry, 27,* 724–727.

Stevenson, S. (1991). Heading off violence with verbal de-escalation. *Journal of Psychosocial Nursing and Mental Health Services, 29,* 6–10.

Stewart, J., & Logan, C. (1997). *Together: Communicating Interpersonally.* New York: McGraw-Hill.

Turner, J. H. (2000). *On the Origins of Human Emotions: A Sociological Inquiry in the Evolution of Human Effect.* Stanford: Stanford University Press.

Turner, J. H. (2002). *Face to Face: Toward a Sociological Theory of Interpersonal Behavior.* Stanford: Stanford University Press.

Van Cleef, G. A., De Dreu, C. K. W., & Manstead, A. S. R. (2004). The interpersonal effects of emotions in negotiations: A motivated information processing approach. *Journal of Personality and Social Psychology, 87,* 510–528.

Watzlawick, P., Beavin, J. H., & Jackson, D. D. (1967). *Pragmatics of Human Communication: A Study of Interactional Patterns.* New York: W.W. Norton & Company.

Welter, R. (1997). Architektur, Gewalt und Aggression in Kliniken. *System Familie, 10,* 88–91.

Whittington, R., & Patterson, R. (1996). Verbal and non-verbal behavior immediately prior to aggression by mentally disordered people: Enhancing the assessment of risk. *Journal of Psychiatric and Mental Health Nursing, 3,* 47–54.

Whittington, R., & Richter, D. (2005). Interactional aspects of violent behavior on acute psychiatric wards. *Psychology, Crime, and the Law, 11,* 377–388.

Whittington, R., & Wykes, T. (1996). Aversive stimulation by staff and violence by psychiatric patients. *The British Journal of Clinical Psychology, 35,* 11–20.

Wong, S. E., Woolsey, J. E., Innocent, A. J., & Liberman, R. P. (1988). Behavioral treatment of violent psychiatric patients. *Psychiatric Clinics of North America, 11,* 569–580.

8

Coercive Measures in the Management of Imminent Violence: Restraint, Seclusion and Enhanced Observation

RICHARD WHITTINGTON, ERIC BASKIND, AND BRODIE PATERSON

1 INTRODUCTION: COERCIVE MEASURES AND THE MANAGEMENT OF IMMINENT VIOLENCE

Even the most effective prediction techniques will not prevent all aggression in mental health care settings and when deescalation alone (see preceding chapter) is ineffective, staff will make the judgment to move toward more intrusive techniques, alongside continued deescalation, to coerce and ultimately control the patient. Such coercive and physical control is fraught with ethical, moral, and legal dilemmas and can be a potent cause of physical injury and psychological harm in both patients and staff. Once the decision to "up the stakes" has been taken, it is difficult to go back down the ladder of coercive interventions and there is a real risk that incompetent coercion can exacerbate the situation and be highly dangerous to the patient. In this chapter we will consider three things. Firstly, we will examine some of the difficult conceptual, ethical, and legal issues around the use of coercive measures in psychiatry. Secondly we will summarize some key, best practice, guidelines with regard to special observation, physical restraint, and seclusion with reference to the relevant sections of the UK National Institute for Clinical and Health Excellence (NICE) Clinical Practice Guidelines for the management of imminent violence. These guidelines are based on one of the most extensive and thorough appraisals of existing research on this issue. Thirdly, since this is a rapidly evolving area, we will examine recent research emerging in the past two to three years which was not included in the NICE review. Special attention will be paid in this section to two high priority questions: What is the service user perspective on the causes of conflict resulting in coercive measures and the actual experience of undergoing them? And, how can mental health services around the world act to reduce their reliance on seclusion and restraint and develop alternative, less coercive interventions?

1.1   Definitions

The term coercive measures will be used here to refer to a cluster of interventions used widely around the world to control behavior which is perceived by staff as indicating that violence by a patient is either already happening or is very imminent. The main focus here is on physical restraint and seclusion. Physical restraint itself has a number of subdivisions. *Manual* or *"hands-on" restraint* is the most fundamental intervention and often underpins or precedes the others. Mechanical restraint, seclusion, and enforced tranquillization often rely on physical restraint as a first step and, in some countries, this is the only form of physical restraint employed in mental health services (see Table 1). *Mechanical restraint*, as defined by Sailas and Wahlbeck (2005), involves the use of belts, handcuffs, or any other equipment which restricts the patient's movements or totally prevents them from moving. This approach is not universally accepted as an intervention and elicits strong disapproval among staff in countries like the UK (Bowers, Alexander, Simpson, Ryan, & Carr-Walker, 2004). *Seclusion*, again as defined by Sailas and Wahlbeck, consists of the "placement and retention of the patient in a bare room" either by locking the door or by stationing staff at the door to ensure the patient remains inside (sometimes referred to as open-area seclusion). There are variations in terms of the type and size of room used for seclusion in that sometimes the patient's bedroom will be used, or a large specially designed area for observation, but the defining characteristics are enforced isolation from the ward community in a bare, unstimulating environment. These interventions, restraint, and seclusion, are the main focus of this chapter but a number of others are worth mentioning and will be discussed in passing below.

Enhanced (or special) observation will also be considered here. This is a coercive technique in that it is initiated by staff as part of their "data-gathering" on the behavior of the patient to assess the risk of imminent violence. Practices vary widely from country to country but there is some move toward consistent definitions. For example, the English NICE (2005) guidelines identify three main levels of enhanced observation: "intermittent" (checked every 15–30 minutes), "within-eyesight" at all times and "within arms-length" levels. The intrusiveness and aversiveness of enhanced observation, especially when it involves two or more staff members within

Table 1. Estimated Use of Coercive Measures in Acute Psychiatry in Selected Countries

	Mechanical Restraint[a]	Manual Restraint	Seclusion	Net bed	Rapid Tranquilization	Pain Compliance[b]
Australia	Occasional	Regular[c]	Regular[c,d]	Never	Regular[c]	Never
Austria	Regular[c]	Occasional[e]	Occasional	Regular[c]	Regular	Never
Canada	Regular[c]	Regular[c,f,g]	Regular[c]	Never	Regular[c]	Never
Czech Republic	Regular[h]	Regular	Regular[h]	Never	Regular	Never
Finland	Regular	Occasional	Regular[i]	Never	Regular	Never
France	Occasional[c]	Regular	Regular[c]	Never	Regular	Never
Germany	Regular[h]	Regular[j]	Regular[j]	Never	Regular[h]	Never
Greece	Regular	Regular	Regular	Never	Regular	Never
Iceland	Never	Regular	Never[k]	Never	Regular	Never
Ireland	Never	Regular[l]	Regular	Never	Regular	Occasional
Italy	Regular	Regular	Never	Never	Regular	Never
Japan	Regular[c]	Regular[m]	Regular[c]	Never	Regular	Never
Netherlands	Occasional	Regular	Regular[c]	Never	Regular[c,n]	Never
New Zealand	Occasional[o]	Regular[c]	Regular	Never	Regular	Not specified
Norway	Regular[p]	Regular[h]	Occasional[q]	Never	Regular[r]	Never
Portugal	Occasional	Regular	Regular	Never	Regular[c]	Never
Slovenia	Occasional	Regular	Never	Never	Regular[c]	Never
Spain	Regular[*]	Regular[j]	Never	Never	Regular[*]	Never
Sweden	Regular	Regular[s]	Occasional	Never	Regular	Never
Switzerland	Regular	Regular	Regular	Never	Regular	Regular
Taiwan	Regular[c]	Regular[c]	Regular[c]	Never	Regular[c]	Never

Compiled from responses by at least one resident expert in each country; the authors gratefully acknowledge the contribution of these experts to the construction of this table.
[a]Defined here as excluding prevention of falls for elderly patients.
[b]Defined here as a formally legitimized technique rather than covert use by individual staff.

(Continued)

Table 1. Estimated Use of Coercive Measures in Acute Psychiatry in Selected Countries—Cont'd

	Mechanical Restraint[a]	Manual Restraint	Seclusion	Net bed	Rapid Tranquilization	Pain Compliance[b]
Thailand	Never	Regular[c]	Regular[c]	Never	Regular[c]	Never
Turkey	Occasional	Occasional	Occasional	Never	Regular	Never
UK: England and Wales	Occasional[c]	Regular[c]	Regular[c]	Never	Regular[c]	Never
UK: Scotland	Occasional	Regular	Regular[h]	Never	Regular	Occasional[l]
USA	Regular[c,j]	Regular[c,j]	Regular[c,j]	Never	Regular	Never

[a]National professional guideline available.
[d]Dependent on setting.
[c]Only used to bring patient to a bed or prevent absconding.
[f]Usually for less than two minutes in preparation for seclusion.
[g]Use of prone restraint actively minimized.
[h]Local hospital guidelines in place.
[i]Banned or occasional use in some hospitals.
[j]Only during involuntary medication or as precursor to mechanical restraint or seclusion.
[k]Time-out in own room, maybe with door open usually for a up to a day.
[l]Only if medication and seclusion not available as options.
[m]Only used to carry out injection or mechanical restraint.
[n]Seclusion preferred.
[o]Special permission of clinical director required.
[p]3% of patients annually (2003).
[q]0.1% of patients annually (2003).
[r]2% of patients annually (2003).
[s]Generally regarded more as self-defense than coercion.
[t]Endorsed in certain circumstances in some settings.

arms length, can approach that of actual restraint but generally observation is viewed by staff as a more therapeutically acceptable intervention. In some countries it is being actively developed both practically and theoretically as a more acceptable and equally effective alternative to seclusion.

Enforced medication (also referred to as rapid tranquillization) is part of the cluster of coercive interventions but is dealt with in some detail in Chapter 9. *Net beds* or cage beds consist of a lockable metal frame bolted to the patient's bed and combine some elements of mechanical restraint and seclusion. They are not widely used around the world and, where they are used, are rapidly being phased out (Tavcar et al., 2005). *Pain compliance* (Paterson, 2005) is a highly controversial technique in which pain is deliberately inflicted by staff on a patient either by actively pressing, or by passively holding, a limb in such a way that any movement by the patient triggers pain. Its usage is often hidden but in some situations it is discussed as an appropriate technique in therapeutic settings.

All of these interventions are quite well defined, widely known, and widely discussed in the psychiatric community, both by patients and staff. It is important to note though, that they represent only the visible tip of the iceberg in terms of the full range of behaviors which staff use to coerce patients. Submerged below the surface are a whole range of unrecorded, unreviewed maneuvers used by staff. Ryan and Bowers (2005) identified numerous types of such coercion which will be recognized by anybody who has ever been on an psychiatric ward as a patient or professional. These include physical techniques (such as "body blocking," leading, imposing, shows of force), nonverbal techniques (such as stern facial expressions), and verbal techniques (e.g., warnings). As the authors note, these maneuvers could be construed as unacceptable coercion or, alternatively, as low-intensity options which may actually prevent the full-blown conflict of a restraint episode. This then raises the issue of what we mean by coercion itself. When do persuasion, manipulation, and influence end and coercion begin? Coercion is generally viewed as a necessary evil, undesirable but justifiable and unavoidable in some situations. Olsen (2003) rightly argues that coercion, like the dangerousness which it seeks to control, is a continuum rather than a simple yes/no dichotomy. Some patient groups argue that a wide range of "persuaders" constitute coercion including pressure and inducements from family and friends to go into hospital, threats of loss of services or other supports if this is refused, and pressure to give informed consent without viable alternatives (NoForceUK, 2006).

1.2   Are Coercive Interventions Effective?

A successful healthcare intervention has to pass at least two tests: does it work (effectiveness), and is it acceptable? Coercive interventions have difficulties on both these tests. The effectiveness of these techniques can be judged in a number of ways. At the most basic level, i.e., stopping violence which is actually occurring, most of them are effective in everyday practice. Any violent individual in an institution will eventually be overwhelmed by the superior force (nurses' bodies, CS spray, riot shields, etc.) which the institution can muster in an emergency and, once overwhelmed, will remain unable to commit physical violence until the belts are removed or the medication is allowed to wear off. But, as we will see below, this process of overwhelming is physically dangerous and psychologically disturbing, for the patient and for the staff, so the success of the intervention comes at a cost. Occasionally this cost is severe but potentially can include patient death (Paterson et al., 2003). Even if no injuries are sustained, a "hangover" of coercion-related anger, resentment, and distrust can linger for many weeks afterward and damage the relationships on the ward.

So if we want to test the effectiveness of coercive interventions it is difficult to know on what outcome to make our judgment, e.g., injuries sustained in the restraint? Verbal aggression while restrained? Physical aggression after release or over the next seven days?. To borrow Wright's (2003) analogy: We do not judge the success of airbags and seat belts in terms of the effect that they have on the rate of car accidents. Increasingly seclusion and restraint are viewed as treatment failures rather than healthcare interventions so their potential for any effectiveness in contributing to the reduction of violence is extremely limited. Also, since the apparently simple terms "seclusion" and "restraint" cover a vast variety of actual interventions by two or more people in a huge range of different physical environments, it is virtually impossible to identify the simple active ingredient which operates and works across all these different situations. Again, as Wright points out, most training in physical restraint is combined with deescalation and conflict management skills so it is difficult to disentangle the relative contributions of each to any improvement. While complex cognitive-behavioral packages are similar in some ways to conflict management interventions and have been successfully "tested," the nature of the latter occurring unpredictably in high-tension emergency interactions makes it nearly impossible to check that an intervention protocol has been adhered to. So, since both the outcome and the intervention are so difficult to tie down, it is little wonder that recent reviews of the literature (Sailas & Fenton, 2002; Sailas & Wahlbeck, 2005) conclude that tightly designed effectiveness studies (i.e., RCTs) are absent from the literature.

1.3   Are Coercive Interventions Ethically Acceptable?

Coercive interventions raise ethical problems that are unique in the field of healthcare. The combination of enforced control and potential danger to the controlled person creates uncomfortable dilemmas for staff and, in some cases, outrage among organized patient groups. An example of patient outrage from the UK is the manifesto of the "Kiss It" campaign which argues that:

> "The methods that are employed by psychiatry, and imposed onto those who experience emotionally vulnerable and volatile states, are often inhuman . . . To ensure individuals do not stray too far from the limited and restricted parameters that define the 'norm', psychiatry implements: incarceration, physical restraints, pain compliance techniques, forced drugging, compulsory electro convulsive 'therapy', psychosurgery, coercion, and brainwashing all of which demonstrate the defectiveness rather than the effectiveness of psychiatric treatment. The

disturbance we may experience in our lives is exacerbated and increased many-fold by the aggressive insensitivity and gross inhumanity of such methods. Those who are subjected to these treatments are often damaged and traumatized by them. We call for urgent and radical reform of the 'mental health' system, and an immediate end to psychiatric assault. This is a human rights issue." (Kiss It, 2006).

It includes testimony from a patient:

"Six of them (psychiatric staff) put me in head and arm locks. I cried out for help. They dragged me to a cell where I was stripped bare and forced face down on the floor. Syringes were inserted in my buttocks and I was injected with extremely powerful drugs. The cell door was bolted and I was left to recede into unconsciousness, utterly alone, terrified and traumatized. This was done to me repeatedly. Rubbing salt in the wound they labeled me paranoid. I am now!" (Kiss It, 2006).

There is a distinction to be drawn between this radical perspective, held by some professionals as well as patients, which rejects any use of coercion in psychiatry and other perspectives which emphasize reform. These approaches represent the consensus within current practice and are based on the acceptance that coercion will always be used in psychiatry, but that its use should be minimized as much as possible. When its use cannot be avoided, the skill and humanity with which it is implemented should be maximized. The reformists recognize serious problems around the world in the quality of how coercion is implemented. The European Committee for the Prevention of Torture and Inhuman or Degrading Treatment or Punishment (CPT) (Niveau, 2004) made 69 visits to psychiatric institutions across Europe between 1989 and 2001 and found that, while there were no cases of torture identified, several substantiated episodes of deliberate ill-treatment did take place. The CPT took the view that secluding a person in a room which is cold, poorly ventilated, unsanitary, unsuitably furnished (e.g., inadequate bedding), or which does not permit communication with staff constitutes ill-treatment and that, anyway, seclusion (though presumably not restraint) is a practice which must be phased out. Of the 22 countries visited more than once only five had no recommendations for improvement in restraint practices imposed on them (Germany, Iceland, Italy, Norway, and Portugal).

Given these issues, and given the inherent conflict within the professional between the need to control and the intention to care, it is no wonder that the ethics of coercion have generated huge debate and controversy among professional groups. Recent attempts have been made to work out the practical ethics to help front-line staff to make the right judgment in very difficult circumstances. Olsen (2003) sets out some criteria for judging the ethics of any particular coercive intervention while O'Brien and Golding (2003), closer to the radical perspective above, argue strongly for a default position in psychiatry where coercive measures are banned as an unjustifiable invasion of patient autonomy while allowing for their use in individual cases. These authors also helpfully provide a seven step hierarchy of coercive practices (from full informed consent with no threats at one end, to physical force at the other) to guide decisions in this area. However, it is sobering to note the findings of Lind et al. (2004), who found that only 11% of their sample of Finnish nurses found seclusion to be an ethically problematic intervention and less than 20% found placing the patient in four-point restraints problematic.

1.4   When are Coercive Measures Legal and Safe?

Coercive interventions, while not in, and of themselves, treatments, must always be seen as being a part of a broader treatment strategy (Olsen, 1998). What is expected by legislation, common law, case law, and/or policy across Europe is the presence of a range and particularly a "hierarchy" such that the extent, nature, and duration of the restriction of liberty used can be matched to the client's behavior. Specific interventions such as seclusion may be precluded by national or local policy guidelines but the general principles involved are illustrated in the comments by The Council of Europe Working Party on Psychiatry on restraint, which emphasized that any:

> "Response to violent behavior by the patient should be graduated, i.e. that staff
> should initially attempt to respond verbally; thereafter, only insofar as required,
> by means of manual restraint; and only in a last resort by mechanical restraint."
> (CEBP, 2000).

Practice must, however, be informed by a knowledge of the risks inherent to certain interventions, notably physical restraint, such that the potential risks involved can be assessed and managed in respect of individual service users. Certain physical procedures particularly *"forceful" prone* (i.e., face down) restraint, in which pressure is exerted on the back, abdomen, or hips to secure the person, particularly when associated with continuing struggle, and *"hyperflexion"* where the service user is bent over at the waist, particularly when seated, have been sources of concern in the UK and US and must be avoided (Paterson & Leadbetter, 1998). Even "supine" restraint, the holding of a service user face up, has however, been reported to be associated with a series of deaths in the US involving aspiration (Morrison et al., 2001). Further research is necessary, however, to establish the relative risks involved in different interventions for individual and/or groups of service users (Brown et al., 2000).

1.5   Policy Around the World

One major tool of reform in this area is to formally identify best practice, disseminate a code of practice to staff and monitor their adherence to the code. Many countries now have national professional guidance on best practice in this area (see Table 1, above) and some of these are easily available on the web (e.g., NICE, 2005). At the same time, many national health agencies around the world have adopted explicit policies to reduce reliance on seclusion and restraint, and replace them with more skilful interventions at the less coercive and intrusive end of the ladder of interventions (Curie, 2005; Glover, 2005). Gradually these national standards are being integrated into local policies and procedures in specific hospitals and units. Lack of a code of practice in some jurisdictions is now considered a breach of international conventions (Dyer, 2003). The CPT takes the view that restraint procedures must be governed by specific local policies which explicitly identify the roles and responsibilities of key staff in the decision-making process, the acceptable duration of the episode and the need for adequate recording (Niveau, 2004). There is evidence that policies are being developed and that many of them incorporate their relevant national guidelines. Zun and Downey (2005) found that 83% of the American Emergency Departments that they contacted had a formal seclusion policy and Cormac et al. (2005) found that all of the seclusion policies they reviewed from UK medium and high secure units followed the relevant national code of practice in terms of guidelines for the decision to use seclusion.

Since such guidelines are now available, it is important to summarize what they recommend as best practice in the area of coercive interventions, especially with regard to seclusion and restraint. We will now turn to one of the most authoritative recent guidelines, that produced by the National Institute of Clinical and Health Excellence (NICE, 2005) for England and Wales.

1.6   Clinical Guidelines on Seclusion and Restraint

The NICE guidelines provide a comprehensive framework on how to assess risk and prevent violence; deescalate and calm down a potentially violent individual; and physically intervene when violence occurs. A comprehensive and detailed literature search and appraisal exercise was conducted for these guidelines, with the main search on seclusion and restraint including all research published up until the early part of 2002. In terms of recommending "what works" in coercive interventions it is important to note that, although many relevant well-designed studies were tracked down, none in this review fitted the criteria for a formal test of effectiveness (i.e., an RCT) so all the recommendations on effectiveness are made in the absence of strong evidence. This confirms the previous finding from the Cochrane review by Sailas and Fenton (2002).

While the focus here is on the specific topics of physical intervention, seclusion, and observation, the guidelines more broadly cover the environment; organization and alarm systems; prediction (antecedents, warning signs, and risk assessment); training; service user perspectives; searching; deescalation techniques; rapid tranquillization; and postincident reviews. A range of care principles are set out as the ideal context in which to implement the recommendations and good practice points contained in the Guidelines. These principles include person-centered care and collaborative interdisciplinary working. Deciding the preferred choice of intervention for the management of violence should involve service users and their carers wherever possible and should be achieved through the use of care plans or advanced directives. As noted above, the Guidelines require the organization to develop a clear strategy and policy, supported by management, which establishes an integrated approach to the problem. There should also be a clear commitment to, and availability of, education and training which ensures that all staff, regardless of their profession or role, are provided with the opportunity to update their knowledge base and are able to implement the recommendations in the Guidelines. From this, it follows that patients should be cared for by persons who have undergone appropriate training and are, therefore, able to initiate and maintain appropriate preventative measures. In practice, this will mean that staffing levels and the skill mix should reflect the needs of the service user and healthcare professional. Care should always be delivered in the context of continuous quality improvement with regular feedback and audit.

A number of *key priorities for implementation* are established by the guidelines. These include recommendations that staff receive training in accordance with an organizational training strategy and, where staff are directly involved in coercive interventions, that this should include ongoing competency training in coping with violence and life support following the use physical intervention or seclusion. The main priorities specific to physical interventions and seclusion are listed in Figure 1.

- Only to be used once deescalation alone has been judged to fail,
- To be considered management rather than treatment strategies,
- Must be justifiable, appropriate, reasonable, and proportionate to the level of risk,
- Must be for as short a duration as possible,
- Safety: support of head and neck, keeping airway open, monitoring vital signs.

Other recommendations:
- the immediate availability of crash bags,
- the quick availability of a doctor,
- awareness and adherence to the relevant Code of Practice,
- respecting the patient's dignity needs,
- explaining the need for the intervention at the earliest opportunity,
- reassessment and reintegration of the patient into the ward milieu as soon as possible afterward,
- enabling the patient to document their perspective,
- maintaining deescalation during physical interventions,
- minimizing the duration of the coercive intervention,
- an absolute ban on placing pressure on the neck, thorax, abdomen, back, or pelvic area during restraint,
- specifying an observation schedule for seclusion,
- minimizing the removal of personal clothing in seclusion,
- enabling the retention of personal objects in seclusion where possible,
- the need for extra vigilance when seclusion and rapid tranquilization are combined if this is absolutely necessary.

Source: NICE (2005).

Figure 1. Some key priorities governing the use of physical interventions and seclusion.

Best practice also involves rigorous documentation. The Guidelines recommend that in all cases following a coercive intervention, a contemporaneous record should be made of the incident using an approved template. As soon as possible following an incident, but in any event within 72 hours, a postincident review should take place with the aim of supporting staff and service users as well as encouraging an improvement in the therapeutic relationship with the service user and their carers. The review should also see what lessons can be learned from the incident. This review should address the incident in as much detail as possible including trigger factors, each person's role in the incident, feelings both during and after the incident as well as inquiring if anything needs to be done to deal with their concerns. It is recommended that the review should be led by a person who was not directly involved in the incident. The contribution of this process of postincident review to reducing the use of restraint and seclusion on wards has been tested in some of the recent studies to be discussed in Section 2.

2 NEW RESEARCH ON SECLUSION AND RESTRAINT

Evidence-based guidelines such as those produced by NICE are essential to the development of best practice in the management of violence and the minimization of coercive interventions. We can be sure that the review underpinning the NICE guidelines represents an accurate summary of the research base at the time the search was concluded. With regard to effectiveness, it is not surprising given the discussion above about research design, that the review was unable to draw any conclusions on the use of physical interventions, seclusion, or pain compliance. With regard to how people view these interventions, it was concluded that staff find it traumatic to implement them and that patients find it degrading to undergo them. Notwithstanding this aversiveness, staff, and to some extent patients, felt that their use was sometimes unavoidable and may be justifiable.

None of the literature discussed in this review was published after 2002 so it is worthwhile now to consider some emerging research to inform our understanding of the issues. We therefore conducted a brief supplementary review for an indication of new developments in this area. This review covered empirical studies published in the period 2002–2005 and replicated elements of the NICE search strategy where possible. Studies from the early part of the period which had been included in the NICE review were excluded.

2.1 How Often are Coercive Measures Used Around the World?

It is increasingly clear that patients in different countries are subjected to coercive interventions at different rates and for different reasons. Table 1 (above) demonstrates that practices acceptable, and even valued, in one country may be banned in a neighboring jurisdiction. In a major review, Nijman et al. (2005) noted in a Dutch study that up to 50% of aggressive episodes were followed by seclusion, compared to none in a UK study. However, since national samples are difficult to recruit, the degree to which this is a national/cultural phenomenon or a reflection of individual studies and ward practices is difficult to tell.

Table 2 illustrates recent studies which have provided estimates of the frequency with which seclusion and restraint are used in nine different countries. Two of the studies are direct international comparisons (Bowers et al., 2005; Hubner-Liebermann et al., 2005), but comparisons across all the listed studies are difficult to make due to the wide range of approaches to data collection (prospective or cross-sectional), data sources (case notes, audit forms, or study questionnaires), settings, definitions of coercive measures, and, most importantly, the format in which the rate is expressed (proportion of patients, number of episodes, etc.). To take the two direct comparisons first, Bowers et al. compared seclusion and restraint rates in three European centers (London, UK; Modena, Italy; and Athens, Greece) and found markedly different patterns of use for coercive interventions over a two-week period. Seclusion was used relatively more often in London, and restraint (both manual and mechanical) was used relatively more often in Athens. The authors noted that minority ethnic patients in each country were more likely to be subjected to coercive measures (including here, intramuscular injection) than the majority population. For instance, minority groups in Italy (mainly North African, Black African, and East European) and Greece (mainly Albanian, Albano-Greek, and Russian Slavic) were more likely to be mechanically restrained. Hubner et al. (2005) conclude that mechanical restraint was used more widely in their Japanese sample (20%) than the German sample (7%).

Daffern et al. (2003) make the important observation that adjacent wards within the same Australian hospital had wildly varying coercive intervention rates and these cannot be wholly explained by differing patient characteristics. This observation is probably true universally and raises important issues about how the "postcode lottery" applies to a patient's likelihood of being coerced on a psychiatric ward. Kaltiala-Heino et al. (2003) noted that seclusion and restraint were implemented for differing reasons. Agitation, disorientation, and actual violence were associated with mechanical restraint while threats were associated with seclusion. There were also significant diagnostic variations with more than 70% of coercive interventions with schizophrenics and substance abusers to manage agitation or disorientation, while most of the interventions with mood disorders were to manage threats.

When comparing coerced and uncoerced patients, Nakajima et al. (2003) found that a small group of multiply secluded Japanese patients ($n = 6$) had more severe psychopathology and lower prolactin levels than unsecluded controls. Similarly, Odawara et al. (2005) report that restrained Japanese patients were older, and more likely to be male, with a prior treatment history, ICD F0/1/2 diagnosis (organic mental disorder, substance use, and schizophrenia), involuntary admission, physical complications, and suicide attempts. Restrained patients were also more commonly admitted at night or during the weekend or holidays. Conversely, with regard to time patterns, Vittengl (2002) found lower odds for physical interventions

Table 2. Estimates of Seclusion and Restraint Use

	Data Source	Reference Period	Country	Setting	Beds	Seclusion Use	Restraint Use	Mean/ Median Duration
Allen and Currier (2004)	Panel survey	Cross-sectional	USA	51 psychiatric EDs	NA		8% patients	3.3 hours (R)
			UK	12 acute wards		5% patients	18% patients*	
Bowers, Douzenis et al. (2005)	PCC/case notes	2 weeks	Italy	3 acute wards		0% patients	10% patients* 10% patients*	
			Greece	11 acute wards		0.5% patients	50% patients* 50% patients*	
Daffern et al. (2003)	Incident audit forms	12 months	Australia	5 forensic wards	80	253 episodes		2.3–5.4 hours (S)
Hubner et al. (2005)	Patient audit system	12 months	Germany	20 acute wards	495		7% patients	
			Japan	3 acute wards	97		20% patients	
Kaltiala et al. (2003)	Case notes and incident audit forms	6 months	Finland	5 acute inpatient clinics		370 episodes	112 episodes	13 hours (S) 9 hours (R)
Leggett and Silvester (2003)	Incident audit forms	4 years	UK	Medium secure forensic hospital	65	58 episodes	33% patients* 557 episodes*	0.2 hours (manual R)
Nakajima et al. (2003)	Incident audit forms	12 months	Japan	1 acute female ward	60	21% patients		
Odawara et al. (2005)	Case notes	4 years	Japan	2 acute wards	50	18% patients		84% > 24 hours (R)
Vittengl (2002)	Incident audit forms	8.6 years	USA	5 acute wards	174	3,293 episodes	2,673 episodes	3.75 hours (S + R)
Wynn (2002)	Incident audit forms	5.5 years	Norway	10 acute wards	107	88 episodes	797 episodes	
Yung et al. (2003)	Case notes	Cross-sectional	Australia	Acute service Early psychosis intervention service	39 16	22% patients 10% patients		

*manual restraint (R) restraint episode (S) seclusion episode.

during weekends in an American hospital with daily peaks at times of high ward activity.

There has been a move to develop statistical models predictive of seclusion and restraint use. Gudjonsson et al. (2004) model predicting restraint use in a UK general psychiatric hospital includes the following variables: attempt to abscond, having a nurse as the target of the aggression, patient agitation, being detained on a civil section (rather than a criminal section or no section at all), and use of violence (rather than threats or property damage). Their seclusion model includes some common variables (nurse target, patient agitation, being on a civil section) and some which are distinct (gender, extent of injury, and patient age). Coutinho et al. (2005) report the development of a predictive model for physical restraint in a Brazilian Emergency Department. Younger age, first attendance, severe aggression, and substance abuse aggression were the significant predictors in this model. More specifically, Riley et al. (2006) found a number of significant differences between incidents in which either prone (face-down) or supine (face-up) restraint on the floor was used, including much higher rates of withdrawn behavior prior to supine restraint.

2.2 What Does It Feel Like to be Restrained or Secluded?

While uncovering the patient's perspective when undergoing coercive interventions has been an important theme for several years (Johnson, 1998), there has been a significant growth of interest in this area recently. This reflects the wider shift to a "service use" model of mental health care delivery which is severely tested when applied to coercive measures. There is a growing (re-)awareness of psychiatric iatrogenesis or "sanctuary harm" and even "sanctuary trauma" (Frueh et al., 2005; Robins et al., 2005), and being subjected to coercive interventions is likely to play a part in this. A number of qualitative studies, often using grounded theory methodologies, have been conducted.

Wynn (2004) interviewed a small group of Norwegian patients in the two weeks after they had been mechanically restrained. Not surprisingly, a wide range of negative reactions were described including fear, anxiety, humiliation, and anger. Disrespect and humiliation was also a theme identified by Robins et al. (2005) in their investigation of sanctuary harm among a group of American patients. Most patients in the Wynn study had no difficulty identifying the reasons why they were restrained, although this is not to say that they agreed it was justified. Some felt unable to become calm while in restraints and were reminded of previous restraint episodes, even those that may have occurred in childhood, including episodes of sexual assault. Some were very afraid of being left alone by staff while restrained and others were unable to sleep after their release for fear that it would happen again, or became more compliant afterwards to avoid recoercion. All the patients felt some physical discomfort during, or after, the episode. One patient viewed it as an act of abuse, most felt it was unfair, and some felt it was little more than a demonstration of power by staff. Commonly there was a feeling of distrust for staff and damage to any existing therapeutic alliance. None of the patients felt it was a positive or fruitful experience. Hoekstra (2004) developed a grounded theory of the seclusion experience through interviews with eight Dutch patients after their discharge. Three main themes were identified centering on issues of autonomy (feelings of dependence, powerlessness, humiliation, being watched, shame, and loss), issues of trust (fear, suspicion, insecurity, oppression, distrust, arbitrariness, safety, acceptance), and issues of loneliness (being alone, boredom). Again, the patients saw it as a largely negative experience but said their feelings of anger declined over time. Interestingly, they said that their relations with carers were not remarkably affected by the seclusion experience. Benson et al. (2003) applied discourse analysis to two incidents involving two professionals and one patient and noted how both parties were very concerned with attributing blame for what had happened. Both parties complained that the other party did not act in the way expected by their role. For the staff, the patient's violence was attributed to her personality rather than a legitimate illness and for the patient, the incident was attributed to staff brutality inappropriate to a caring professional.

Chien et al. (2005) study is unusual and somewhat provocative for all sides in the debate on coercive measures since this team found both positive and negative responses among a group of Chinese (Hong Kong) patients who had been restrained. While over half the sample reported negative responses revolving around a lack of staff concern and empathy, failure to provide information, powerlessness, and uncertainty, a larger number reported positive feelings toward the staff involved and guidance on how to minimize the distress associated with restraint. They emphasized that it was possible to have feelings of safety and trust in staff, with staff expressing care and concern during the episode, using explanations and frequent interactions and overall conveying a sense of respect to the patient despite the circumstances.

Using a more structured approach, Meehan et al. (2004) surveyed patient views in Australia on the effects of seclusion. Only a tiny minority of patients (4%) believed seclusion to be often beneficial to the secluded patient (compared to 60% of staff in this sample). An overwhelming majority (>80%) said that it makes the patient feel frustrated, punished, or angry with staff. But, as with the study above, there were high levels of agreement with some potentially positive gains such as "it helps the patient to behave better when let out" (89% sometimes or often), "it helps the patient get away from people who upset them" (71%), "it helps the patient calm down" (67%), and "it allows nondisruptive expression of feelings" (64%). There was also some recognition that staff are not entirely punitive when implementing seclusion. Over 70% of patients agreed that staff feel they are being helpful to the patient, that they are relieved the problem is dealt with, that they feel safer, that they are annoyed that prevention has failed, and are satisfied there are no alternatives. Less than a third of patients, though, agreed that seclusion "helps the patient feel better."

A number of studies have contacted patients after they have left hospital and asked them to reflect on their experience of coercive measures. Frueh et al. (2005) found that 46% of those patients who had been "taken down," 34% of those who had witnessed somebody else being "taken down," 48% of those placed in seclusion, and 52% of those placed in restraints, were severely or extremely distressed a week after the event had taken place. Cusack et al. (2003) investigated the prevalence of sanctuary trauma (defined as diagnosable Post-Traumatic Stress Disorder and distinct from the less severe sanctuary harm). Thirty nine percent of 57 American patients in their sample had undergone coercive measures. Being put in seclusion was categorized as harmful, or capable of producing, or exacerbating symptoms from previous traumas, but it was not categorized as traumatic. Lessing and Beech (2004) surveyed patient satisfaction following discharge from an American psychiatric hospital. It is very noticeable in this study, as the authors point out, that hospital factors were stronger predictors of satisfaction than patient factors (e.g., age). They argue that this finding undermines the tendency in some organizations to discount complaints because they reflect "variations in patient attributes" (i.e., "difficult" individuals) rather than actual issues in the quality of care received. While personal experience of restraint was not a significant predictor of satisfaction, the unit restraint rate was a significant predictor. Surprisingly, furthermore, it was a positive predictor suggesting that high unit restraint rates were associated with high satisfaction. The authors looked into this apparently paradoxical finding in more detail by examining some open-ended responses and found that the patients who were supporting more controlling interventions on wards often cited their own feelings of danger while on the ward. Obviously, some patients are afraid of other patients on the ward and want staff to control them effectively, albeit humanely. In turn, this reminds us that, contrary to the radical view of coercive measures mentioned above, psychiatry is not a simple "us (staff) and them (patients)" dichotomy, and that different patients have different needs in terms of feeling safe and secure in hospital.

2.3   What Do Staff Think and Believe About Coercive Measures?

Alongside the growth of interest in the patient perspective, a number of recent studies have attempted to gain a more sophisticated and detailed picture of how staff think about these measures. We have already considered a survey above on the ethical views of staff (Lind et al., 2004), but we will now consider views on the clinical aspects of restraint and seclusion. There is general agreement on the indicators for seclusion and restraint revolving around issues of controlling actual or imminent violence to self, people or property but, as we have already seen, there are varying views on the acceptability of the procedure. The Attitudes to Containment Measures Questionnaire (ACMQ) was used by Bowers et al. (2004) to examine approval rates among UK nurses for various types of intervention. In this UK sample, there was low approval for seclusion, physical restraint, and mechanical restraint as techniques for managing conflict and relatively high approval for special observation. Seventy-five percent of nurses in Meehan et al.'s (2004) study rated seclusion as "highly therapeutic" and 60% considered it often beneficial but, at the same time, a small group (8%) rated it as "highly punitive." Divisions like this between staff on the value of coercive measures mirror the division among patient groups noted above, indicating that straightforward "pro-" and "anti-" camps on each side do not exist. Overall, nurses tended to be aware of both the positive and negative potential effects of seclusion and had a more optimistic view of their benefits than the patient sample, who completed the same scale. There was awareness among UK staff in Lee et al.'s (2003) survey that restraint could damage patient well being and their relationship with staff without alleviating any underlying psychopathology or disorder. At the same time it was demeaning to the patient. Huge attitudinal differences are revealed when staff in two countries with psychiatric systems which might be considered comparable and historically linked (UK and Australia) are considered. Seventy percent of staff in Duxbury's (2002) survey using the MAVAS agreed that seclusion should be discontinued but only 2% of Australian nurses in Meehan et al.'s (2004) survey agreed with this. As with so many of these comparisons though, it is impossible to deduce whether these reflect genuine national cultural differences or simply the local cultures of the two settings examined.

The decision to restrain or seclude is ultimately subjective, albeit informed by evidence and best practice, and any subjective decision will be influenced by personal beliefs and attitudes. Some of the respondents to Lee et al.'s (2003) survey of UK nurses said they were worried about the attitudes of some of their colleagues which reflected a "bouncer" mentality in which they intended to "deck them first." Leggett and Silvester (2003) have demonstrated how incidents of manual restraint, where the staff considered the patient had control over their actions leading up to the restraint, were associated with subsequent placement in seclusion. There was also a gender effect in that nurses were more likely to say they had no explanation for aggressive patient behavior when the patient was female. We must also remember that participating in a restraint episode is, at best, emotionally challenging and, at worst, highly distressing for staff. Apart from the risk of injury there is the sharp sense of contravening personal beliefs about the need to care for vulnerable patients. Three percent of nurses in Lee et al.'s (2003) survey found their last restraint episode very difficult and stressful and required sick leave afterward.

Crichton (Crichton, 2002; Leadbetter et al., 2005) demonstrated that staff responses to patient aggression in mental health settings are significantly influenced by the process of moral judgment. Such judgments contain three inseparable dimensions: containment of the unsafe, underlying pathology, and moral censure. Patient behaviors judged by staff to result from causal factors outwith the patient's control (e.g., psychosis) were more likely to be considered "mad," while those patients judged capable of exercising increased self-control (such as personality disordered patients) were more likely to be regarded as "bad." In turn, such judgments shaped the nature of staff responses with "bad" behavior attracting an increased likelihood of punitive responses while "mad" behavior attracted more helpful or therapeutic responses. As Towell (1975) suggests:

"Where the medical treatment ideology was a dominant influence, patients who are not regarded as 'ill' thereby lost their claim to receive help. Instead the deviant behavior of such patients was likely to seem as intentioned, the deviant judged responsible and attempts made to control the behavior through the application of negative sanctions."

2.4   How Can Alternatives to Coercive Measures be Introduced?

Given the undoubted harmful effects on patients and staff of implementing seclusion and restraint, there is a growing movement among professionals and policy-makers to consider their use as "treatment failures" and to replace them with less coercive measures. The questions are: What can replace these measures and, how can change be successfully achieved?

One obvious approach is to ask patients themselves about possible alternatives. The Norwegian patients interviewed by Wynn (2004) were also asked about how restraint could have been avoided in their particular episode. They recommended a variety of staff approaches such as more positive attention and more open communication before the conflict intensified. They wanted an approach which emphasized their security, but in an unthreatening way. Some felt that the episode had got out of hand because they were pushed into a corner and felt provoked by staff. None of them felt that improved pharmacotherapy would have helped.

So what initiatives can mental health services adopt if they want to reduce their reliance on coercive measures? Sailas and Wahlbeck's (2005) review identified a number of interventions which were found useful in one or more studies including sensory approaches, early identification and management, self-diagnosis of stress triggers by patients, enhanced patient coping strategies, staff training in deescalation and nonviolent intervention, identification of high risk patients, crisis intervention teams, daily review of restraints, incentive systems, and patient advocates. Fisher (2003) also describes a number of case studies in which success has been achieved in this area based on trauma theory.

A number of empirical studies have been conducted in the past few years to look for associations between changes in how a mental health service is delivered and reductions in seclusion and restraint rates (Curie, 2005). These studies are summarized in Table 3. The methodological criticisms of work in this area (Sailas & Fenton, 2002; Sailas & Wahlbeck, 2005; Wright, 2003) continue to be valid, with only one very recent study (Needham, 2004) meeting the criteria for a randomized controlled trial, and most of the others either prospectively observing changes in a single environment following the introduction of a new initiative, or just opportunistically relying post hoc on associations between observed reductions and ongoing service changes. However, as discussed above, it will always be difficult to establish effectiveness in this area and the problem is too urgent to wait for conclusive "proof"; in any case, there is much that can be learned practically from the initiatives discussed in these studies. A number of common themes are identifiable as occurring among these initiatives.

The most common approach is some form of enhanced and/or individualized patient risk assessment (see also Chapter 6). Some services used structured

Table 3. Pre–Post Studies of Changes in Seclusion and Restraint

Study	Country	Setting	Staff Education/ Training for Managing Incidents	Individualized Risk Assessment	Other	Post-Intervention Assessment Period (months)	% Reduction Pre-Post			Other Benefits/ Comments
							Seclusion	Restraint	Coercive Measures	
(Bols, et al., 2004)	Belgium	Rehabilitation ward	X			60	97%			Achieved alongside large increase in involuntary patients
Donat (2003)	USA	General psychiatric hospital		X	X	60			75%	Changes to administrative review procedures was the best predictor of reduction
D'Orio et al. (2004)	USA	Psychiatric ED	X	X	X	9			39%	
Goodness and Renfro (2002)	USA	High security forensic unit		X		24			50%	Intervention based on social learning theory
Jonikas et al. (2004)	USA	3 acute wards	X	X		6		98%		

(Continued)

Table 3. Pre–Post Studies of Changes in Seclusion and Restraint—Cont'd

Study	Country	Setting	Staff Education/ Training for Managing Incidents	Individualized Risk Assessment	Other	Post-Intervention Assessment Period (months)	% Reduction Pre-Post Seclusion	% Reduction Pre-Post Restraint	Coercive Measures	Other Benefits/ Comments
Khadivi et al. (2004)	USA	3 acute wards	X	X	X	12			52%	Assaults on staff increased significantly
LeBel and Goldstein (2005)	USA	Adolescent unit			X	12		91%		92% reduction in financial costs and significant drop in other employer costs as well
Needham (2004) RCT	Switzerland	3 acute wards (treatment)	X	X		3			+4%	After the removal of outliers severe aggressive incidents and coercive measures dropped significantly in the treatment group. Mild aggressive incidents and attacks toward persons remained stable in both groups
		3 acute wards (control)				3			+55%	

Smith et al. (2005)	USA	9 general psychiatric hospitals		X	NA	93%	65%	Reduced duration: 88% seclusion, 84% restraint
Sullivan et al. (2005)	USA	General psychiatric hospital	X	X	NA		70%	82% drop in hours confined
Tavcar et al. (2005)	Slovenia	General psychiatric hospital	X	X	12		50%	Main innovation introduced was phasing out of net beds

instruments like the Broeset Violence Checklist (Needham, 2004), or adaptations of the Overt Aggression Scale (D'Orio et al., 2004), while others refer to individualized patient plans often including identification of potential aggression triggers and advanced directives on preferred interventions when feeling agitated (Sullivan et al., 2005). Khadivi et al. (2004), approach of flagging a history of violence on admission forms is another example. Collaboration with the patient, when exploring life history and identifying triggers, is vital to this process and enables personal preferences in the management of angry and aroused behavior to be established.

The second most common approach was some form of staff education or training. It is likely that most studies included some form of staff training as well, since few initiatives can be introduced without such training, but the focus here is on specific improved incident management training. Usually the emphasis of training was on improved prediction, deescalation and aggression minimization skills as requested by the patients in Wynn's (2004) study, to emphasize prevention and avoid forcing both patient and staff up the ladder of coercion. Some (e.g. Needham, 2004) provide details on the content of the training and references to training manuals for further information. Training is widely advocated as a solution to the problem of aggression in health care settings and, as a by-product, can offer reductions in the use of coercive measures. Since it is widely advocated and has now to some extent been shown to be effective, and since there is a huge diversity of training packages available, it is necessary to identify which components of training are actively contributing to success and incorporate these into a core training syllabus (see also Chapter 11).

Both of these initiatives, risk assessment and training, are focused on the skills of individual staff and patients but it is widely recognized that organizational changes are essential as well (Leather et al., 1999). A number of studies (e.g. Smith et al., 2005) discuss more structural (and potentially expensive) ward-level changes such as improved staff–patient ratios, increased activity, and off-ward programs and positive reinforcement contingency programs. Another major theme in these initiatives is postincident debriefing (Jonikas et al., 2004), and postincident review (Khadivi et al., 2004). Debriefing with both staff and, in some cases patients, is an obvious opportunity to learn alternatives generally, or specifically relating to a particular patient. Donat (2003) enhanced institutional incident review procedures by recruiting department heads to give the review committee more "clout," increasing the speed with which incidents were considered by the committee and lowering the threshold so that more low-level incidents were considered. This might enable consideration of successfully defused incidents to inform future practice.

Alongside this, several initiatives included enhanced access to expertise either in the emergency situation (D'Orio et al., 2004), or in terms of longer-term prevention measures (LeBel & Goldstein, 2005). Technological and pharmacological "fixes" were not prominent, although electronic information systems increase speed of incident reporting (Donat, 2003), and D'Orio et al. (2004) mention CCTV surveillance for monitoring patent behavior and thus improved risk assessment.

It is important to emphasize the environmental nature of all of these innovations. New drugs may play a role in some successful reduction programs (Smith et al., 2005) but the management of external factors is a priority, whether at the individual or organizational levels.

3 ENHANCED OBSERVATION

As initiatives to reduce restraint and seclusion bite, more acceptable alternatives are being promoted and one of these approaches is enhanced or "special" observation. Much consideration is given in the NICE (2005) guidelines to the effective use of this intervention. The primary aim of observation is seen here as being to provide an opportunity to engage positively with the patient, so it is recommended that its operation should be meaningful, grounded in trust, and therapeutic for the patient. The minimum acceptable level for all in-patients is "general observation" in which a designated member of staff is at least aware of the location of a patient at all times, without the requirement to be within view. As part of this general observation, at least once every shift each patient's mental state should be assessed by a nurse who should also engage positively with him or her so as to develop a positive, caring, and therapeutic relationship. The nurse should also assess, and record in the notes, the service user's moods and behaviors in relation to the risks of disturbed and/or violent behavior during this assessment. When observation is stepped up to the intermittent level (15 minute checks) because the patient is felt to be potentially at risk of violent behavior but this is not imminent, or where the patient is in the process of recovery postincident, it is felt important that the patient's sensitivity is respected, and as little intrusion as possible is caused. Again, the nurse should engage positively with the service user during the checks. Within-eyesight observation should be initiated when it is judged that violence is imminent and, at this stage, it may be necessary to carry out a search of their belongings and remove any dangerous objects. Again, and even more than before, positive engagement with the patient is essential at this level of observation. The highest level of observation, within arms-length, should be reserved for those patients who are deemed to be at the highest risk of violence. Obviously it involves close proximity supervision and, in view of the elevated level of risk, it may be necessary for more than one member of staff to conduct the observation. As always, positive engagement with the patient is essential at this level of observation.

A research base for enhanced observation exists but is only in its infancy. Bowers and Park (2001) report that nearly 20% of admissions to acute inpatient psychiatric care will be placed on some form of intervention involving enhanced supervision. While the exact terminology will vary and a variety of terms may be used e.g., special, close, maximum, continuous, and/or constant observation (Bowers & Park, 2001) the procedure reported is essentially a form of increased level of supervision of the patient in order to manage and decrease patient care-related risks (Moore et al., 1995). Such risks commonly include self harm and suicide but increased observation can be and is, also used as part of wider attempts to manage and reduce the potential for violence particularly that associated with acute illness (Neilson & Brennan, 2001).

Notwithstanding the potential benefits, there are concerns that the intrusive nature of higher levels of observation, potentially involving staff being at arms length at all times, may for some patients be counterproductive. This may be especially true where the patient presents with paranoid ideation (Yonge & Sterwin, 1992). Enhanced observation in such circumstances may increase both the probability of violence and the risks of staff suffering injury due to issues of proximity (Clinical Resource Audit Group (CRAG), 2002). There remains, however, a limited research base on the use of enhanced observation to manage the potential for violence. Mackay et al. (2005), in a small qualitative study involving six nurses, identified that a range of skills were employed including "intervening"; "maintaining the safety of the patient and others"; "prevention, deescalation and management of aggression"; "assessing"; "communication"; and "therapy." There remains, however, a need for further research on the role of enhanced supervision in the prevention of violence, particularly comparing the practice in different settings, and with different patient populations.

4   CONCLUSION

We have seen that coercive measures are widely used in mental health services around the world and that their use creates enormous problems for the patients who are subjected to them, or simply witness them, and for the staff who have to implement them. Reframing them as treatment failures and mere temporary crisis management, rather than legitimate therapeutic interventions, is changing the culture in a way that all patients and many staff will welcome. Boosting "quality" by enforcing strict adherence to good practice guidelines on their appropriate use when they become unavoidable will not satisfy those who will always view psychiatric coercion as an abuse of inalienable human rights, but is the best that can be offered in a world where the safety and security of everybody on the ward must be protected. Research efforts to define best practice in this troubling area must continue to listen to both patients and staff to ensure that we preserve as much of the humanity of psychiatric care as possible at a time when it is easily experienced as simply inhumane.

5   APPENDIX: A SELECTION OF NEW RESEARCH AND CLINICAL INSTRUMENTS USED IN THE LITERATURE REVIEWED HERE

Attitudes to Containment Scale (Bowers et al., 2004): an attitude scale which elicits approval rates for 11 different types of containment measure.

Attitudes to Seclusion Questionnaire (Meehan et al., 2004): an attitude scale with established psychometric properties which elicits views on seclusion use and changes to the seclusion process.

Broeset Violence Checklist (Needham, 2004): a six-item violence risk assessment tool with established psychometric properties (Almvik).

Ethical Views on Coercive Measures (Lind et al., 2004): a six-item attitude scale listing psychiatric interventions and eliciting views on how ethically problematic they are.

Management of Violence and Aggression Scale (Duxbury, 2002): an attitude scale with established psychometric properties which elicits views on controlling, deescalating, and noncontrolling approaches to the management of violence.

Nursing Assessment Tool (Sullivan et al., 2005): a three-part structured instrument for violence assessment focusing on personal history, predictors, and preferred agitation management options.

Patient–staff Conflict Checklist (Bowers et al., 2005): a behavioral checklist of 21 conflict types and nine containment measures providing a frequency count per patient, ward, and/or shift.

Psychiatric Experiences Questionnaire (Cusack et al., 2003; Frueh et al., 2005): a 26-item scale listing traumatic or harmful experiences that may occur in psychiatric settings and eliciting experience and responses to such experiences.

Patient Satisfaction Questionnaire (Lessing & Beech, 2004): a 29-item scale with three factors (treatment effectiveness, staff competence, and environment).

Seclusion Survey (Zun & Downey, 2005): a 15-item practice and service audit tool relating particularly to Emergency Departments.

REFERENCES

Allen, M. H., & Currier, G. W. (2004). Use of restraints and pharmacotherapy in academic psychiatric emergengy services. *General Hospital Psychiatry, 26*(1), 42–49.

Benson, A., Secker, J., Balfe, E., Lipsedge, M., Robinson, S., & Walker, J. (2003). Discourses of blame: Accounting for aggression and violence on an acute mental health inpatient unit. *Social Science and Medicine, 57,* 917–926.

Bols, W., Kempe, P., Abrahams, F., De Hert, M., & Peuskens, J. (2004). Use of a seclusion room in a rehabilitation setting for schizophrenic patients, a ten-year prospective study. *Schizophrenia Research, 67,* 142–142.

Bowers, L., Alexander, J., Simpson, A., Ryan, C., & Carr-Walker, P. (2004). Cultures of psychiatry and the professional socialization process: The case of containment methods for disturbed patients. *Nurse Education Today, 24,* 435–442.

Bowers, L., Douzenis, A., Galeazzi, G., Forghieri, M., Tsopelas, C., Simpson, A., et al. (2005). Disruptive and dangerous behavior by patients on acute psychiatric wards in three European centers. *Social Psychiatry and Psychiatric Epidemiology, 40,* 822–828.

Bowers, L., & Park, A. (2001). Special observation in the care of psychiatric patients: Literature review. *Issues in Mental Health Nursing, 22,* 769–786.

Brown, R., Genel, M., & Riggs, J. (2000). American Medical Association Council of Scientific Affairs Position Statement: Use of seclusion and restraint in children and adolescents. *Archives of Pediatric Adolescent Medicine, 154,* 653–656.

CEBP (2000). *The protection of the human rights and dignity of people suffering form mental disorder; especially those placed as involuntary patients in a psyhciatric establishment.* Strasbourg: Council of Europe Steering Committee on Bioethics (CEBP) Working Party on Psychiatry.

CRAG (2002). Engaging people: Observation of people with acute mental health problems, Scottish Office, Edinburgh.

Chien, W. T., Chan, C. W. H., Lam, L. W., & Kam, C. W. (2005). Psychiatric inpatients' perceptions of positive and negative aspects of physical restraint. *Patient Education And Counseling, 59,* 80–86.

Cormac, L., Russell, I., & Ferriter, M. (2005). Review of seclusion policies in high secure hospitals and medium secure units in England, Scotland and Wales. *Journal of Psychiatric and Mental Health Nursing, 12,* 380–382.

Coutinho, E. S., Hut, G., Allen, M. H., & Adams, C. E. (2005). Physical restraints for agitated patients in psychiatric emergency hospitals in Rio de Janeiro, Brazil: A predictive model. *Schizophrenia Bulletin, 31,* 220–220.

Crichton, J, and Calgie, J (2002). Responding to Inpatient Violence at a Psychiatric Hospital of Special Security: A Pilot project. *Medicine Science and the Law, 42*(1), 30–33.

Curie, C. G. (2005). Special section on seclusion and restraint: Commentary: SAMHSA's commitment to eliminating the use of seclusion and restraint. *Psychiatric Services, 56,* 1139–1140.

Cusack, K. J., Frueh, B. C., Hiers, T., Suffoletta-Maierle, S., & Bennett, S. (2003). Trauma within the psychiatric setting: A preliminary empirical report. *Administration and Policy in Mental Health, 30,* 453–460.

Daffern, M., Mayer, M. M., & Martin, T. (2003). A preliminary investigation into patterns of aggression in an Australian forensic psychiatric hospital. *Journal of Forensic Psychiatry and Psychology, 14,* 67–84.

Donat, D. C. (2003). An analysis of successful efforts to reduce the use of seclusion and restraint at a public psychiatric hospital. *Psychiatric Services, 54,* 1119–1123.

D'Orio, B. M., Purselle, D., Stevens, D., & Garlow, S. J. (2004). Reduction of episodes of seclusion and restraint in a psychiatric emergency-service. *Psychiatric Services, 55,* 581–583.

Duxbury, J. (2002). An evaluation of staff and patient views of an strategies employed to manage inpatient aggression and violence on one mental health unit: A pluralistic design. *Journal of Psychiatric and Mental Health Nursing, 9,* 325–337.

Dyer, C. (2003). Unjustified seclusion of psychiatric patients is breach of human rights. *British Medical Journal, 327,* 183–183.

Fisher, J. A. (2003). Curtailing the use of restraint in psychiatric settings. *Journal Of Humanistic Psychology, 43,* 69–95.

Frueh, B. C., Knapp, R. G., Cusack, K. J., Grubaugh, A. L., Sauvegeot, J. A., Cousins, V. C., et al. (2005). Special section on seclusion and restraint: Patient reports of traumatic or harmful experiences within the psychiatric setting. *Psychiatric Services, 56,* 1123–1133.

Goodness, K. R., & Renfro, N. S. (2002). Changing a culture: A brief program analysis of a social learning program on a maximum-security forensic unit. *Behavioral Sciences & The Law, 20*(5), 495–506.

Glover, R. W. (2005). Special section on seclusion and restraint: Commentary: Reducing the use of seclusion and restraint: A NASMHPD priority. *Psychiatric Services, 56,* 1141–1142.

Gudjonsson, G., Rabe-Hesketh, S., & Szmukler, G. (2004). Management of psychiatric in-patient violence: Patient ethnicity and use of medication, restraint, and seclusion. *The British Journal of Psychiatry, 184,* 258–262.

Hoekstra, T., Lendemeijer, H., & Jansen, M. (2004). Seclusion: the inside story. *Journal of Psychiatric & Mental Health Nursing, 11*(3), 276–283.

Hubner-Liebermann, B., Spiessl, H., Iwai, K., & Cording, C. (2005). Treatment of schizophrenia: Implications derived from an intercultural hospital comparison between Germany and Japan. *The International Journal of Social Psychiatry, 51,* 83–96.

Johnson, M. (1998). Being restrained: A study of power and powerlessness. *Issues in Mental Health Nursing, 19,* 191–206.

Jonikas, J. A., Cook, J. A., Rosen, C., Laris, A., & Kim, J. B. (2004). A program to reduce use of physical restraint in psychiatric inpatient facilities. *Psychiatric Services, 55,* 818–820.

Kaltiala-Heino, R., Tuohimaki, C., Korkeila, J., & Lehtinen, V. (2003). Reasons for using seclusion and restraint in psychiatric inpatient care. *International Journal Of Law And Psychiatry, 26,* 139–149.

Khadivi, A. N., Patel, R. C., Atkinson, A. R., & Levine, J. M. (2004). Association between seclusion and restraint and patient-related violence. *Psychiatric Services, 55,* 1311–1312.

Kiss It (2006). "Protest against the inhumanity of psychiatric assault: Have a heart." Retrieved 6/2/06, from http://www.kissit.org/.

Leadbetter, D., Paterson, B., & Crichton, J. (2005). From moral panic to moral action: Social policy, violence and physical interventions in human services. *International Conference on High Risk Interventions.* New York: Cornell University.

Leather, P., Brady, C., Lawrence, C., Beale, D., & Cox, T. (Eds.). (1999). *Work-related Violence. Assessment and Intervention.* London: Routledge.

LeBel, J., & Goldstein, R. (2005). Special section on seclusion and restraint: The economic cost of using restraint and the value added by restraint reduction or elimination. *Psychiatric Services, 56,* 1109–1114.

Lee, S., Gray, R., Gournay, K., Wright, S., Parr, A.-M., & Sayer, J. (2003). Views of nursing staff on the use of physical restraint. *Journal of Psychiatric and Mental Health Nursing, 10,* 425–430.

Leggett, J., & Silvester, J. (2003). Care staff attributions for violent incidents involving male and female patients: A field study. *The British Journal Of Clinical Psychology, 42,* 393–406.

Lessing, E. E., & Beech, R. P. (2004). Use of patient and hospital variables in interpreting patient satisfaction data for performance improvement purposes. *The American Journal of Orthopsychiatry, 74,* 376–382.

Lind, M., Kaltiala-Heino, R., Suominen, T., Leino-Kilpi, H., & Valimaki, M. (2004). Nurses' ethical perceptions about coercion. *Journal of Psychiatric and Mental Health Nursing, 11,* 379–385.

Mackay, I., Paterson, B., & Cassells, C. (2005). Constant or special observations of inpatients presenting a risk of aggression or violence: Nurses' perceptions of the rules of engagement. *Journal of Psychiatric and Mental Health Nursing, 12,* 464–471.

Meehan, T., Bergen, H., & Fjeldsoe, K. (2004). Staff and patient perceptions of seclusion: Has anything changed? *Journal of Advanced Nursing, 47,* 33–38.

Moore, P., Berman, K., Knight, M., & Devine, J. (1995). Constant observation: Implications for nursing practice. *Journal of Psychosocial Nursing, 33,* 46–50.

Morrison, L., Duryea, P., & Moore, C. (2001). The lethal hazard of prone restraint. Oakland, California: Protection and Advocacy Inc. Investigations Unit.

Nakajima, M., Terao, T., & Nakamura, J. (2003). Characteristics of repeatedly secluded elderly female schizophrenic inpatients. *Progress in Neuro-Psychopharmacology and Biological Psychiatry, 27,* 771–774.

Needham, I. (2004). *A nursing intervention to handle patient aggression: The effectiveness of a training course in the management of aggression,* Maastricht. PhD thesis.

Neilson, O., & Brennan, W. (2001). The use of special observations: An audit within a psychiatric unit. *Journal of Psychiatric and Mental Health Nursing, 8,* 147–155.

NICE (2005). *Clinical Practice Guidelines for the violence: The short term management of disturbed/ violent behavior in psychiatric in-patient settings and emergency departments.* National Institute for Clinical Excellence, London, England.

Nijman, H., Palmstierna, T., Almvik, R., & Stolker, J. (2005). Fifteen years of research with the Staff Observation Aggression Scale: A review. *Acta Psychiatrica Scandinavica, 111,* 12–21.

Niveau, G. (2004). Preventing human rights abuses in psychiatric establishments: The work of the CPT. *European Psychiatry, 19,* 146–154.

NoForceUK (2006). "What is coercion?" Retrieved 18/7/06, from http://quicksitebuilder.cnet.com/ insight/noforceuk/id8.html

O'Brien, A., & Golding, C. E. A. (2003). Coercion in mental healthcare: The principle of least coercive care. *Journal of Psychiatric and Mental Health Nursing, 10,* 167–173.

Odawara, T., Narita, H., Yamada, Y., Fujita, J., Yamada, T., & Hirayasu, Y. (2005). Use of restraint in a general hospital psychiatric unit in Japan. *Psychiatry And Clinical Neurosciences, 59,* 605–609.

Olsen, D. (1998). Toward an ethical standard for coerced mental health treatment: Least restrictive or most therapeutic. *The Journal of Clinical Ethics, 9,* 235–245.

Olsen, D. (2003). Influence and coercion: Relational and rights-based ethical approaches to forced psychiatric treatment. *Journal of Psychiatric and Mental Health Nursing, 10,* 705–712.

Paterson, B. (2005). Thinking the unthinkable: A role for pain compliance and mechanical restraint in the management of violence. *Mental Health Practice, 8,* 18–23.

Paterson, B., Bradley, P., Stark, C., Saddler, D., Leadbetter, D., & Allen, D. (2003). Deaths associated with restraint use in health and social care in the UK: The results of a preliminary survey. *Journal of Psychiatric and Mental Health Nursing, 10,* 3–16.

Paterson, B., & Leadbetter, D. (1998). Restraint and sudden death from asphyxia. *Nursing Times 94,* 62–64.

Riley, D., Meehan, C., Whittington, R., Lancaster, G., & Lane, S. (2006). Patient restraint positions in a psychiatric inpatient service. *Nursing Times, 102,* 42–45.

Robins, C. S., Sauvageot, J. A., Cusack, K. J., Suffoletta-Maierle, S., & Frueh, B. C. (2005). Special section on seclusion and restraint: Consumers' perceptions of negative experiences and "sanctuary harm" in psychiatric settings. *Psychiatric Services, 56,* 1134–1138.

Ryan, C., & Bowers, L. (2005). Coercive maneuvers in a psychiatric intensive care unit. *Journal of Psychiatric and Mental Health Nursing, 12,* 695–702.

Sailas, E., & Fenton, M. (2002). Seclusion and restraint for people with serious mental illnesses (Cochrane Review). *The Cochrane Library,* Issue 1, 2002. Oxford: Update Software.

Sailas, E., & Wahlbeck, K. (2005). Restraint and seclusion in psychiatric inpatient wards. *Current Opinion In Psychiatry, 18,* 555–559.

Smith, G. M., Davis, R. H., Bixler, E. O., Lin, H. M., Altenor, A., Altenor, R. J., et al. (2005). Special section on seclusion and restraint: Pennsylvania state hospital system's seclusion and restraint reduction program. *Psychiatric Services, 56,* 1115–1122.

Sullivan, A. M., Bezmen, J., Barron, C. T., Rivera, J., Curley-Casey, L., & Marino, D. (2005). Reducing restraints: Alternatives to restraints on an inpatient psychiatric service utilizing safe and effective methods to evaluate and treat the violent patient. *The Psychiatric Quarterly, 76,* 51–65.

Tavcar, R., Dernovsek, M. Z., & Grubic, V. N. (2005). Use of coercive measures in a psychiatric intensive care unit in Slovenia. *Psychiatric Services, 56,* 491–492.

Towell, D. (1975). Understanding Psychiatric Nursing. London: Royal College of Nursing, London.

Vittengl, J. R. (2002). Temporal regularities in physical control at a state psychiatric hospital. *Archives of Psychiatric Nursing, 16,* 80–85.

Wright, S. (2003). Control and restraint techniques in the management of violence in inpatient psychiatry: A critical review. *Medicine, Science, and the Law, 43,* 31–38.

Wynn, R. (2004). Psychiatric inpatients' experiences with restraint. *Journal of Forensic Psychiatry and Psychology, 15,* 124–144.

Yonge, O., & Sterwin, L. (1992). What psychiatric nurses say about constant care. *Clinical Nursing Research, 1,* 80–90.

Yung, A. R., & Harris, B. (2003). Management of early psychosis in a generic adult mental health service. *Australian and New Zealand Journal of Psychiatry, 37*(4), 429–436.

Zun, L. S., & Downey, L. (2005). The use of seclusion in emergency medicine. *General Hospital Psychiatry, 27,* 365–371.

9

The Pharmacological Management of Aggression

LAURETTE E. GOEDHARD, JOOST J. STOLKER, EIBERT
R. HEERDINK, HENK L.I. NIJMAN, BEREND OLIVIER,
AND TOINE C.G. EGBERTS

1 INTRODUCTION

The occurrence of aggressive incidents in psychiatric care has a great impact on the well being of staff and patients, and is associated with considerable costs (Cole, 2005; Hunter & Carmel, 1992; Nijman, Bowers, Oud, & Jansen, 2005). Considering the high impact of aggression in mental health care, prevention, and management of aggression should have high priority (Palmer, 1996).

Several treatment approaches to manage aggressive behavior exist, including psychopharmacological and behavioral approaches (Morrison, 2003). Observational research has shown that aggressive patients more often use psychotropics compared to nonaggressive patients (Soliman & Reza, 2001; Stolker, 2002). Because in animal and human models of aggression, several neurotransmitters appeared to be implicated in the modulation of aggressive behavior (Miczek, Fish, De Bold, & De Almeida, 2002), it is not surprising that a broad range of psychotropics has been investigated for their antiaggressive properties. However, despite the high prevalence of psychotropic drug use in aggressive patients, evidence for the efficacy of the pharmacological management of aggressive behavior is currently lacking. Lack of evidence is reflected by the existence of a variety of guidelines for the emergency management of aggression, and was stressed in two recent systematic reviews for the maintenance of the pharmacotherapy of aggression dating from 1996 to 1997 (Fava, 1997; Pabis & Stanislav, 1996).

In this chapter, a brief overview of the neurotransmitters targeted by psychotropics, based upon the neurobiology of aggression, will be presented. Subsequently, an overview will be given of published randomized controlled trials (RCTs) addressing the pharmacotherapy of aggression in general adult psychiatry. Finally, guidelines for pharmacotherapy in the management of aggressive behavior and recommendations for the conduct of future research will be proposed.

2 PSYCHOPHARACOTHERAPY FOR AGGRESSION: NEUROTRANSMITTERS TARGETED

The role of neurotransmitters in the modulation of aggressive behavior has been a subject of many studies in both animals and humans in the last few decades. Results indicate that serotonin, GABA and dopamine play a key role in the modulation and pathology of aggressive behavior (Miczek et al., 2002).

Serotonin has been investigated most extensively. This neurotransmitter can interact with 14 different serotonergic receptors and the regulation of its activity also uses a very efficient 5-HT transporter system (Olivier, 2004). Psychotropics acting on various aspects of the serotonin system include the serotonergic antidepressants (SSRIs), the atypical antipsychotics, and the 5-HT_{1A} receptor agonist buspirone. Although the 5-HT_{1A} and 5-HT_{1B} receptors are postulated as potential important modulators of aggression (Olivier), several other serotonergic receptors can still play an important role.

Drugs acting on $GABA_A$ receptors may have aggression heightening but also aggression suppressing effects, which are likely to be determined by the specific subunit of the $GABA_A$ benzodiazepine receptor complex on which the drugs are acting (Miczek et al., 2002). Furthermore, inhibition or disinhibition appears to be dose related. In laboratory settings benzodiazepines in low doses increase aggressive behavior, whereas high doses cause sedation (Miczek et al.). Besides benzodiazepines, some anticonvulsants are also acting through the GABA-ergic system.

Aggression modulation through the dopaminergic system is likely to be mediated through the D_2 receptor family. The typical antipsychotics, and to a lesser extent the atypical antipsychotics, are the drugs targeting the dopamine D_2 receptors.

3 RANDOMIZED CONTROLLED TRIALS ADDRESSING THE PHARMACOTHERAPY OF AGGRESSION

3.1 Study Selection

As previously stated, the aim of this chapter is to review the available evidence for the pharmacotherapy of aggression. For this review, only published randomized controlled trials (RCTs) are considered, as these are seen as the gold standard for obtaining evidence for drug effects (Starfield, 1998). For the RCTs included, an acceptable methodological quality was required, which was defined by a Jadad score of three or more (Jadad et al., 1996). The Jadad scale is an instrument to adjudicate methodological quality. Criteria used for this instrument comprises the quality of randomization, the quality of blinding, and a description of dropouts and withdrawals.

There are different theoretical concepts of aggression. Symptoms associated with aggression include hostility, agitation, violence, and anger (Baumeister, Smart, & Boden, 1996; Lindenmayer, 2000; McNiel & Binder, 1994; Troisi, Kustermann, Di Genio, & Siracusano, 2003). Because these symptoms are closely related to aggression, it is assumed that influencing them will also have an impact on any aggressive behavior displayed. Therefore, we included all RCTs that also assessed the pharmacological management of those symptoms.

Trials assessing the pharmacotherapy for the management of aggression have been conducted in different psychiatric and nonpsychiatric settings. Given the heterogeneity of these populations, it seems likely that study results might not be directly comparable to each other. Therefore, this review is restricted to general adult psychiatry, meaning that studies conducted in nonpsychiatric settings and specialized psychiatric settings, i.e., organic brain diseases and mental retardation, were not included, as were studies that evaluated only children or elderly patients.

3.2 Pharmacotherapy in an Acute Situation vs. Maintenance Pharmacotherapy

Pharmacotherapy of aggression in an acute situation and maintenance pharmacotherapy of aggression will be addressed separately. This distinction is useful, as the aim of pharmacotherapy in the two situations is different. In the acute situation, drugs are administered to stop a dangerous situation by sedation or motor interference such as muscle weakness. However, for maintenance therapy, i.e., pharmacotherapy for patients to whom aggression is an ongoing problem, long-term sedation might be considered an undesired effect as it hampers adequate psychiatric examination, as well as the therapeutic patient relationship. Furthermore, habituation to sedation is likely to occur. Therefore, for pharmacotherapy in the case of aggressive behavior as an ongoing problem, drugs with other antiaggressive properties are used. Ideally such drugs act on neurotransmitter pathways specifically implicated in the modulation of aggression.

3.2.1 Management of Aggressive Behavior in an Acute Situation

From previous studies it is known that most aggressive incidents in mental health care occur during the first days of admission (Binder & McNiel, 1990; Davis, 1991). Therefore, most available trials addressing the pharmacological management of acutely aggressive patients have been conducted at acute admission wards and psychiatric emergency departments. Most trials used the "rapid tranquillization strategy" in which antipsychotics or benzodiazepines are administered in a compressed time-frame, titrating dosage against symptoms to control assaultive, hyperactive, and hostile patients (Menuck & Voineskos, 1981). Ideally, the goal of this strategy is to calm down disturbed patients to such an extent that communication is possible, thereby enabling health workers to evaluate the psychiatric status. In some cases, putting a patient to sleep can also be an appropriate goal (Battaglia, Lindborg, Alaka, Meehan, & Wright, 2003; TREC Collaborative Group, 2003).

The studies evaluated are represented in Figure 1 (Alexander et al., 2004; Battaglia et al., 1997; Bieniek, Ownby, Penalver, & Dominguez, 1998; Breier et al., 2002; Chin et al., 1998; Chouinard, Annable, Turnier, Holobow, & Szkrumelak, 1993; Chouinard, Safadi, & Beauclair, 1994; Currier et al., 2004; Dorevitch, Katz, Zemishlany, Aizenberg, & Weizman, 1999; Fruensgaard, Korsgaard, Jorgensen, & Jensen, 1977; Kinon, Ahl, Rotelli, & McMullen, 2004; van Leeuwen et al., 1977; Meehan et al., 2001; Reschke, 1974; Resnick & Burton, 1984; Stotsky, 1977; Taymeeyapradit & Kuasirikul, 2002; TREC Collaborative Group, 2003; Wright et al., 2001). The study population predominantly comprised schizophrenic patients experiencing an acute exacerbation. Other diagnoses included mania and substance abuse. However, in most of the trials, substance abuse was an exclusion criterion. Another frequently established "diagnosis" was acute agitation.

Outcome measures most frequently used to assess changes in aggressive behavior included subscales of the BPRS (Overall & Gorham, 1962) and the PANNS (Kay, Fiszbein, & Opler, 1987). Other outcome measures include sedation-scales and additional number of injections needed to calm the patient down.

Pharmacological agents used in the evaluated RCTs comprised antipsychotic agents, benzodiazepines, combination therapy of benzodiazepines and antipsychotics, and promethazine. In most studies, drugs were administered parenterally; one study also assessed the efficacy of oral doses (Breier et al., 2002).

Typical Antipsychotics. Typical antipsychotics can be classified into high-potency and low-potency antipsychotics (Schwartz & Brotman, 1992). Low-potency antipsychotics, like chlorpromazine, are historically used for the management of acute agitation and aggression. However, because low-potency antipsychotics are more likely to inflict serious adverse events, e.g., excessive sedation and hypotension, compared to high-potency antipsychotics, preference is given to the latter (Buckley, 1999; Man & Chen, 1973; Reschke, 1974).

Haloperidol, a high-potency antipsychotic, is the most frequently used drug in the evaluated RCTs. In one of the first placebo-controlled trials in this field, conducted in 1974, haloperidol in doses of 1, 2, and 5 mg was compared to chlorpromazine and placebo (Reschke, 1974). Benefit for haloperidol in dosages of 2 and 5 mg over placebo and chlorpromazine was reported. Other typical antipsychotics investigated included droperidol, thiotixene, loxapine, and zuclopenthixol (Chin et al., 1998; Chouinard et al., 1994; Fruensgaard et al., 1977; Resnick & Burton, 1984; Stotsky, 1977; Taymeeyapradit & Kuasirikul, 2002). These antipsychotics were compared to haloperidol. Droperidol was also compared to the placebo (van Leeuwen et al., 1977). The observed differences in efficacy between the different typical antipsychotics predominantly rest on differences in pharmacokinetic properties of the

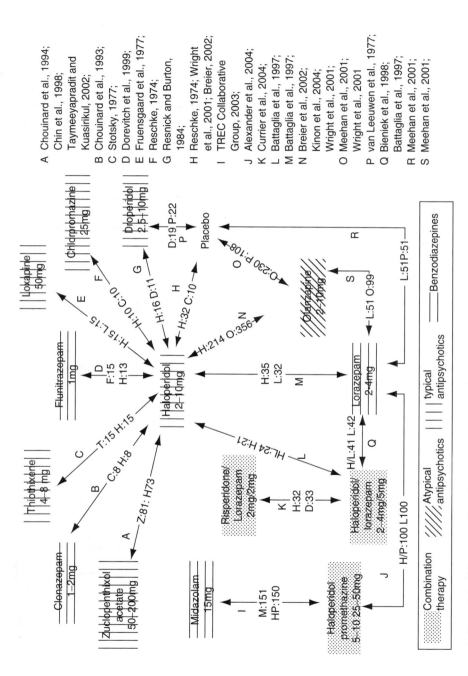

Figure 1. Drugs joined by arrows have been compared to each other (in one or more studies); numbers along the arrows indicate the total number of study participants in each treatment arm of the RCT(s). Dosages per administration are indicated under the drug name.

different drugs. Droperidol induced a quicker onset of action than haloperidol (Resnick & Burton); these results were approved by two randomized controlled trials conducted in emergency departments (Richards, Derlet, & Duncan, 1998; Thomas, Schwartz, & Petrilli, 1992). These studies were not included in Figure 2, because they were not conducted in a study population consisting solely of psychiatric patients. The advantage of using zuclopenthixol over haloperidol was that, over a period of seven days, fewer injections were required to obtain the same effect, as zuclopenthixol acts as a short-acting depot (Taymeeyapradit & Kuasirikul). However, more extrapyramidal symptoms and sedation were reported for zuclopenthixol compared to haloperidol.

Benzodiazepines. Because of their anxiolytic and sedative properties, benzodiazepines are extremely suitable to tranquillize aggressive patients, especially when the underlying psychiatric disorder is a substance-induced psychosis.

The benzodiazepines studied in the RCTs retrieved comprised lorazepam (Alexander et al., 2004; Battaglia et al., 1997; Bieniek et al., 1998; Meehan et al., 2001), flunitrazepam (Dorevitch et al., 1999), and clonazepam (Chouinard et al., 1993). The short-acting lorazepam is the most extensively studied benzodiazepine. Lorazepam has been compared to haloperidol (Battaglia et al.; Bieniek et al.), placebo and olanzapine (Alexander et al.), and combination therapy of haloperidol and promethazine (Alexander et al.). No significant differences between haloperidol and lorazepam were observed in the trials. However, combination therapy of haloperidol and lorazepam was superior over monotherapy of haloperidol or lorazepam in that the onset of action was more rapid (Battaglia et al.; Bieniek et al.). Furthermore, heavier sedation was reached with combination therapy when

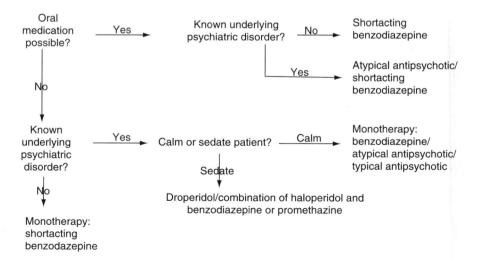

Figure 2. Advised strategy for pharmacotherapy in an acute situation.

compared to monotherapy. Other benzodiazepines in the evaluated studies were midazolam and clonazepam. Midazolam was found to be more rapid a sedative than the combination of haloperidol and promethazine (TREC Collaborative Group, 2003). No difference in agitation scores was observed between haloperidol and clonazepam (Chouinard et al.).

Atypical Antipsychotics. At the beginning of the 1990s risperidone, the second atypical antipsychotic in the market after clozapine, was introduced, followed by olanzapine, quetiapine, ziprasidone, and aripiprazole. Recently, intramuscular forms of the atypical antipsychotics olanzapine and ziprasidone and an oral concentrate of risperidone became available. We will not discuss ziprasidone, because in Europe at the moment this drug is only registered for use in clinical trials, due to its association with cardiac side-effects. Whereas the calming and sedating effect of typical antipsychotics is principally mediated through dopaminergic mechanisms, the sedating and calming effect of olanzapine is likely to be mediated through histaminergic mechanisms (Collaborative Working Group on Clinical Trial Evaluations 1998; Richelson & Souder, 2000).

Olanzapine, after both oral and intramuscular administration, was at least as effective as haloperidol in a population of mildly agitated patients (Breier et al., 2002; Kinon et al., 2004; Wright et al., 2001). An advantage of the use of olanzapine over haloperidol was the decreased risk of extra-pyramidal symptoms in the case of olanzapine (Wright et al.). Oral risperidone combined with lorazepam has been compared to intramuscular administration of haloperidol and lorazepam (Currier et al., 2004). For both treatments a similar effect was reached, with a shorter time of onset for the intramuscular therapy. The observed difference in onset time was about 20 minutes. In accordance with the Dubin, Waxman, Weiss, Ramchandani, and Tavani-Petrone study (1985), in which oral administration of haloperidol and thioridazine were compared to intramuscular administration, patients randomized on oral therapy did not refuse the oral medication. These study results suggest that in certain circumstances, probably in the case of mild aggressive behavior, oral therapy can be a good alternative to parenteral tranquillization.

3.2.2 Maintenance Pharmacotherapy of Aggressive Behavior

For a detailed review of the maintenance pharmacotherapy of aggression we refer to Goedhard et al. (2006). We identified 31 RCTs that assessed the use of medication as maintenance therapy for the management of aggression (Allan et al., 1996; Alpert et al., 1990; Blin, Azorin, & Bouhours, 1996; Caspi et al., 2001; Citrome et al., 2001, 2004; Coccaro & Kavoussi, 1997; Davidson, Landerman, Farfel, & Clary, 2002; Davidson, McLeod, Turnbull, & Miller, 1981; Dorrego, Canevaro, Kuzis, Sabe, & Starkstein, 2002; Frankenburg & Zanarini, 2002; de la Fuente & Lotstra, 1994; Hollander et al., 2001, 2003; van der Kolk et al., 1994; Lipman et al., 1986; Maoz et al., 2000; Marder, Davis, & Chouinard, 1997; McDougle et al., 1996; Min, Rhee, Kim, & Kang, 1993; Monnelly, Ciraulo, Knapp, & Keane, 2003; Nickel et al., 2005; Peuskens, 1995; Ratey et al., 1992; Rinne, van den Brink, Wouters, & van Dyck, 2002; Salzman et al., 1995; Soloff et al., 1989, 1993; Vartiainen et al., 1995; Zanarini & Frankenburg, 2001; Zanarini, Frankenburg, & Parachini, 2004). Most studies were conducted in a schizophrenic population (Allan et al.; Alpert et al.; Blin et al.; Caspi et al.; Citrome et al., 2001, 2004; Maoz et al.; Marder et al.; Min et al.; Peuskens; Ratey et al.; Vartiainen et al.) or in cluster B personality disordered patients (Coccaro & Kavoussi; Frankenburg & Zanarini; de la Fuente & Lotstra; Hollander et al., 2001, 2003; Nickel et al.; Rinne et al.; Salzman et al.; Soloff et al., 1989, 1993; Zanarini & Frankenburg; Zanarini et al.). Other diagnoses included PTSD (Davidson et al., 2002; Monnelly et al.), autistic disorder (McDougle et al.), intermittent explosive disorder (Mattes, 1990), ADHD (Dorrego et al.), anorexia nervosa (Fassino et al., 2002), and depressive disorder (Davidson et al., 1981; Fava et al., 1997; Lipman et al.).

A whole range of different outcome measures—21 in total—have been used in the RCTs included and involved observational as well as self-report scales. Furthermore, some scales were especially constructed for measuring aggression, while others were subscales measuring items related to aggression in a broader perspective, for example the anger scale of the Profile of Mood State (McNair, Lorr, & Doppleman, 1981). The use of different outcome scales hampered the assessment of efficacy across these studies. The most frequently used specific aggression scales were different versions of the Overt Aggression Scale (OAS) (Yudofsky, Silver, Jackson, Endicott, & Williams, 1986). As most studies were conducted in an outpatient setting, the "OAS-Modified for outpatients" was used more often. Other outcome measures included diagnosis-related scales, like subscales of the PANNS (Kay et al., 1987) and SCL-90 (Lipman, Covi, & Shapiro, 1979).

Antipsychotic Agents. When patients with schizophrenia are treated with antipsychotics, a reduction in aggressive behavior is found (Steinert, Sippach, & Gebhardt, 2000). This effect of antipsychotics might be due to the treatment of the acute illness, as other studies have shown that patients with unstable mental illness are at increased risk of displaying aggressive behavior (McNiel, Binder, & Greenfield, 1988). However, theoretically, antipsychotic agents might also be effective in reducing aggressive behavior independently from the effect on psychosis, as both typical and atypical antipsychotics act on dopaminergic mechanisms and the atypical antipsychotics additionally on the serotonergic receptors.

Nine RCTs investigating antipsychotics (Blin et al., 1996; Citrome et al., 2001; Marder et al., 1997; Min et al., 1993; Monnelly et al., 2003; Peuskens, 1995; Soloff et al., 1989, 1993; Zanarini & Frankenburg, 2001) were retrieved and evaluated. In two of the three RCTs comparing haloperidol to placebo (Marder et al.; Soloff et al., 1989, 1993), haloperidol was superior over the placebo in reducing hostility (Soloff et al., 1989, 1993). These two studies were conducted in a borderline personality disordered outpatient population. However, the follow-up period was relatively short, lasting only five weeks. Seven studies compared the efficacy of atypical antipsychotics in reducing aggressive behavior to typical antipsychotics or a placebo in schizophrenic patients, female borderline outpatients, and posttraumatic-stress disordered patients (Blin et al.; Citrome et al.; Marder et al.; Min et al.; Monnelly et al.; Peuskens; Zanarini & Frankenburg). Study results indicate that atypical antipsychotics are superior to typical antipsychotics in reducing aggressive behavior. One study showed that clozapine was significantly superior over haloperidol, risperidone, and olanzapine in a schizophrenic population resistant to previous neuroleptic treatment (Citrome et al.). The antiaggressive mechanism of clozapine in this study appeared unrelated to the overall psychopathological improvement.

Antidepressants. At the beginning of the 1990s antidepressants were suspected of having paradoxical effects, in that they might enhance aggressive behavior (Heiligenstein, Beasley, & Potvin, 1993). Heilligenstein and colleagues conducted a metaanalytic study on fluoxetine to investigate this (Heiligenstein et al.). In their metaanalysis, fluoxetine did not increase aggressive behavior. In contrast to prior findings, results from this study indicated that antidepressants decrease aggressive behavior. Furthermore, neurobiological studies indicated the importance of serotonin in the modulation of aggressive behavior. Consequently, in the last decade, serotonergic antidepressants have been investigated for their antiaggressive properties.

With reference to the general adult psychiatric population we found one RCT comparing imipramine to phenelzine (Davidson et al., 1981) and ten RCT's comparing antidepressants to a placebo (Coccaro & Kavoussi, 1997; Davidson et al., 2002; Lipman et al., 1986; McDougle et al., 1996; Rinne et al., 2002; Salzman et al., 1995; Soloff et al., 1993; Soloff et al., 1989; van der Kolk et al., 1994; Vartiainen et al., 1995). In the study comparing imipramine to phenelzine, superiority of imipramine was observed (Davidson et al., 1981). Antidepressants which were found to be superior over a placebo included fluoxetine, fluvoxamine, sertraline, and citalopram (Coccaro & Kavoussi; Davidson et al.; McDougle et al.; Soloff et al., 1989; Vartiainen et al.). These RCTs have been conducted with different study populations, namely autism, post traumatic stress disorder, schizophrenia, and cluster B personality disorder. The total study follow-up of these five studies with positive results was 12 or 13 weeks. In five other studies, no benefit was found for antidepressants over a placebo. However, in four of the five studies the follow-up period ranged from five to eight weeks, which may, as a follow-up period, be too short. Furthermore, in some of the studies not showing the benefit of antidepressants, baseline aggression levels were low and thus only a small reduction in aggressive behavior can be achieved using pharmacotherapy.

On the basis of the RCTs evaluated it can be concluded that there is some evidence that serotonergic antidepressants are effective in reducing aggressive behavior in several psychiatric diseases.

Betaadrenergic Blockers. Betaadrenergic blockers have been shown to be effective in decreasing aggression in organic brain diseases (Fava, 1997). The mechanism by which betaadrenergic blocking drugs might reduce aggression is not fully understood, as both betaadrenergic blockers passing the blood–brain-barrier, and betaadrenergic blockers hardly passing the blood–brain-barrier, were found effective.

For the general adult psychiatric population, we found five studies, all of which have been conducted in a schizophrenic population (Allan et al., 1996; Alpert et al.,

1990; Caspi et al., 2001; Maoz et al., 2000; Ratey et al., 1992). In three studies, a benefit from the use of nadolol and propranolol was reported (Caspi et al.; Ratey et al.). The study population in two of those studies comprised chronic schizophrenic patients, while in the other two studies that did not show positive results in favor of the betaadrenergic blockers, the study population comprised schizophrenic patients experiencing an acute exacerbation. Acute psychiatric illness is associated with aggression. Since, in most acutely ill patients, aggression will not remain an ongoing problem after the stabilization of their illness, we think that the antiaggressive effects of drugs is difficult to demonstrate in such RCTs, as aggressive behavior is likely to decrease in the active treatment group and also in the placebo group.

Overall, it may be concluded that betaadrenergic blockers can be useful in reducing aggressive behavior in schizophrenic patients. However, it is unclear whether these benefits outweigh the observed adverse events like syncope and bronchospasm, which were observed in the RCTs evaluated.

Anticonvulsants. Anticonvulsants are frequently used in the management of aggressive behavior (Citrome, 1995). A possible rationale for this is the association of aggression and EEG abnormalities or seizures (Monroe, 1989; Stone, McDaniel, Hughes, & Hermann, 1986). Furthermore some anticonvulsants, including valproate and topiramate, have GABA-ergic properties.

We found six RCTs that assessed the efficacy of anticonvulsants in reducing aggressive behavior (Citrome et al., 2004; de la Fuente and Lotstra, 1994; Frankenburg and Zanarini, 2002; Hollander et al., 2001, 2003; Nickel et al., 2005). Studied anticonvulsants comprised valproate sodium, carbamazepine, and topiramate.

One of these studies was conducted in schizophrenic patients with an acute exacerbation (Citrome et al., 2004). The other five studies were conducted in borderline personality disordered (out)patients. In three of these five studies, anticonvulsants were superior over placebo (Frankenburg & Zanarini, 2002; Hollander et al., 2003; Nickel et al., 2005). In the three studies not favoring anticonvulsants over a placebo, either the sample-size was small or the population consisted of patients with an acute exacerbation of mental illness, a population in which it is difficult to investigate the effect of maintenance therapy as mentioned in the previous paragraph.

Overall, based upon these six trials, we conclude that anticonvulsants can be effective in reducing aggressive behavior in cluster B personality disordered outpatients. No serious adverse events were observed or mentioned in the different studies.

Others. Besides trials comparing an active drug to placebo, or another active drug of the same class, we found three trials comparing two different types of drugs. Zanarini, Frankenburg, & Parachini (2004) compared the combination of olanzapine and fluoxetine vs. monotherapy in a study population of female borderline outpatients. Combination therapy and monotherapy of olanzapine were superior to fluoxetine monotherapy in reducing impulsive aggressive behavior. Furthermore,imipramine was found to be superior over chlordiazepoxide in a population consisting of depressed and anxious outpatients (Lipman et al., 1986). In a randomized crossover trial no differences were observed between lithium and methylphenidate in reducing aggressive behavior (Dorrego et al., 2002).

3.2.3 Limitations of the Evaluated RCTs

Although RCTs are considered a gold standard for testing the efficacy of medical interventions (Starfield, 1998), they also have limitations. The main methodological issues that were encountered in this review concerned the generalizability to daily clinical practice and a low statistical power for detecting differences in efficacy between the treatment groups.

Poor generalizability from clinical trial populations to patients seen in daily practice is one of the limitations particularly associated with RCTs (Dieppe, Bartlett, Davey, Doyal, & Ebrahim, 2004). Previous studies have shown that psychiatric patients with comorbid disorders are frequently excluded from RCTs (March et al., 2005; Heerdink, Stolker, Meijer, Hugenholtz, & Egberts, 2004; Zarin, Young, & West, 2005). There are indications that the aggressive patient, as seen in daily clinical practice, was excluded from the RCTs evaluated in this review. Firstly, recruitment procedures that depend on voluntary participation (Edlund, Craig, & Richardson, 1985) are likely to result in the exclusion of highly aggressive patients. Indeed, aggression at baseline was frequently low. Also, the application of strict study inclusion and exclusion criteria is likely to result in the exclusion of aggressive patients. For example, patients with substance abuse, which is associated with aggression, were frequently excluded from the RCTs we analyzed (Steadman et al., 2000). Concomitant use of psychotropics was also frequently used as an exclusion criterion.

The statistical power for detecting differences between treatment groups was usually small, due to the small number of patients included in the trials, as can also be seen in Figure 1. Besides reducing the ability to detect treatment efficacy, studies with small sample sizes will also have a limited value in detecting adverse effects. Furthermore, the baseline aggression level was frequently low. As a consequence, only a small reduction of aggressive behavior can be achieved using pharmacotherapy and, to detect small changes, large sample sizes are required.

Additional limitations of the evaluated RCTs addressing the maintenance pharmacotherapy of aggressive behavior were short follow-up times, and the use of numerous outcome scales. The latter issue hampered the assessment of efficacy across studies.

3.2.4 Advised Pharmacological Approach of Acutely Aggressive Patients

Taking into account the limitations of the evaluated studies, a pharmacological treatment strategy as depicted in Figure 2 is proposed. As different studies suggest that the difference between oral and parenteral medication is not the effect reached, but the shorter time of onset when using parenteral administration, oral therapy should be considered first. If the patient is unwilling to accept oral medication, or if a short time of onset is desired, intramuscular medication is the therapy of choice. One should choose between the administration of antipsychotics, atypical or typical, benzodiazepines, or a combination therapy of typical antipsychotics and benzodiazepines or promethazine. The choice between these agents depends on the objective of the pharmacotherapy, i.e., very quick vs. quick response, sedative vs. calming effect, as well as the characteristics of the individual patient, for instance the underlying psychiatric disorder and the risk of adverse events.

If the underlying psychiatric disorder is unknown, the use of benzodiazepines seems to be the safest option as benzodiazepines interfere less with the diagnostic process, e.g., differentiation between substance-induced psychosis and chronic psychosis. However, sometimes monotherapy with benzodiazepines might be insufficient. In those cases, combination therapy of benzodiazepines or promethazine with antipsychotics could be used (see also Figure 2). If the underlying psychiatric disorder is known, the following strategy is advised. If the reduction of aggressive behavior has to be reached as soon as possible and if there are no somatic contraindications, one could opt for the administration of droperidol.

There are some concerns regarding the association between droperidol and cardiac adverse events—fatal QTc prolongations. However, reports are inconsistent. Based upon postmarketing case reports the USA's Food and Drug Administration (FDA) added a "black box" warning to the use of droperidol, which means that prescribers should consider alternative medication for patients at high risk for cardiac arrhythmias (USA Food and Drug Administration, 2001). In contrast, three reviews showed that there is no clear evidence about the increased risk of fatal cardiac adverse events (Chase & Biros, 2002; Kao, Kirk, Evers, & Rosenfeld, 2003; Shale, Shale, & Mastin, 2004).

A second choice of treatment, when reduction of aggressive behavior is urgently needed, is the use of combination therapy of a typical antipsychotic and a benzodiazepine. Because haloperidol and lorazepam have been most extensively studied, we recommend the combined use of these. If the goal of therapy is of calming the patient rather than sedating or getting them to sleep, one could opt for monotherapy of an antipsychotic agent—typical or atypical—or a benzodiazepine. The lower incidence of extrapyramidal adverse events in atypical antipsychotics compared to typical antipsychotics might favor the choice of atypical antipsychotics. However, if the choice of therapy in the acute situation determines the choice of long-term therapy, as Hugenholtz, Stolker, Heerdink, Nolen, and Leufkens (2003) recently showed, the long-term side-effects associated with the use of antipsychotics should be considered; including, in the case of atypical antipsychotics, the metabolic syndrome (American Diabetes Association, American Psychiatric Association, American Association of Clinical Endicrinologists, and North American Association for the Study of Obesity, 2004), and tardive dyskinesia in the case of typical antipsychotics. Furthermore, eight cases of fatal adverse events have been reported after the use of intramuscular olanzapine in excessive dosages or in a combination with benzodiazepines and/or other antipsychotics (Eli Lilly and Company Limited, 2004).

When choosing benzodiazepines, paradoxical reactions, i.e., disinhibition, can occur (Cole & Kando, 1993). However, this side effect is rare. Other known side-effects include the risk of dependence, withdrawal, and tolerance, as well as respiratory arrest.

3.2.5 Advised Strategy for the Maintenance Therapy of Aggression

As unstable psychiatric illness has been found to be associated with aggression, the maintenance pharmacotherapy of aggressive behavior should focus firstly on the underlying disease. If aggressive behavior is still present after adequate pharma-cotherapy for the underlying psychiatric disorder has been established, a number of different drugs can be administered. As previously mentioned, drugs used for the maintenance therapy of aggression should ideally have a specific antiaggressive pro-file, without adversely affecting nonaggressive behavior. The most likely system through which this effect could be reached is serotonin. At this time, drugs specifi-cally acting on aggressive behavior are not available. Because the evidence of effi-cacy from the evaluated RCTs is incomplete, maintenance therapy of aggressive behavior should be applied with reserve. Furthermore, if maintenance therapy is applied, good monitoring of the effect, i.e., assessment of aggressive behavior at baseline, and during follow-up, is essential. Currently, it is not possible to give a conscious choice for a particular drug in the case of repetitively aggressive behavior. Therefore, we advise to start any treatment with the safest drugs, as previously suggested by Eichelmann and Tardiff (1999).

4 RECOMMENDATIONS FOR FUTURE RESEARCH

This chapter shows that the evidence obtained by RCTs is incomplete. We found that in quite a substantial number of RCTs, statistical power was rather small. Furthermore, generalizability of study results to daily clinical practice is question-able. For future research, we recommend the conduct of large-scale pragmatic trials (Zarin et al., 2005). In addition to these trials, observational study designs should be used to study the effectiveness and safety of drugs used to treat aggressive patients (Heerdink et al., 2004; Stolker, 2002).

REFERENCES

Alexander, J., Tharyan, P., Adams, C., John, T., Mol, C., & Philip, J. (2004). Rapid tranquillisation of violent or agitated patients in a psychiatric emergency setting. Pragmatic randomised trial of intra-muscular lorazepam v. haloperidol plus promethazine. *The British Journal of Psychiatry, 185*, 63–69.

Allan, E. R., Alpert, M., Sison, C. E., Citrome, L., Laury, G., & Berman, I. (1996). Adjunctive nadolol in the treatment of acutely aggressive schizophrenic patients. *The Journal of Clinical Psychiatry, 57*(10), 455–459.

Alpert, M., Allan, E. R., Citrome, L., Laury, G., Sison, C., & Sudilovsky, A. (1990). A double-blind, placebo-controlled study of adjunctive nadolol in the management of violent psychiatric patients. *Psychopharmacology Bulletin, 26*(3), 367–371.

American Diabetes Association, American Psychiatric Association, American Association of Clinical Endicrinologists, & North American Association for the Study of Obesity (2004). Consensus development conference on antipsychotic drugs and obesity and diabetes. *The Journal of Clinical Psychiatry, 65*(2), 267–272.

Battaglia, J., Lindborg, S., Alaka, K., Meehan, K., & Wright, P. (2003). Calming versus sedative effects of intramuscular olanzapine in agitated patients. *The American Journal of Emergency Medicine, 21*(3), 192–198.

Battaglia, J., Moss, S., Rush, J., Kang, J., Mendoza, R., Leedom, L., et al. (1997). Haloperidol, lorazepam, or both for psychotic agitation? A multicenter, prospective, double-blind, emergency department study. *The American Journal of Emergency Medicine, 15*(4), 335–340.

Baumeister, R. F., Smart, L., & Boden, J. M. (1996). Relation of threatened egotism to violence and aggression: The dark side of high self-esteem. *Psychological Review, 103*(1), 5–33.

Bieniek, S. A., Ownby, R. L., Penalver, A., & Dominguez, R. A. (1998). A double-blind study of lorazepam versus the combination of haloperidol and lorazepam in managing agitation. *Pharmacotherapy, 18*(1), 57–62.

Binder, R. L., & McNiel, D. E. (1990). The relationship of gender to violent behavior in acutely disturbed psychiatric patients. *The Journal of Clinical Psychiatry, 51*(3), 110–114.

Blin, O., Azorin, J. M., & Bouhours, P. (1996). Antipsychotic and anxiolytic properties of risperidone, haloperidol, and methotrimeprazine in schizophrenic patients. *Journal of Clinical Psychopharmacology, 16*(1), 38–44.

Breier, A., Meehan, K., Birkett, M., David, S., Ferchland, I., Sutton, V., et al. (2002). A double-blind, placebo-controlled dose-response comparison of intramuscular olanzapine and haloperidol in the treatment of acute agitation in schizophrenia. *Archives of General Psychiatry, 59*(5), 441–448.

Buckley, P. F. (1999). The role of typical and atypical antipsychotic medications in the management of agitation and aggression. *The Journal of Clinical Psychiatry, 60*(Suppl. 10), 52–60.

Caspi, N., Modai, I., Barak, P., Waisbourd, A., Zbarsky, H., Hirschmann, S., et al. (2001). Pindolol augmentation in aggressive schizophrenic patients: A double-blind crossover randomized study. *International Clinical Psychopharmacology, 16*(2), 111–115.

Chase, P. B., & Biros, M. H. (2002). A retrospective review of the use and safety of droperidol in a large, high-risk, inner-city emergency department patient population. *Academic Emergency Medicine, 9*(12), 1402–1410.

Chin, C. N., Hamid, A. R., Philip, G., Ramlee, T., Mahmud, M., Zulkifli, G., et al. (1998). A double blind comparison of zuclopenthixol acetate with haloperidol in the management of acutely disturbed schizophrenics. *The Medical Journal of Malaysia, 53*(4), 365–371.

Chouinard, G., Annable, L., Turnier, L., Holobow, N., & Szkrumelak, N. (1993). A double-blind randomized clinical trial of rapid tranquilization with I. M. clonazepam and I. M. haloperidol in agitated psychotic patients with manic symptoms. *Canadian Journal of Psychiatry, 38*(Suppl. 4), S114–S121.

Chouinard, G., Safadi, G., & Beauclair, L. (1994). A double-blind controlled study of intramuscular zuclopenthixol acetate and liquid oral haloperidol in the treatment of schizophrenic patients with acute exacerbation. *The Journal of Clinical Psychopharmacology, 14*(6), 377–384.

Citrome, L. (1995). Use of lithium, carbamazepine, and valproic acid in a state-operated psychiatric hospital. *The Journal of Pharmacy Technology, 11*(2), 55–59.

Citrome, L., Casey, D. E., Daniel, D. G., Wozniak, P., Kochan, L. D., & Tracy, K. A. (2004). Adjunctive divalproex and hostility among patients with schizophrenia receiving olanzapine or risperidone. *Psychiatric Services, 55*(3), 290–294.

Citrome, L., Volavka, J., Czobor, P., Sheitman, B., Lindenmayer, J. P., McEvoy, J., et al. (2001). Effects of clozapine, olanzapine, risperidone, and haloperidol on hostility among patients with schizophrenia. *Psychiatric Services, 52*(11), 1510–1514.

Coccaro, E. F., & Kavoussi, R. J. (1997). Fluoxetine and impulsive aggressive behavior in personality-disordered subjects. *Archives of General Psychiatry, 54*(12), 1081–1088.

Cole, A. (2005). Four in five nurses on mental wards face violence. *British Medical Journal, 330*(7502), 1227.

Cole, J. O., & Kando, J. C. (1993). Adverse behavioral events reported in patients taking alprazolam and other benzodiazepines. *The Journal of Clinical Psychiatry, 54*(Suppl. 49–61), 62–63.

Collaborative Working Group on Clinical Trial Evaluations (1998). Measuring outcome in schizophrenia: Differences among the atypical antipsychotics. *The Journal of Clinical Psychiatry, 59*(Suppl. 12), 3–9.

Currier, G., Chou, J., Feifel, D., Bossie, C., Turkoz, I., Mahmoud, R., et al. (2004). Acute treatment of psychotic agitation: A randomized comparison of oral treatment with risperidone and lorazepam versus intramuscular treatment with haloperidol and lorazepam. *The Journal of Clinical Psychiatry, 65*(3), 386–394.

Davidson, J. R., Landerman, L. R., Farfel, G. M., & Clary, C. M. (2002). Characterizing the effects of sertraline in post-traumatic stress disorder. *Psychological Medicine, 32*(4), 661–670.

Davidson, J. R., McLeod, M. N., Turnbull, C. D., & Miller, R. D. (1981). A comparison of phenelzine and imipramine in depressed inpatients. *The Journal of Clinical Psychiatry, 42*(10), 395–397.

Davis, S. (1991). Violence by psychiatric inpatients: A review. *Hospital and Community Psychiatry, 42*(6), 585–590.

Dieppe, P., Bartlett, C., Davey, P., Doyal, L., & Ebrahim, S. (2004). Balancing benefits and harms: The example of non-steroidal anti-inflammatory drugs. *British Medical Journal, 329*, 31–34.

Dorevitch, A., Katz, N., Zemishlany, Z., Aizenberg, D., & Weizman, A. (1999). Intramuscular flunitrazepam versus intramuscular haloperidol in the emergency treatment of aggressive psychotic behavior. *The American Journal of Psychiatry, 156*(1), 142–144.

Dorrego, M. F., Canevaro, L., Kuzis, G., Sabe, L., & Starkstein, S. E. (2002). A randomized, double-blind, crossover study of methylphenidate and lithium in adults with attention-deficit/hyperactivity disorder: Preliminary findings. The Journal of Neuropsychiatry and Clinical Neurosciences, *14*(3), 289–295.

Dubin, W. R., Waxman, H. M., Weiss, K. J., Ramchandani, D., & Tavani-Petrone, C. (1985). Rapid tranquilization: The efficacy of oral concentrate. *The Journal of Clinical Psychiatry, 46*(11), 475–478.

Edlund, M. J., Craig, T. J., & Richardson, M. A. (1985). Informed consent as a form of volunteer bias. *The American Journal of Psychiatry, 142*(5), 624–627.

Eichelmann, B. S., & Tardiff, K. (1999). Long-term medication for violent patients. In: K. Tardiff (Ed.). *Medical management of the violent patient* (pp. 255–276) New York: Marcel Dekker, Inc.

Eli Lilly and Company Limited (2004). *Letter to the healthcare professionals.* Basingstoke, Hampshire, UK: Eli Lilly and Company Limited.

Fassino, S., Leombruni, P., Daga, G., Brustolin, A., Migliaretti, G., Cavallo, F., et al. (2002). Efficacy of citalopram in anorexia nervosa: A pilot study. *European Neuropsychopharmacology, 12*(5), 453–459.

Fava, M. (1997). Psychopharmacologic treatment of pathologic aggression. *The Psychiatric Clinics of North America, 20*(2), 427–451.

Fava, M., Nierenberg, A. A., Quitkin, F. M., Zisook, S., Pearlstein, T., Stone, A., et al. (1997). A preliminary study on the efficacy of sertraline and imipramine on anger attacks in atypical depression and dysthymia. *Psychopharmacology Bulletin, 33*(1), 101–103.

Frankenburg, F., & Zanarini, M. (2002). Divalproex sodium treatment of women with borderline personality disorder and bipolar II disorder: A double-blind placebo-controlled pilot study. *The Journal of Clinical Psychiatry, 63*(5), 442–446.

Fruensgaard, K., Korsgaard, S., Jorgensen, H., & Jensen, K. (1977). Loxapine versus haloperidol parenterally in acute psychosis with agitation. A double-blind study. *Acta Psychiatrica Scandinavica, 56*(4), 56–64.

de la Fuente, J. M., & Lotstra, F. (1994). A trial of carbamazepine in borderline personality disorder. *European Neuropsychopharmacology, 4*(4), 479–486.

Goedhard, L. E., Stolker, J. J., Heerdink, E. R., Nijman, H. L. I., Olivier, B., & Egberts, A. C. G. (2006). Pharmacotherapy for the treatment of aggressive behavior in general adult psychiatry: A systematic review. *The Journal of Clinical Psychiatry.*

Heerdink, E. R., Stolker, J. J., Meijer, W. E., Hugenholtz, G. W., & Egberts, A. C. (2004). Need for medicine-based evidence in pharmacotherapy. *The British Journal of Psychiatry, 184*(5), 452.

Heiligenstein, J. H., Beasley, C. M., Jr., & Potvin, J. H. (1993). Fluoxetine not associated with increased aggression in controlled clinical trials. *International Clinical Psychopharmacology, 8*(4), 277–280.

Hollander, E., Allen, A., Lopez, R. P., Bienstock, C. A., Grossman, R., Siever, L. J., et al. (2001). A preliminary double-blind, placebo-controlled trial of divalproex sodium in borderline personality disorder. *The Journal of Clinical Psychiatry, 62*(3), 199–203.

Hollander, E., Tracy, K. A., Swann, A. C., Coccaro, E. F., McElroy, S. L., Wozniak, P., et al. (2003). Divalproex in the treatment of impulsive aggression: Efficacy in cluster B personality disorders. *Neuropsychopharmacology, 28*(6), 1186–1197.

Hugenholtz, G. W., Stolker, J. J., Heerdink, E. R., Nolen, W. A., & Leufkens, H. G. (2003). Short-acting parenteral antipsychotics drive choice for classical versus atypical agents. *European Journal of Clinical Pharmacology, 58*(11), 757–760.

Hunter, M., & Carmel, H. (1992). The cost of staff injuries from inpatient violence. *Hospital and Community Psychiatry, 43*, 586–588.

Jadad, A. R., Moore, R. A., Carroll, D., Jenkinson, C., Reynolds, D. J., Gavaghan, D. J., et al. (1996). Assessing the quality of reports of randomized clinical trials: Is blinding necessary? *Controlled Clinical Trials, 17*(1), 1–12.

Kao, L. W., Kirk, M. A., Evers, S. J., & Rosenfeld, S. H. (2003). Droperidol, QT prolongation, and sudden death: What is the evidence? *Annals of Emergency Medicine, 41*(4), 546–558.

Kay, S. R., Fiszbein, A., & Opler, L. A. (1987). The positive and negative syndrome scale (PANSS) for schizophrenia. *Schizophrenia Bulletin, 13*(2), 261–276.

Kinon, B. J., Ahl, J., Rotelli, M. D., & McMullen, E. (2004). Efficacy of accelerated dose titration of olanzapine with adjunctive lorazepam to treat acute agitation in schizophrenia. *The American Journal of Emergency Medicine, 22*(3), 181–186.

van der Kolk, B. A., Dreyfuss, D., Michaels, M., Shera, D., Berkowitz, R., Fisler, R., et al. (1994). Fluoxetine in posttraumatic stress disorder. *The Journal of Clinical Psychiatry, 55*(12), 517–522.

van Leeuwen, A. M., Molders, J., Sterkmans, P., Mielants, P., Martens, C., Toussaint, C., et al. (1977). Droperidol in acutely agitated patients. A double-blind placebo-controlled study. *The Journal of Nervous and Mental Disease, 164*(4), 280–283.

Lindenmayer, J. P. (2000). The pathophysiology of agitation. *The Journal of Clinical Psychiatry, 61*(Suppl. 14), 5–10.

Lipman, R. S., Covi, L., Rickels, K., McNair, D. M., Downing, R., Kahn, R. J., et al. (1986). Imipramine and chlordiazepoxide in depressive and anxiety disorders. I. Efficacy in depressed outpatients. *Archives of General Psychiatry, 43*(1), 68–77.

Lipman, R. S., Covi, L., & Shapiro, A. K. (1979). The Hopkins Symptom Checklist (HSCL)—factors derived from the HSCL-90. *Journal of Affective Disorders, 1*(1), 9–24.

Man, P. L., & Chen, C. H. (1973). Rapid tranquilization of acutely psychotic patients with intramuscular haloperidol and chlorpromazine. *Psychosomatics, 14*(1), 59–63.

Maoz, G., Stein, D., Meged, S., Kurzman, L., Levine, J., Valevski, A., et al. (2000). The anti-aggressive action of combined haloperidol-propranolol treatment in schizophrenia. *European Psychologist, 5*(4), 312–325.

March, J. S., Silva, S. G., Compton, S., Shapiro, M., Califf, R., & Krishnan, R. (2005). The case for practical clinical trials in psychiatry. *The American Journal of Psychiatry, 162*(5), 836–846.

Marder, S. R., Davis, J. M., & Chouinard, G. (1997). The effects of risperidone on the five dimensions of schizophrenia derived by factor analysis: Combined results of the North American trials. *The Journal of Clinical Psychiatry, 58*(12), 538–546.

Mattes, J. A. (1990). Comparative effectiveness of carbamazepine and propranolol for rage outbursts. *The Journal of Neuropsychiatry and Clinical Neurosciences, 2*(2), 159–164.

McDougle, C. J., Naylor, S. T., Cohen, D. J., Volkmar, F. R., Heninger, G. R., & Price, L. H. (1996). A double-blind, placebo-controlled study of fluvoxamine in adults with autistic disorder. *Archives of General Psychiatry, 53*(11), 1001–1008.

McNair, D. M., Lorr, M., & Doppleman, L. F. (1981). *Edits Manual for the Profile of Mood States (POMS)*. San Diego, USA: Educational and Industrial Testing Service.

McNiel, D. E., & Binder, R. L. (1994). The relationship between acute psychiatric symptoms, diagnosis, and short-term risk of violence. *Hospital and Community Psychiatry, 45*(2), 133–137.

McNiel, D. E., Binder, R. L., & Greenfield, T. K. (1988). Predictors of violence in civilly committed acute psychiatric patients. *The American Journal of Psychiatry, 145*(8), 965–970.

Meehan, K., Zhang, F., David, S., Tohen, M., Janicak, P., Small, J., et al. (2001). A double-blind, randomized comparison of the efficacy and safety of intramuscular injections of olanzapine, lorazepam, or placebo in treating acutely agitated patients diagnosed with bipolar mania. *Journal of Clinical Psychopharmacology, 21*(4), 389–397.

Menuck, M., & Voineskos, G. (1981). Rapid parenteral treatment of acute psychosis. *Comprehensive Psychiatry, 22*(4), 351–361.

Miczek, K. A., Fish, E. W., De Bold, J. F., & De Almeida, R. M. (2002). Social and neural determinants of aggressive behavior: Pharmacotherapeutic targets at serotonin, dopamine and gamma-aminobutyric acid systems. *Psychopharmacology, 163*(3–4), 434–458.

Min, S. K., Rhee, C. S., Kim, C. E., & Kang, D. Y. (1993). Risperidone versus haloperidol in the treatment of chronic schizophrenic patients: A parallel group double-blind comparative trial. *Yonsei Medical Journal, 34*(2), 179–190.

Monnelly, E. P., Ciraulo, D. A., Knapp, C., & Keane, T. (2003). Low-dose risperidone as adjunctive therapy for irritable aggression in post-traumatic stress disorder. *The Journal of Clinical Psychopharmacology, 23*(2), 193–196.

Monroe, R. R. (1989). Dyscontrol syndrome: Long-term follow-up. *Comprehensive Psychiatry, 30*(6), 489–497.

Morrison, E. F. (2003). An evaluation of four programs for the management of aggression in psychiatric settings. *Archives of Psychiatric Nursing, 17*(4), 146–155.

Nickel, K. M., Nickel, C., Kaplam, P., Lahmann, C., Mühlbacher, M., Tritt, K., et al. (2005). Treatment of aggression with topiramate in male borderline patients: A double-blind, placebo-controlled study. *Biological Psychiatry, 57*(5), 495–499.

Nijman, H., Bowers, L., Oud, N., & Jansen, G. (2005). Psychiatric nurses' experiences with inpatient aggression. *Aggressive Behavior, 31*, 217–227.

Olivier, B. (2004). Serotonin and aggression. *Annals of the New York Academy of Sciences, 1036*, 382–392.

Overall, J., & Gorham, D. (1962). The brief psychiatric rating scale. *Psychological Reports, 10*, 799–812.

Pabis, D. J., & Stanislav, S. W. (1996). Pharmacotherapy of aggressive behavior. *The Annals of pharmacotherapy, 30*(3), 278–287.

Palmer, C. (1996). Clinical practice guidelines: The priorities. *Psychiatric bulletin (London, England), 20*, 40–42.

Peuskens, J. (1995). Risperidone in the treatment of patients with chronic schizophrenia: A multinational, multi-centre, double-blind, parallel-group study versus haloperidol. Risperidone Study Group. *The British Journal of Psychiatry, 166*(6), 712–726.

Ratey, J. J., Sorgi, P., O'Driscoll, G. A., Sands, S., Daehler, M. L., Fletcher, J. R., et al. (1992). Nadolol to treat aggression and psychiatric symptomatology in chronic psychiatric inpatients: A double-blind, placebo-controlled study. *The Journal of Clinical Psychiatry, 53*(2), 41–46.

Reschke, R. (1974). Parenteral haloperidol for rapid control of severe, disruptive symptoms of acute schizophrenia. *Diseases of the Nervous system 35*, 112–115.

Resnick, M., & Burton, B. T. (1984). Droperidol vs. haloperidol in the initial management of acutely agitated patients. *The Journal of Clinical Psychiatry, 45*(7), 298–299.

Richards, J. R., Derlet, R. W., & Duncan, D. R. (1998). Chemical restraint for the agitated patient in the emergency department: Lorazepam versus droperidol. *The Journal of Emergency Medicine, 16*(4), 567–573.

Richelson, E., & Souder, T. (2000). Binding of antipsychotic drugs to human brain receptors focus on newer generation compounds. *Life Sciences, 68*(1), 29–39.

Rinne, T., van den Brink, W., Wouters, L., & van Dyck, R. (2002). SSRI treatment of borderline personality disorder: A randomized, placebo-controlled clinical trial for female patients with borderline personality disorder. *The American Journal of Psychiatry, 159*(12), 2048–2054.

Salzman, C., Wolfson, A. N., Schatzberg, A., Looper, J., Henke, R., Albanese, M.,et al. (1995). Effect of fluoxetine on anger in symptomatic volunteers with borderline personality disorder. *Journal of Clinical Psychopharmacology, 15*(1), 23–29.

Schwartz, J. T., & Brotman, A. W. (1992). A clinical guide to antipsychotic drugs. *Drugs, 44*(6), 981–992.

Shale, J. H., Shale, C. M., & Mastin, W. D. (2004). Safety of droperidol in behavioral emergencies. *Expert Opinion on Drug Safety, 3*(4), 369–378.

Soliman, A. E., & Reza, H. (2001). Risk factors and correlates of violence among acutely ill adult psychiatric inpatients. *Psychiatric Services, 52*(1), 75–80.

Soloff, P. H., Cornelius, J., George, A., Nathan, S., Perel, J. M., & Ulrich, R. F. (1993). Efficacy of phenelzine and haloperidol in borderline personality disorder. *Archives of General Psychiatry, 50*(5), 377–385.

Soloff, P. H., George, A., Nathan, S., Schulz, P. M., Cornelius, J. R., Herring, J., et al. (1989). Amitriptyline versus haloperidol in borderlines: Final outcomes and predictors of response. *Journal of Clinical Psychopharmacology, 9*(4), 238–246.

Starfield, B. (1998). Quality-of-care research: Internal elegance and external relevance. *JAMA : The Journal of the American Medical Association, 280*(11), 1006–1008.

Steadman, H. J., Silver, E., Monahan, J., Appelbaum, P. S., Robbins, P. C., Mulvey, E. P., et al. (2000). A classification tree approach to the development of actuarial violence risk assessment tools. *Law and Human Behavior, 24*(1), 83–100.

Steinert, T., Sippach, T., & Gebhardt, R. P. (2000). How common is violence in schizophrenia despite neuroleptic treatment? *Pharmacopsychiatry, 33*(3), 98–102.

Stolker, J. J. (2002). *Struggles in prescribing: Determinants of psychotropic drug use in multiple clinical settings.* Utrecht: Universiteit Utrecht.

Stone, J. L., McDaniel, K. D., Hughes, J. R., & Hermann, B. P. (1986). Episodic dyscontrol disorder and paroxysmal EEG abnormalities: Successful treatment with carbamazepine. *Biological Psychiatry, 21*(2), 208–212.

Stotsky, B. A. (1977). Relative efficacy of parenteral haloperidol and thiothixene for the emergency treatment of acutely excited and agitated patients. *Diseases of the Nervous System, 38*, 967–973.

Taymeeyapradit, U., & Kuasirikul, S. (2002). Comparative study of the effectiveness of zuclopenthixol acetate and haloperidol in acutely disturbed psychotic patients. *Journal of the Medical Association of Thailand = Chotmaihet thangphaet, 85*(12), 1301–1308.

Thomas, H., Jr., Schwartz, E., & Petrilli, R. (1992). Droperidol versus haloperidol for chemical restraint of agitated and combative patients. *Annals of Emergency Medicine, 21*(4), 407–413.

TREC Collaborative Group (2003). Rapid tranquillisation for agitated patients in emergency psychiatric rooms: A randomized trial of midazolam versus haloperidol plus promethazine. *British Medical Journal, 327*(7417), 708–713.

Troisi, A., Kustermann, S., Di Genio, M., & Siracusano, A. (2003). Hostility during admission interview as a short-term predictor of aggression in acute psychiatric male inpatients. *The Journal of Clinical Psychiatry, 64*(12), 1460–1464.

USA Food and Drug Administration (2001). FDA strengthens warnings for droperidol. *FDA Talk Paper*, T01–T62.

Vartiainen, H., Tiihonen, J., Putkonen, A., Koponen, H., Virkkunen, M., Hakola, P., et al. (1995). Citalopram, a selective serotonin reuptake inhibitor, in the treatment of aggression in schizophrenia. *Acta Psychiatrica Scandinavica, 91*(5), 348–351.

Wright, P., Birkett, M., David, S., Meehan, K., Ferchland, I., Alaka, K., et al. (2001). Double-blind, placebo-controlled comparison of intramuscular olanzapine and intramuscular haloperidol in the treatment of acute agitation in schizophrenia. *The American Journal of Psychiatry, 158*(7), 1149–1151.

Yudofsky, S. C., Silver, J. M., Jackson, W., Endicott, J., & Williams, D. (1986). The Overt Aggression Scale for the objective rating of verbal and physical aggression. *The American Journal of Psychiatry, 143*(1), 35–39.

Zanarini, M. C., & Frankenburg, F. R. (2001). Olanzapine treatment of female borderline personality disorder patients: A double-blind, placebo-controlled pilot study. *The Journal of Clinical Psychiatry, 62*(11), 849–854.

Zanarini, M. C., Frankenburg, F. R., & Parachini, E. A. (2004). A preliminary, randomized trial of fluoxetine, olanzapine, and the olanzapine-fluoxetine combination in women with borderline personality disorder. *The Journal of Clinical Psychiatry, 65*(7), 903–907.

Zarin, D. A., Young, J. L., & West, J. C. (2005). Challenges to evidence-based medicine: A comparison of patients and treatments in randomized controlled trials with patients and treatments in a practice research network. *Social Psychiatry and Psychiatric Epidemiology, 40*, 27–35.

IV

IMPROVING STAFF SKILLS IN HANDLING MANAGEMENT

10

Aggression Management Training Programs: Contents, Implementation, and Organization

Nico E. Oud

1 INTRODUCTION

"Workplace violence — be it physical or psychological — has become a global problem crossing borders, work settings, and occupational groups. For long a forgotten issue, violence at work has dramatically gained momentum in recent years and is now a priority concern in both industrialized and developing countries" (International Labor Office (ILO), International Council of Nurses (ICN), World Health Organization (WHO), & Public Services International (PSI), 2002).

Assaults represent a serious safety and health hazard for healthcare institutions, and violence against their employees continues to increase. Workplace violence in the health care sector gains, therefore, increasing recognition as an issue of great concern, as it affects staff morale, recruitment, retention, and direct health care budgets (Beech & Leather, 2003).

Workplace violence may affect more than half of health care workers, and the negative consequences of such widespread aggression and violence impact heavily on the delivery of health care services. Evidence clearly indicates that workplace violence is far too high and interventions are urgently needed (ILO et al., 2002). Unfortunately, especially for nurses, aggression and violence is an all-too-familiar syndrome as, professionally, nurses have not only to deal with the terrible outcomes of violence in caring for victims of violence, they are also threatened with aggression and violence themselves in their workplace. In fact, nurses are three times more likely to experience aggression and violence than other health care professionals (International Council of Nurses (ICN), 1999).

According to the Study of Work Related Violence, a report by the North Eastern Health Board the recognition of work-related violence is placed as a specific occupational service hazard. Therefore, a legislative and moral imperative on health care organizations to implement whatever interventions are necessary to reduce the inherent risks to staff. One measure that has been shown to significantly decrease risks to staff is the provision of training in the prevention, recognition, and management of work related aggression and violence (North Eastern Health Board (NEHB), 2004). Staff need to have the appropriate competencies to manage aggressive and violent behavior in all kind of in- and outpatient settings. However, staff training may be advocated as the appropriate managerial response, but identifying appropriate content and duration of training and trainers is difficult and there is little evidence of training effectiveness (Beech & Leather, 2003), and only very few training programs are based on evidence of either the effectiveness of training or the benefits perceived by staff and/or service users (National Institute for Clinical Excellence (NICE), 2005).

Recently, however, some documents addressing this matter have been published, namely:

- Framework guidelines for addressing workplace violence in the health care sector (ILO et al., 2002).
- Mental health policy implementation guide regarding developing positive practice to support the safe and therapeutic management of aggression and violence in mental health in-patient settings (National Institute for Mental Health in England (NIMHE), 2004).
- Clinical guidelines for the short-term management of disturbed/violent behavior in in-patient psychiatric and emergency settings (NICE, 2005).

It is recommended to all international and national professional organizations and health care institutions to look carefully at these publications in order to develop their own (inter)national/institutional guidelines for addressing workplace aggression, violence, and sexual harassment in the health care sector. These guidelines should be, at least, advisory in nature, informational in content, and intended to be used and implemented by all stakeholders in the health care sector. The aim should be to reassure health care service users and staff about the effectiveness of the process of the recognition, prevention, and management of workplace aggression, violence, and sexual harassment. A further objective could be to promote positive, evidence-based practice initiatives to train and protect service users, staff, and visitors who are exposed to aggression, violence, and sexual harassment through auditing, monitoring, benchmarking, and clinical governance of services (NIMHE, 2004), in order to provide a safe, therapeutic, and healthful workplace for all stakeholders in the health care system.

Currently there are no formal regulations governing training for the short-term management of disturbed/violent behavior in Europe. There are, however, already over 700 training providers in the United Kingdom (NICE, 2005) and it is recommended that in the UK a national approach to training should be set up as soon as possible. The National Institute for Mental Health in England (NIMHE) is currently mapping the various training packages on offer and in conjunction with the National Health Service Security and Management Service (SMS) is drawing up a core training curriculum for the UK and setting up an accreditation scheme for trainers. Correctly the NICE report states that, as training is expensive, it is necessary that services are able to measure the benefits of this training, and that without such an evidence-base there is a danger that beneficial and, possibly life-saving, training will be neither sought nor offered.

With regard to the content and duration of this training, there are relatively few guidelines or criteria presented in the above-mentioned, recommended guidelines. This chapter provides some statements and recommendations regarding the content and duration of (basic) training and of the education of trainers for such (basic) courses.

2 REACHING A SAFE AND SECURE WORKPLACE ENVIRONMENT

A safe and secure workplace environment for all health care workers should be a basic right. It is an essential element not only for the provision of quality and safe patient care, but also for safe and therapeutic management of aggression, violence, and sexual harassment in health care settings and, of course, for the health care workers' well-being, as well as for the well-being of the patient within the health care system. It is believed that patient and health care worker safety should be the new standard for quality care; care that, in any setting in which it is delivered, is free from aggression, violence, sexual harassment, and unintended injury. The United Kingdom Central Council for Nursing, Midwifery and Health Visiting (UKCC) states that violence directed toward staff, patients, and visitors is completely unacceptable, and that a position of Zero Tolerance should be the starting point (UKCC, 2002).

Current thinking on workplace aggression and violence stresses the need to address this problem more and more in terms of the total organizational dimensions of workplace aggression and violence. The assertion is that a total organizational response to this phenomenon must reflect the ideas of a learning organization. An organization that is able to reflect from top down and from bottom to top, and continually learn from its current experiences can meet existing, and future, demands more readily (Senge et al., 1999). Such learning, according to Paterson and Leadbetter (2004) requires detailed attention to the nature of the problem of aggression and violence in terms of both individual and organizational dimensions. It requires managers to move beyond the management of individual instances and the prevalence culture of victim-blaming and embrace approaches such as the root cause analysis which seeks to identify causal factors at all levels (Paterson, Leadbetter, & Miller, 2004). Responding in this way to, and managing, aggression and violence is one of the major missions of the health care services. Therefore, the problem of workplace aggression, violence, and sexual harassment in the health care system must be addressed at a variety of levels, and should lead to a consistent and coordinated organizational response.

The development of an incident of aggression, violence, or sexual harassment can never be attributed to one single factor or cause. It is always a result of various biological, genetic, sociological, and psychological factors, as well as the personalities of the involved actors (health care workers, patients, relatives), staff–patient interaction, and environmental and organizational factors such as ward/hospital structure and atmosphere. The problem of aggression, violence, and sexual harassment is not a problem concerning only the patient, nor a mono-disciplinary problem for, for example, the nursing profession alone. It is an interdisciplinary and total organizational problem of the health care system. The solution to this joint problem needs a comprehensive, integrated approach, directed at all the influencing factors and stakeholders mutually and not just to one of them (Oud, 1997). Here a number of themes and factors reoccur in the literature, and from the perspective of organizational development, these themes and factors are interactive. With regard to reducing the use of restraint and seclusion, Colton (2004) identified specific actions/factors that need to occur, or be addressed, in order to achieve a reduction of the use of restraint and seclusion: leadership, orientation and training, staffing, environmental factors, programmatic structure, timely and responsive treatment planning, processing after the incident, communication, consumer involvement, systems evaluation, and quality improvement. He states that, although no theme is paramount, a number of studies suggest that without effective leadership, efforts to reduce aggression, violence, and sexual harassment and consequently the use of restraint and seclusion will be unfocused, unsupported, and ultimately less effective, which is also the case if the focus is only on one factor, for example training only nursing staff.

Staff training should be comprehensive and Colton's study (2004) states clearly that those programs (training) that appear to be most effective tend to cover a range of topics, rather than focusing primarily on behavioral interventions such as the proper technique for implementing a physical hold. Comprehensive (interdisciplinary) educational training of all staff members should orient them to the goal, structure, and content of a comprehensive safety and health program for the recognition, prevention, and management of workplace aggression, violence, and sexual harassment, in order to be effective. It should provide staff with the knowledge, skills, and competencies to implement such programs consistently across their work shifts. Colton states that only in this way, may progress in addressing one factor result in progress in achieving another factor as well.

It is also a matter of common knowledge that the actual number of incidents with regard to workplace aggression, violence, and sexual harassment is often not known, as incidents of this kind are likely to be underreported, or not reported at all (National Audit Office, 2003). This may, according to the Occupational Safety and

Health Administration (OSHA, 2004), be due, in part, to the persistent perception within the health care industry that assaults are part of the job. The OSHA states that underreporting may reflect a lack of institutional reporting policies; an employee believes that reporting will not be of benefit to them or an employee fears that employers may deem assaults a result of employee negligence, or poor job perform-ance. In a study into the content of violence policy management documents in the United Kingdom's acute inpatient mental health services (Noak et al., 2001) it was found that policies varied widely in their content, and serious shortcomings were noted in the extent to which policies included information regarding their status and review, advice on the prevention of violence, the management of violent incidents, and postincident action.

3   GENERAL GUIDELINES REGARDING TRAINING

According to the OSHA (2004) guidelines—for preventing workplace violence for health care workers—an effective safety and health program for the recognition, pre-vention, and management of workplace aggression, violence, and sexual harassment should contain five main components:

- Management commitment and employee involvement
- Workplace analysis
- Hazard prevention and control
- Health and safety training
- Record-keeping and program evaluation, to ensure that all staff are aware of potential risk factors and how to protect patients, themselves, and their coworkers through established policies and procedures (OSHA, 2004)

Although it is, indeed, very important that all five components are part of an overall comprehensive, consistent, coordinated, organizational health and safety program, this chapter addresses, more specifically, some matters regarding component four, namely health and safety training. In a culture that seeks to minimize the risk of its occurrence through effective systems of organizational, environmental, and clinical risk assessment, the primary focus in dealing with aggression, violence, and sexual harassment should be that of recognition, prevention, and deescalation. This approach should also promote therapeutic engagement, collaboration with service users (patients/clients), and the use of advanced directives (NIMHE, 2004). A col-laborative approach, and engagement by staff and patients, in planning care in order to minimize aggression, violence, and sexual harassment, and consequently com-pulsion and coercion, should be the first health and safety standard in health care institutions. All stakeholders have the right to work, or to be treated, in the safest and least restrictive health care setting. A possible solution to the problem of aggression, violence, and sexual harassment can never be found without taking the service user seriously into account and having them actively involved. It is becoming clear that the problem of aggression and violence needs to be managed with a multifaceted approach, but it is also clear that simply training staff to manage aggressive and violent behavior only, will not resolve the overall problem (Beech & Bowyer, 2004).

However, even where such a program exists, and best practice in the recognition, prevention, and management of workplace aggression, violence, and sexual harassment is implemented, it is unlikely that all types of this behavior will be eliminated. When physical violence or other dangerous behavior is foreseeable, training in reactive behavioral management strategies including theoretical models of aggression, violence, sexual harassment, de-escalation, and physical interventions strategies and procedures is necessary. But, as stated earlier, training in the recognition, prevention, postincident care, and management of workplace aggression, violence, and sexual harassment should always form one component of a total strategy by the health care organization in achieving a safe, healthy, and therapeutic environment for all the involved stakeholders of such an environment. This is also stated by the NEHB study (2004), which says that the issue of providing staff training is a complex one and should not be limited only to issues of staff safety. Also required is the compassionate and skilful care of patients, and staff should be fully competent and skilled in the management of aggression, violence, and sexual harassment. The same study noted that training has shown to dramatically reduce the number of assaults toward staff, diminish the severity of any injuries as a consequence of such assaults, and to significantly reduce costs from occurrence of work related violence.

Considerable debate remains, however, regarding the content and duration of such training programs, especially as to how physical interventions, as part of wider training, should appear in respect of procedures, overall course content, and duration (Paterson & Leadbetter, 2004). With the emphasis only on, for example, physical restraint and interventions as an instrument for controlling patients, health care workers (nurses) are being armed only with those physical techniques as a possible solution when faced with violence, and not with alternatives (Tucker, 2004). Instead, it should be compulsory that preventive strategies like verbal deescalation, influencing workplace setting, postincident care, debriefing, etc., are being taught as well. The regulation of physical restraint training and training in the recognition, prevention, postincident care, and management of workplace aggression, violence, and sexual harassment and effective accreditation schemes should be the number one priority on the agenda for national health care worker (nurse) organizations, national health care employer organizations, national service user organizations, and national health care political policies.

4   RECOMMENDED CONTENT OF TRAINING

According to Paterson and Leadbetter (2004), there is some agreement on the potential core constituents of such training and, in accordance with the proposed curriculum for aggression management by the American Psychiatric Association (APA, 1993), the NMC (formerly the UKCC) report regarding "the recognition, prevention, and therapeutic management of violence in mental health care" (UKCC, 2002), and the ENTMA letter (2005), it is suggested that such training should, at least, address the following elements:

- The recommended essential components of training in the recognition, prevention, and therapeutic management of violence: theoretical aspects, deescalation strategies, breakaway techniques, and restraint techniques (UKCC, 2002—Appendix 5).
- Promotion of an explicit core values-base that is compatible with the ethos of caring services and relevant professional ethics, e.g., service user involvement and collaboration with service users in order to achieve the safest, least restrictive, and least oppressive health care setting possible, and showing the willingness and ability to enhance/improve staff and service user safety.
- Integration of primary, secondary, and tertiary prevention strategies, not just crisis management skills.
- Provision of tailored solutions to local problems based on risk assessment (Doyle & Dolan, 2002), detailed incident analysis, and environmental assessment rather than a standard one-size-fits-all program, and teaching only those procedures that, on the basis of this assessment, are actually foreseeable in the workplace rather than worst-case scenarios.
- Demonstration of a hierarchical approach to the problem of aggression, violence, and sexual harassment allowing graduated responses to the level of risk in any given situation compatible with the principle of least restrictive intervention, the relevant practice setting, and the legal context.
- Provision of interventions that are capable of being mastered and used by the majority of staff with the majority of service users, and only those physical interventions/techniques that are described fully in writing, and have been subjected to independent biomechanical evaluation, and in accordance with the recommendations regarding physical interventions described in the NICE Guidelines (NICE, 2005).
- Physical contact skills/interventions in relation to life support techniques, and the application of safe and therapeutic breakaway techniques, and restraint/seclusion techniques.
- Identification of the risks involved in physical interventions during training and to actively work toward the reduction and/or elimination of procedures associated with higher risks of adverse consequences. These include prone and supine restraint, basket holds, and procedures which involve pressure across a joint and/or deliberate application of pain. With regard to the latter, every effort must be made to use techniques that do not rely upon the deliberate application of pain, as this distorts the therapeutic relationship and may lead to a worsening of an already highly charged situation. This should, therefore, be avoided unless absolutely necessary (NICE, 2005).
- Content that is based upon regular evaluation of, and grounded in, the systematic collection of evidence and regular audit, and in accordance with the NICE guidelines.

- Demonstrating commitment to service user involvement in the development, implementation, and evaluation of the training.
- The use of assessment instruments e.g., the Brøset Violence Checklist (Abderhalden et al., 2004), the Staff Observation Aggression Scale—Revised (SOAS-R) (Nijman, 1999), and the Perception of Prevalence of Aggression Scale (POPAS) (Nijman, Bowers, Oud, & Jansen, 2005) (see Nijman chapter, this volume).
- Definitions and theoretical models of aggression, violence, and sexual harassment, whereby from the theoretical perspective of the interaction model, the classical role allocation of perpetrator and victim is rejected, and participants engaged in aggressive/violent behavior are perceived as actors in a social interaction. Both parties (staff and service users) are actively encouraged to reflect on their own contribution to the genesis, the prevention, the management, and the aftermath of aggression/violence (course description in Needham, 2004). Aggression and violence is recognized as multifactory, with a number of potential contributory sources/actors, and therefore the problem has also no single solution, such as only training staff in restraint procedures (Beech & Bowyer, 2004).
- Information regarding a safe working environment, or systems of work, in relation to design and layout, use of alarms, security procedures, reporting procedures, setting conditions and triggers, etc.
- Information in relation to particular service user groups: children, elderly people, people experiencing mental illness, learning disabilities, acquired brain injury, etc., and taking into account minority ethnic groups, gender, pregnancy, racial, cultural, social, religious/spiritual, and other special concerns.
- Deescalation techniques, effective interpersonal communication skills, theoretical (aggression, violence, and conflict) models, and practice strategies and training/applying specific communication skills, in order to prevent, deescalate, apply postincident care, and/or manage safely and therapeutically incidents of aggression, violence, and sexual harassment. The main task of the health care worker should be to develop and maintain a therapeutic professional contact with the service user, or to restore this kind of relationship as soon as possible during and after an incident whereby, if necessary, only the "behavior" of the service user could be condemned, but never the person themselves (see Richter chapter, this volume).
- Legal and ethical issues (see Hatling et al. chapter, this volume).
- Identification of the dimensions and practice of staff and service user support before and after incidents of aggression, violence, or sexual harassment (see Needham chapter and Conclusion, this volume).
- Use of a variety of teaching approaches, such as classical lessons, but also role playing, reflection, live demonstrations, and practice sessions, and it is strongly recommended that this is coupled with mentoring and coaching on the job (Colton, 2004).

- Orientation to organizational as well as regional, national, and international policies, procedures, and programs, such as for example organizational values and norms, clinical treatment pathways, instructions with regard to the use of seclusion and restraint, pre and post incident care, and instructions with regard to documentation and assessment requirements.
- All health care workers or staff working directly with service users should take part in such basic courses, and these should be looked on as an interdisciplinary task. The American Psychiatric Association (APA) is also recommending that psychiatrists receive training so as to be able to assist in emergency situations in which their assistance is crucial. Seclusion and restraint clinicians should be familiar with the standards for seclusion and restraint, including the indications, contraindications, and alternatives to seclusion and restraint, and the criteria for release from this.
- All health care workers should regularly take part in refresher courses.

The detailed recommendations recently published by NICE (2005) with regard to training can be found in the appendix of this chapter.

5 TRAINING COURSE AIMS

An example for training course aims might be the one described in the draft guidelines, regarding the implementation of a national syllabus, by the NHS Security Management Service for Promoting Safer and Therapeutic Services (Miller, 2005). These state that a training program for mental health and learning disability services in the nonphysical prevention and management of violence should have the following course aims, where a participant is able to:

- Describe the role of the security management director and local security management specialist in relation to the management of violence in mental health or learning disability settings, as defined by directions issued by the Department of Health to all health bodies.
- Describe theoretical, pathological, and environmental explanations for aggression within mental health or learning disability settings.
- Demonstrate an understanding of the application of risk management interventions and the requirements for the effective assessment of danger with reference to prevention planning.
- Demonstrate an understanding of restraint-related risks, as outlined in the Independent Inquiry into the death of David Bennett and NICE guidelines, with a view to incorporating risk reduction strategies into practice.
- Demonstrate an understanding of the need for, and scope of, postincident review procedures. How to identify strategies and interventions for future prevention, and identify spheres of influence in relation to the individual, team, and organizational change required to achieve a reduction in aggression and violence.

- Identify and demonstrate aspects of nonverbal deescalation, verbal strategies, and conflict resolution styles.
- Identify and reflect upon the effect of functional and dysfunctional coping strategies on people's lives and behavior, and be able to relate this to mental health or learning disability settings.
- Demonstrate an understanding of the positive contributions service users can make to prevention strategies, including awareness of how issues relating to culture, race, disability, sexuality, and gender can enhance this process.
- Describe individual and organizational responsibilities in relation to legal, ethical, and moral frameworks relating to the use of force.

In addition, according to the above-mentioned draft guidelines, the following interventions and related topics should be addressed during a basic training course:

- Environment, organization, and alarm systems
- Prediction (antecedents, warning signs, and risk assessment)
- Training
- Service user perspectives, including those relating to ethnicity, gender, and other special concerns
- Searching.
- Deescalation techniques
- Observation
- Physical intervention
- Seclusion
- Rapid tranquillization
- Postincident reviews
- Emergency departments

6   FOCUS, DURATION, AND EFFECTS OF TRAINING

Taking into account the necessary comprehensiveness of the training and the broad range of topics, it is clear that such training programs should be at least four to six days in length, longer if necessary, with a minimum of four days (32 hours) for a course. According to ENTMA (2005), supported by Tucker (2004) and Colton (2004), it is also clear that if the training is less than four days, physical restraint techniques should not be taught at all, and also never restricted to teaching or training of only breakaway techniques. Training programs can only be effective if they cover a range of topics, rather than focusing primarily, or only, on behavioral interventions such as the proper techniques for physical holds or restraints. The effect of a comprehensive, five-day, training course in aggression management was tested in a multicenter randomized controlled clinical trial in Switzerland. The study showed a statistically significant reduction of severe aggressive incidents and coercive measures, and a substantial reduction of the subjective severity of aggressive incidents after the training course in the intervention group (three teams/wards) in comparison to the control group (three teams/wards) (Needham, 2004). In other words, the study results suggest that the training course has contributed to a reduction of severe aggression, the subjective perception of aggression by the nurses, and coercion. However, no statistically significant changes were found regarding the overall aggressive incidents, attacks against staff, which is probably due to the fact that the measurement was taken too soon after the training, and that for cultural change and quality improvement, more implementation time and follow-up is needed.

Another example of basic training is described by Sjøgreen, Jensen, and Kielberg (2003). This training course was developed in 1994 and is compulsory for the majority of professionals employed in the mental health services in Denmark (see Appendix).

Next to basic training for direct service staff working in the field, there is also a need to focus on the training of at least two other major staff groups (Paterson & Leadbetter, 2004):

- *Management*: Managers' requirements tend to differ from direct service workers and the more senior the manager, the less likely they may be to experience violence. Their primary needs, therefore, are to understand their legal obligations for worker and service user safety, and to develop an awareness of effective organizational approaches to the management of aggression, violence, and sexual harassment. This does not mean, however, that they do not require basic personal safety training.
- *Support and administration staff*: These roles may vary in terms of the degree of contact they have with service users. They may have no contact, limited direct service user contact or substantial contact. Their need for training will therefore vary.

The reader is referred to the chapter in this volume about the effects of aggression management programs by Richter, Needham, and Kunz for details of the outcomes of such training courses.

7 TRAINING TRAINERS

According to the Mental Health Policy Implementation Guide, regarding the development of positive practice to support the safe and therapeutic management of aggression and violence in mental health inpatient settings of the National Institute for Mental Health in England (NIMHE, 2004), it is essential that education and training in the safe and therapeutic management of aggression and violence is developed and delivered by trainers who have expertise and practice credibility. The trainers within the ENTMA (2005) are such trainers and, based upon their experience in their respective countries (United Kingdom, Norway, Denmark, Germany, Finland, Switzerland, Netherlands, and Austria), recommend that such training courses for trainers should preferably be an integral part of the educational system for health care professionals and also linked to a university. However, in all European countries, there are no formal regulations or systematic evidence regarding the background, qualifications, status, and practice credibility of trainers of trainers. The NIMHE have, therefore, stated some positive practice standards in the absence of a mandatory accreditation and regulation scheme, and will be developing proposals for a national accreditation scheme for both trainers, and education and training. It is recommended that such developments be set up in all European countries and, according to ENTMA, the preparation of trainers should comprise an absolute minimum of 400–500 study hours, of which about one-third would be face-to-face contact, a third for supervised practice, and a third for self-study and for carrying out some work toward a thesis as an written end product of such study. Attending such a trainer program should only follow after the candidate trainer has themselves attended a basic training, so that they already have some experience, skills, and knowledge regarding the possible role of a trainer. Examples of such studies are the validated course "Preparation of Trainers in the Management of Actual or Potential Aggression" at Keele University in Staffordshire, UK, which consists of 40 study days, and the "Trainer for aggression management course" at the SBK Bildungszentrum, Zurich, Switzerland, which comprises 36 days and 100 hours for self study, and 80 hours for working on a thesis. Both examples are representative of the content of such courses.

It is recommended to take initiatives to set up such training programs for trainers in the recognition, prevention, postincident care, and therapeutic management of aggression, violent behavior, and sexual harassment in health care, and to develop mandatory accreditation and regulation schemes for those programs. According to NIMHE guidelines (2004), appropriate programs should develop standards for training and practice, assess the competencies of trainers, and demonstrate regular review and evaluation. It further states that all trainers:

- Must attend an annual update/refresher course which incorporates a reassessment of the trainer's competencies to practice
- Must have extensive knowledge and understanding of the challenges and implications for clinical practice in health service provision, which can be demonstrated via a portfolio of evidence, or a relevant professional qualification (health/social care/teaching)
- Must have a recognized teaching or assessment qualification
- Remain professionally accountable for what they teach and its influence on practice, and must promote the highest standards of professionalism to those they teach
- Need to remain clinically up-to-date and clinically credible
- Must maintain a portfolio of evidence to support continuous professional development and life-long learning
- Internal trainer portfolios should be reviewed annually by the employing organization

8 CONCLUSION

This chapter outlines the issues pertaining to training and the training of trainers in the recognition, prevention, postincident care, and therapeutic management of aggressive, violent behavior, and sexual harassment in health care. Assuming that many official (inter)national organizations have vague knowledge of these issues, the author saw it as a duty to inform the reader about them. After all, the first step in developing and facilitating policies regarding this subject is to become familiar with the existing knowledge and expertise on this matter. A second, more important, step will be for national and international professional organizations to start developing strategies and policies regarding guidelines for the training of staff and other trainers in the recognition, prevention, postincident care, and therapeutic management of aggressive, violent behavior, and sexual harassment in health care.

9 APPENDIX

9.1 NICE Recommendations on Training Programs

9.1.1 Training

Staff need to have the appropriate skills to manage disturbed/violent behavior in psychiatric inpatient settings. Training in the interventions used for the short-term management of disturbed/violent behavior safeguards both staff and service users. Training that highlights awareness of racial, cultural, social, and religious/spiritual needs, and gender differences, along with other special concerns, also mitigates against disturbed/violent behavior. Such training should be properly audited to ensure its effectiveness.

Policy
All service providers should have a policy for training employees and staff-in-training in relation to the short-term management of disturbed/violent behavior. This policy should specify who will receive what level of training (based on risk assessment), how often they will be trained, and also outline the techniques in which they will be trained.

All service providers should specify who the training provider is and ensure consistency in terms of training and refresher courses.

Training relating to the management of disturbed/violent behavior should be subject to approved national standards.

If participants on training courses demonstrate inappropriate attitudes then trainers should pass this information onto the relevant line manager for appropriate action.

Specific Staff Training Needs
There should be an ongoing program of training for all staff in racial, cultural, spiritual, social and special needs issues to ensure that staff are aware of and

know how to work with diverse populations and do not perpetuate stereotypes. Such courses should also cover any special populations, such as migrant populations, and asylum seekers, that are relevant to the locality.

All staff whose need is determined by risk assessment should receive ongoing competency training to recognize anger, potential aggression, antecedents and risk factors of disturbed/violent behavior and to monitor their own verbal and non-verbal behavior. Training should include methods of anticipating, de-escalating or coping with disturbed/violent behavior.

Staff members responsible for carrying out observation and engagement should receive ongoing competency training in observation so that they are equipped with the skills and confidence to engage with service users.

All staff involved in administering or prescribing rapid tranquillization, or monitoring service users to whom parenteral rapid tranquillization has been administered, should receive ongoing competency training to a minimum of Immediate Life Support (ILS — Resuscitation Council UK) (covers airway, cardiopulmonary resuscitation [CPR], and use of defibrillators).

Staff who employ physical intervention or seclusion should, as a minimum, be trained to Basic Life Support (BLS — Resuscitation Council UK).

All staff whose level of need is determined by risk assessment should receive training to ensure current competency in the use of physical intervention which should adhere to approved national standards.

Service providers should ensure that staff's capability to undertake physical intervention and physical intervention training courses is assessed.

All staff whose level of need is determined by risk assessment should receive ongoing competency training in the use of seclusion. Training should include appropriate monitoring arrangements for service users placed in seclusion.

All staff involved in rapid tranquillization should be trained in the use of pulse oximeters.

Prescribers and those who administer medicines should be familiar with and have received training in rapid tranquillization, including:

- The properties of benzodiazepines; their antagonist, flumazenil; antipsychotics; antimuscarinics; and antihistamines
- The risks associated with rapid tranquillization, including cardiorespiratory effects of the acute administration of these drugs, particularly when the service user is highly aroused and may have been misusing drugs; is dehydrated or possibly physically ill
- The need to titrate doses to effect

All staff involved in undertaking of searches should receive appropriate instruction which is repeated and regularly updated.

Incident Recording. Training should be given to all appropriate staff to ensure that they are aware of how to correctly record any incident using the appropriate local templates.

Refresher Courses. Services should review their training strategy annually to identify those staff groups that require ongoing professional training in the recognition, prevention and de-escalation of disturbed/violent behavior and in physical intervention to manage disturbed/violent behavior.

Evaluating Training

All training should be evaluated, including training in racial, cultural, religious/spiritual and gender issues, along with training that focuses on other special service user concerns.

Independent bodies/service user groups should, if possible, be involved in evaluating the effectiveness of training.

Service User Training/Involvement in Training. Service users and/or service user groups should have the opportunity to become actively involved in training and setting the training agenda, for example groups with potential vulnerabilities such as:

- Service users with a sensory impairment
- Black and minority ethnic service users
- Service users with a physical impairment
- Service users with a cognitive impairment
- Female service users
- Service users with communication difficulties

9.2 Training Program Description of Courses in Switzerland (Needham, 2004)

The five day aggression management training course under investigation was developed by N. Oud in the Netherlands. It is a skill-oriented, action-centered, and problem-centered, participating learning package and includes aspects such as the nature and prevalence of aggression, violence, and sexual harassment, the use of aggression scales, preventive measures, and strategies, deescalation techniques, ethical aspects of violence management, and safety management. The primary goal of the course is the prevention and deescalation of aggression. However, techniques are also offered for aiding patients who are manifestly aggressive. Such skills include break-away techniques, control and restraint, and postincident care. Course participants are introduced to the concept of "actors" in social interaction in order to avoid the "perpetrator vs. victim" dichotomy. Another important content of the course is the coordination of nurses or other carers in handling patient aggression. This training course has received anecdotal praise from participants but this is the first scientific investigation on its effects.

9.3 Training Contents of a Danish program (Sjögreen et al., 2003)

The course offered at Aarhus consists of three main elements (1) theory, (2) control and restraint techniques, and (3) role-play. Within each of these elements the focus is on preliminary preparation, response to specific situations, and supplementary work. Participants attending the course express an increased understanding of their own and others' roles, and that the tools acquired are useful in their future work with conflict management and prevention of violence.

1. *Theory*: The first main element consists of imparting knowledge and sharing experience in the forms of lectures followed by dialogue and assignments. All the topics outlined in the theoretical framework are covered thoroughly (culture of workplace, psychosocial work environment, structure of workplace, procedure for prevention of violence, professional and personal development, and physical work environment). Within all areas dialogue and cooperation between patients, staff, and management is necessary in order to create a workplace where you sure to be taken care of if violence should occur.

2. *Control and Restraint Techniques*: The second main element of the program is a training component closely worked with a group of psychosocial consultants. Those consultants have developed a number of control and restraint holds which enables staff to maintain the respect for, and care of, the patient, and at the same time ensure, staff safety. These very simple holds do not require great strength, only the use of proper techniques. These are taught to the participants who are then given the opportunity for daily repetition and training. Apart from physical techniques also considered are: body language, boundaries, co-operation, and communication. These verbal and nonverbal aspects of communication between patient and staff are very important. Specifically the relationship between words, body, and tone is being considered. All these factors play a role in defusing violent or threatening incidents.

3. *Role Play*: The third element is role play, which is based on work situations. The role play mimics realistic situations and some participants undergo strong emotions as anger, fear, or anxiety. Some have described experiencing palpitations or tunnel vision. Of course one is very careful not to push participants either too far or too little. Learning situations are created which can then be discussed and reviewed. Nevertheless participants should be confronted by sufficiently difficult challenges to develop their skills. The aim of the role play is thus to give each participant a chance to work in difficult situations and improve their ability to respond to conflict while maintaining as much of their self-esteem and dignity as possible. The role play provides instructors with a possibility of working realistically with signals, interpretations, preparation, cooperation, communication, reactions, possible actions, etc. The role play is an educational tool which greatly increases the understanding of the essential areas within conflict management and prevention of violence.

The success of the course lies in its ability to create a learning environment where the participants can work, learn, and develop in an atmosphere of appreciation and respect. This environment allows people to achieve a better understanding of themselves, gain insight into their own and other people's motives, signals, and reactions in conflict situations.

REFERENCES

Abderhalden, C., Needham, I., Miserez, B., Almvik, R., Dassen, T., Haug, H. J., et al. (2004). Predicting inpatient violence in acute psychiatric wards using the Brøset-Violence-Checklist: A multicentre prospective cohort study. *Journal of Psychiatric and Mental Health Nursing, 11*, 422–427.

American Psychiatric Association (APA). (1993). *Clinician Safety — Task force report 33 on clinician safety*. (edited by William R. Dubin, M. D. and John R. Lion, M. D) Washington: APA.

Beech, B., & Bowyer, D. (2004). Management of aggression and violence in mental health settings. *Mental Health Practice, 7*(7), 31–37.

Beech, B., & Leather, P. (2003). Evaluating a management of aggression unit for student nurses. *Journal of Advanced Nursing, 44*(6), 603–612.

Colton, D. (2004). *Checklist for assessing your organization's readiness for reducing seclusion and restraint*. Staunton: Commonwealth Center for Children and Adolescence.

Doyle, M., & M. Dolan, M. (2002). Violence risk assessment: Combining actuarial and clinical information to structure clinical judgments for the formulation and management of risk. *Journal of Psychiatric and Mental Health Nursing, 9*, 649–657.

ENTMA (The European Network of Trainers and educators of trainers in the recognition, prevention, post-incident care, and therapeutic Management of Aggression, violent behavior, and sexual harassment in health care) (2005). *Letter to the European National Nurses Organizations: Recommendations regarding the content and duration of (basic) training in the recognition, prevention, post-incident care, and therapeutic management of aggression, violent behavior, and sexual harassment in health care, and about the regulation, content, and duration of educating trainers for such courses*. Amsterdam: Connecting, Partnership for Training and Consult.

International Council of Nurses (ICN). (1999). *Guidelines on coping with violence in the workplace*. Geneva: International Council of Nurses.

International Labor Office (ILO), International Council of Nurses (ICN), World Health Organization (WHO), and Public Services International (PSI). (2002). *Framework guidelines for addressing workplace violence in the health sector*. Geneva: International Labor Office.

Miller, G. (2005). Familiarization Seminar. *A training program for mental health and learning disability services in the non-physical prevention and management of violence*. Presentation at the 2005 Study days of Connecting in Amsterdam: *Implementing a National Syllabus: Promoting Safer and Therapeutic Services*, Sunday, 6 November 2005, Amsterdam.

National Audit Office. (2003). *A safer place to work: Protecting NHS hospital and ambulance staff from violence and aggression*. London: The Stationary Office.

National Institute for Clinical Excellence (NICE). (2005). *Violence: The short-term management of disturbed/violent behavior in in-patient psychiatric settings and emergency departments. Clinical Practice Guideline 25*. London: NICE.

National Institute for Mental Health in England (NIMHE). (2004). *Mental health policy implementation guide: Developing positive practice to support the safe and therapeutic management of aggression and violence in mental health in-patient settings*. Leeds: NIMHE.

Needham, I. (2004). *A nursing intervention to handle patient aggression — The effectiveness of a training course in the management of aggression*. PhD dissertation. Maastricht: Universitaire Pers.

Nijman, H. (1999): *Aggressive behavior of psychiatric inpatients — Measurement, prevalence, and determinants*. PhD dissertation. Maastricht: Universitaire Pers.

Nijman, H., Bowers, L., Oud, N., & Jansen, G. (2005). Psychiatric nurses' experiences with inpatient aggression. *Aggressive Behavior, 31*, 217–227.

Noak, J., Wright, S., Sayer, J., Parr, A., Gray, R., Southern, D., et al. (2001). The content of management of violence policy documents in United Kingdom acute inpatient mental health services. *Journal of Advanced Nursing, 37*(4), 394–401.

North Eastern Health Board Committee on Work-place Violence. (2004). *Study of work-related violence.* Kells Co. Meath, Ireland: Health Service Executive North Eastern Area, Administrative Head Office.

Occupational Safety and Health Administration (OSHA). (2004). *Guidelines for preventing workplace violence for health care and social service workers.* Washington: OSHA.

Oud, N.E. (1997). *Aggression and psychiatric nursing.* Information brochure. Amsterdam: Broens & Oud, partnership for consult & training (Connecting, maatschap voor consult & training).

Paterson, P., & Leadbetter, D. (2004). *Only when there is no alternative: Improving the physical and psychological safety of physical interventions used in care settings.* Available at http://www.nm.stir.ac.uk/diploma/managing_violence.htmPaterson, P., Leadbetter, D., & Miller, G. (2004). *Workplace violence in health and social care as an international problem: A public health perspective on the 'total organizational response'.* (personal note: Draft article, available at b.a.paterson@stir.ac.uk) (via: http://www.nm.stir.ac. uk/diploma/managing_violence.htm).

Senge, P., Kleiner, A., Roberts, C., Ross, R., Roth, G., & Smith, B. (1999). *The dance of change: The challenges of sustaining momentum in learning organizations.* New York: Doubleday/Currency.

Sjögreen, V., Jensen, A., & Kielberg, P. (2003). Education for violence prevention — A Danish example. In: M. Habermann & L. R. Uys (Eds.). *Violence in Nursing: International Perspectives* (pp. 217–236). Frankfurt am Main: Peter Lang.

Tucker, R. (2004). *The regulator's perspective.* Paper presented at the conference "The management of violence — Changing a culture", Liverpool University, 21–22 April 2004.

United Kingdom Central Council for Nursing, Midwifery and Health Visiting (UKCC). (2002). The recognition, prevention and therapeutic management of violence in mental health care — A summary. London: UKCC.

11

The Effects of Aggression Management Training for Mental Health Care and Disability Care Staff: A Systematic Review

DIRK RICHTER, IAN NEEDHAM, AND STEFAN KUNZ

1   SUMMARY

1.1   Background

Aggression management training for staff has been implemented in many organizations of mental health and disability care. The efficacy of such programs has rarely been analyzed.

1.2   Methods

A systematic review was conducted which contains all published evaluation studies on aggression management training. Inclusion criteria were randomized controlled trails, control group designs, or pre–post measurement studies.

1.3   Results

Thirty nine published studies were included. The quality of the studies included was deemed as generally low. No clear trend regarding a reduction of violent incidents resulted. However, the studies revealed clear positive effects on staff knowledge about violence and their confidence to cope with aggressive situations.

1.4 Conclusions

Sensitization effects of staff after training probably lead to reporting bias. Although the results on the number of violent incidents remain unclear, it is recommended to conduct comprehensive aggression management training in mental health and disability care institutions.

2 INTRODUCTION

The way of dealing with aggression and violence is one of the most prominent characteristics of the quality of psychiatric hospitals. This applies to the security of carers (Richter & Berger, 2001; Steinert, Vogel, Beck, & Kehlmann, 1991) and of patients (Fähndrich & Ketelsen, 2004; Steinert, 2004) alike. In the last few years, training programs for workers in institutions for mental health care and disability care have been implemented, mainly at the instigation of nurses. Initially such courses included exclusive training in physical defense, and methods for applying coercive measures (Fuchs, 1998; Mason & Chandley, 1999). At a later stage deescalation techniques, which logically precede defense techniques, were incorporated (for details see the chapter on deescalation by Richter, this volume). Currently combinations of these techniques are generally used. Various approaches used in German-speaking countries have been described (Anke, Bojack, Krämer, & Seißelberg, 2003; Richter, Fuchs, & Bergers, 2001) and for a synopsis of contents employed in English speaking regions see Farrell and Cubit (2005).

The diversity and variability of such training invites the question of their effectiveness. In German-speaking regions, little empirical work has been done to test such training. This systematic literature review offers a summary of research results on this theme.

2.1 Research Question and Method

Due to the differing quality and the heterogeneity of available research reports a metaanalysis was not possible. We therefore chose to conduct a systematic review on the theme. The following themes regarding training courses in aggression management were identified:

- Knowledge (on aggression/violence and aggression management)
- Subjective feelings by staff of security in dealing with aggression
- Incident rates
- Injuries inflicted on carers
- Lost work days

- Coercive measures: mechanical restraint, seclusion, or involuntary medication
- Miscellaneous. For example techniques, satisfaction with the training course, or the relevance of the training for work on the ward.

Unfortunately the publications meeting these criteria are quite heterogeneous, rendering comparisons difficult. Only one of the studies complied to the "gold standard" of a randomized controlled trial. Thus, we cannot exclude the possibility of bias in the population under scrutiny.

2.2   Inclusion Criteria and Data Search

All published articles which reported quantitative effects of specific training programs in aggression management and which included either a control group or a pre–post measure were included. We excluded research results employing only effectiveness data after the training course (Grube, 2001; Weisman & Lamberti, 2002) or studies focusing solely on situations in which deescalation is effective (Jambunathan & Bellaire, 1996). We also neglected epidemiological studies which compared trained and untrained carers' exposition to aggression but reported no details on training programs (Lee, Gerberich, Waller, Anderson, & McGovern, 1999). Studies published between 1976 and 2004 were included. We found no relevant publications prior to 1976. In order to ameliorate the data base, publications from neighboring domains of psychiatry (institutions for the care of the disabled or for aged residents) were included. This decision was supported by the fact that such patients—at least in Germany—are treated on wards that are similar to psychiatric hospitals.

Electronic data searching was conducted employing PubMed, the Cumulative Index to Nursing and Allied Health Sciences Literature (CINAHL), and PsychInfo. The search strategy included the terms "violence," "aggression," "training," "mental," and "psychiatric." Because of the poor results of the electronic search (on this subject, see Allen, 2001), complementary search strategies were employed. These included the hand search of references quoted in relevant texts, e.g., a report of the United Kingdom Central Council for Nursing, Midwifery and Health Visiting (UKCC, 2001) or of the British Institute for Learning Disabilities (BILD) (Allen) and the consulting of experts in the domain (predominantly members of the European Violence in Psychiatry Research Group).

2.3   Design and Relevance of Study Results

The relevance attributed to the primary studies was judged on the grounds of the research design. Programs aiming at reducing injuries on carers using a control group received a higher rating than pre–post measure designs without a control group (Robson, Shannon, Goldenhar, & Hale, 2001). On considering pre–post designs without control groups it becomes increasingly difficult to exclude the possibility that observed changes might be due to extraneous variables other than the training program in aggression management. Also, studies comparing the frequencies of aggressive incidents received a higher ranking than survey studies or other research reporting the subjective experiences of staff.

For the purpose of this systematic review the following hierarchy of studies was defined:

- Randomized controlled trials (RCT)
- Studies comparing frequencies of aggressive incidents employing control groups
- Studies comparing staff knowledge/confidence by means of interviews employing control groups
- Studies comparing aggressive incidents employing a pre–post measure
- Studies comparing staff knowledge/confidence by means of interviews employing a pre-post measure

These study groups were further divided into sub-categories according to the type of training intervention used: deescalation training, defense technique training, combinations of deescalation and defense technique training. This allowed the distinction and the evaluation of possible effects in each training sub-category. Although training in deescalation differs from training in defense techniques, empirical studies show that self-defense training may have "positive" aggression–prevention side effects by promoting participants' self-esteem which in turn may help to reduce aggressive incidents (Philips & Rudestam, 1995; Poster, 1996).

In spite of similarities in study design and the type of training (deescalation, defense techniques, or combinations thereof) the studies are difficult to compare due to the investigation in differing populations and settings (e.g., acute psychiatry, geropsychiatry, forensic psychiatry, services for the disabled). The training also differs considerably in duration and content. Furthermore, the time between the intervention and the measurement of the effect varies between one week and several years. A further difficulty is the partially inadequate description of the training courses in the studies, especially regarding the contents, the duration, and the number or types of participants. Another limitation to the quality of the publications is the fact that the evaluation of the effectiveness of the training was often conducted by the persons offering or administrating the courses. Thus, some publication bias, e.g., the nonpublication of nonpositive results can be expected.

2.4 Results

Of the 39 published studies employed in this review, three were conducted in nursing homes (Feldt & Ryden, 1992; Fitzwater & Gates, 2002; Hagan & Sayers, 1995) and one in a school for persons with intellectual limitations (Perkins & Leadbetter, 2002). All the other studies were conducted in psychiatric settings or in institutions for the disabled. Nineteen studies included only the training of nurses.

2.4.1 Randomized Controlled Trials (RCT)

The only primary study using a "gold standard" design reported a decrease in the severity of aggressive episodes. However, no reduction in the number of violent incidents could be observed. In the experimental group, where a combination of self-defense and deescalation techniques was introduced, a decrease in the use of coercive measures occurred (Needham, Abderhalden, Haug et al., 2004) (Table 1).

2.4.2 Studies Comparing Aggressive Incidents Employing Control Groups

In the studies examining the effects of deescalation training only one (Whittington & Wykes, 1996) out of three (Nijman, Merckelbach, Allertz, & à Campo, 1997; Smooth & Gonzales, 1995; Whittington & Wykes) reported a significant decrease in aggressive incidents. No studies focusing solely on the effect of self-defense techniques were found. For studies which used a combination of deescalation interventions and self-defense techniques the outcomes were mixed. In two studies, aggressive incidents in the intervention group decreased (Fitzwater & Gates, 2002; Infantino & Musingo, 1985), two studies reported increases (Ore, 2002; Rice, Helzel, Varney, & Quinsey, 1985), and two studies found no significant difference (Carmel & Hunter, 1990; van Rixtel, Nijman, & Jansen, 1997). Because of the low number of retrievable studies focusing on injuries (Carmel & Hunter; Infantino & Musingo) and lost days of work (Ore; Rice et al.) as an outcome and because of their contradictory results it was not possible to summarize any tendencies for these study types. Coercive measures were subject to examination in only one study, where deescalation training was the preferred intervention (Smooth & Gonzales). One single study examined the effects of deescalation training versus a combination of deescalation training plus defense techniques versus an untrained control group (Philips & Rudestam, 1995). A combination of de-escalation and defense techniques seemed to be most effective.

2.4.3 Studies Comparing Staff Knowledge/Confidence by Means of Interviews Employing Control Groups

Study designs using interviews to establish participants' knowledge and subjective feelings of security for handling aggressive situations tended to detect an advantage for the intervention groups. The majority of the studies found that trained employees did report increased confidence compared to untrained colleagues. These findings were valid for defense technique interventions (McGowan, Wynaden, Harding, Yassine, & Parker, 1999) as well as for training courses which combined defense techniques and deescalation interventions (Allen & Tynan, 2000; Fitzwater & Gates, 2002; Hurlebaus & Link, 1997; Infantino & Musingo, 1985; Rice et al., 1985; Thackrey, 1987). In two studies the confidence level did not vary between the groups (Hurlebaus & Link; van Rixtel et al., 1997). No study reported any confidence reduction in the intervention group after the training sessions.

Table 1. Studies Included in the Systematic Review

Type of Study	Authors	Country	Setting	Participants	N	Knowledge	Feelings of Security	Incidents	Injuries	Lost Work Days	Coercive Measures	Miscellaneous
RCT—combination	Needham, Abderhalden, Haug et al. (2004)	CH	Psychiatric hospitals	Nurses wards	6 acute			$-^a$			−	
Control—deescalation	Nijman et al. (1997)	NL	Psychiatric hospitals	All professionals	n.k.			=				
Control—deescalation	Smooth and Gonzales (1995)	US	Psychiatric hospitals	All professionals	72			=			−	
Control—deescalation	Whittington and Wykes (1996)	UK	Psychiatric hospitals	Nurses	155			−				
Control—defense	McGowan et al. (1999)	AUS	Psychiatric hospitals	Nurses	70		+					
Control—combination	Ore (2002)*	AUS	Disability care institutions	Professionals employed in disability care institutions	358			+		+		Costs+
Control—combination	van Rixtel et al. (1997)	NL	Psychiatric hospitals	Not known	38		=	=				Perceived security+

Comparison	Reference	Country	Setting	Participants	N					Other outcomes
Control—combination	Infantino and Musingo (1985)	US	Psychiatric hospitals	Nurses	96	+	−	=		Relevance for job+
Control—combination	Hurlebaus and Link (1997)	US	Psychiatric hospitals	Nurses	23	+	=			
Control—combination	Allen and Tynan (2000)	UK	Disability care institutions	Professionals employed in disability care institution	109	+	+			Aggressiveness of workers−
Control—combination	Thackrey (1987)	US	Psychiatric hospitals	All professionals	106	+				
Control—combination	Carmel and Hunter (1990)	US	Psychiatric hospitals	All professionals	744	=	−			
Control—combination	Rice et al. (1985)	CDN	Psychiatric wards	Nurses	88	+	+	=		Skills+
Control—combination	Fitzwater and Gates (2002)	US	Nursing homes	Nurses	20	+	−			
Control—de-escalation Combination No intervention	Philips and Rudestam (1995)	US	Psychiatric hospitals	Not known	24	−[b]				Aggressiveness of workers− Skills+

(Continued)

Table 1. Studies Included in the Systematic Review—Cont'd

Type of Study	Authors	Country	Setting	Participants	N	Knowledge	Feelings of Security	Incidents	Injuries	Lost Work Days	Coercive Measures	Miscellaneous
Pre–post—deescalation	Wilkinson (1999)	US	Geronto-psychiatric wards	Nurses	32			+	−			
Pre–post—deescalation	Colenda and Hamer (1991)	US	Geronto-psychiatric hospitals	All professionals	n.k.			−				
Pre–post—deescalation	Hoeffer et al. (1997)	US	Geronto-psychiatric nursing homes	Nurses	n.k.			−				
Pre–post—deescalation	Maxfield et al. (1996)	US	Geronto-psychiatric hospitals	Nurses	96	+		−				
Pre–post—deescalation	Shah and De (1998)	UK	Geronto-psychiatric ward	Nurses	15			−				Aggression rate—
Pre–post—deescalation	Feldt and Ryden (1992)	US	Nursing homes	Nurses	17	=						
Pre–post—defense	St. Thomas Psychiatric Hospital (1976)	CDN	Psychiatric hospitals	All professionals	n. k.			−		−		

Design	Study	Country	Setting	Population	N					Costs	Injury induced absenteeism
Pre–post— defense	Forster et al. (1999)	US	Psychiatric hospitals	All professionals	n. k.				–		
Pre–post— defense	Mortimer (1995)	UK	Locked acute wards	All professionals	23		–				
Pre–post— defense	Parkes (1996)	UK	Psychiatric wards	Nurses	n. k.			+[c]			
Pre–post— combination	Martin (1995)	US	Psychiatric hospitals	Nurses	n. k.		+	–		–	
Pre–post— combination	Sjöström et al. (2001)	SWE	Psychiatric hospitals	All professionals	185		=[d]				=
Pre–post— combination	Hagan and Sayers (1995)	CDN	Nursing homes	Nurses	134		–				
Pre–post— combination	Gertz (1980)	US	Psychiatric hospitals	All professionals	317		–				
Pre–post— combination	Lehmann et al. (1983)	US	Psychiatric hospitals	All professionals	144	+	+				
Pre–post— combination	Allen et al. (1997)	UK	Disability care institutions	Professionals employed in disability care institution	n. k.		–[e]	–			
Pre–post— combination	Calabro et al. (2002)	US	Psychiatric hospitals	Nurses	118	+	–				

(Continued)

Table 1. Studies Included in the Systematic Review—Cont'd

Type of Study	Authors	Country	Setting	Participants	N	Knowledge	Feelings of Security	Incidents	Injuries	Lost Work Days	Coercive Measures	Miscellaneous
Pre–post—combination	Baker and Bissmire (2000)	UK	Disability care institutions	Professionals employed in disability care institution	13	+	+	=				
Pre–post—combination	Needham, Abderhalden, Meer et al. (2004)	CH	Psychiatric hospitals	Nurses	n.k.			=			—	
Pre–post—combination	Perkins and Leadbetter (2002)	UK	School for children with an intelligence deficiency	Employees of a school	14	+	+					
Pre–post—combination	Paterson et al. (1992)	UK	Not known	Nurses	25	+						Job stress- Skills+
Pre–post—combination	McDonnell (1997)	UK	Disability care institutions	Professionals employed in disability care institution	21	+	+					
Pre–post—combination	Ilkiw-Lavalle et al. (2002)	AUS	Psychiatric wards	All professionals	103	+						Satisfaction with training+

[a]Decrease of severe incidents not included in the total sum
[b]Only combination training vs. deescalation, where combination training yielded more favorable results
[c]Increase statistically insignificant
[d]Divergent results on using two different questionnaires
[e]Trend statistically not significant

Legend

Study type
RCT—randomized controlled trial
Control—control group design
Pre–post—pre–post-test study design
Defense—training of physical defense techniques
Deescalation—training of deescalation techniques
Combination—combined training of defense and deescalation techniques

Signs employed
+ Increase
– Decrease
= No change

Abbreviations
N = Number; n.k. = not known

2.4.4 Studies Comparing Aggressive Incidents Employing a Pre–Post Measure

The majority of studies examining defense techniques (Mortimer, 1995; St. Thomas Psychiatric Hospital, 1976) and deescalation strategies (Colenda & Hamer, 1991; Hoeffer, Rader, McKenzie, Lavelle, & Stewart, 1997; Maxfield, Lewis, & Cannon, 1996; Shah & De, 1998) registered a decrease in aggressive incidents. The same phenomenon could be observed for staff injuries (except Parkes, 1996), lost working days and coercive measures (Forster, Cavness, & Phelps, 1999; St. Thomas Psychiatric Hospital; Wilkinson, 1999). However, this trend was not confirmed in programs combining deescalation and defense training as evidenced by the heterogeneous results. Several studies reported a decline (Allen, McDonald, Dunn, & Doyle, 1997; Calabro, Mackey, & Williams, 2002; Gertz, 1980; Hagan & Sayers, 1995) whereas others came to the contrary conclusion (Lehmann, Padilla, Clark, & Loucks, 1983; Martin, 1995) or could not detect any change at all (Baker & Bissmire, 2000; Needham, Abderhalden, Meer et al., 2004; Sjöström, Eder, Malm, & Beskow, 2001).

2.4.5 Studies Comparing Staff Knowledge/Confidence by Means of Interviews Employing a Pre–Post Measure

All reviewed studies of this type, with one exception, reporting no significant changes (Feldt & Ryden, 1992), registered positive effects of training programs on staff knowledge and confidence (Baker & Bissmire, 2000; Calabro et al., 2002; Ilkiw-Lavalle, Grenyer, & Graham, 2002; Lehmann et al., 1983; Maxfield et al., 1996; McDonnell, 1997; Paterson, Turnbull, & Aitken, 1992; Perkins & Leadbetter, 2002).

3   DISCUSSION

From a methodological point of view the quality of the studies regarding aggression management in health care institutions and in services for the disabled is rather poor. As remarked on elsewhere (Allen, 2001; NICE, 2005; UKCC, 2001), institutions and clinicians are forced to draw practical conclusions on the basis of poor empirical evidence. However, it must be noted that investigations of high quality are very intensive in terms of costs and resources. Furthermore, training programs in aggression management are complex interventions and cannot be standardized in the same manner as interventional studies in other domains (e.g., pharmacological trials).

Local policy and conditions, e.g., the support of the intervention offered by stakeholders in the institutions, play an important role. Due to the fact that training courses are offered at the institutional level, strong study designs such as randomized controlled trials are difficult to conduct because the unit of randomization is an organizational unit (the hospital or ward) giving rise to a small number of "participants" and thus prone to bias (Needham, Abderhalden, Haug et al., 2004).

Interestingly, no major differences were found between case control and pre–post-test studies. However, studies employing questionnaires produced more positive results than studies providing more "hard" data such as incidence rates and effects of aggression on carers. This finding is corroborated by other reviews (Allen, 2001; NICE, 2005; UKCC, 2001).

In spite of these methodological difficulties two trends can be detected. Many studies employing different interventions, study designs, and settings come to the same conclusion that training courses seem to enhance participants' knowledge and subjective feelings of security for handling aggressive situations. Thus, it seems reasonable to interpret this finding as relatively sound. The second trend is that no robust conclusions can be drawn on aggression rates and the consequences of aggression, e.g., lost days of work or injuries. However, the first randomized controlled trial in this area (Needham, Abderhalden, Haug et al., 2004) demonstrated slightly positive results which may infer that the effects of training courses may lead to a reduction of severe attacks and coercive measures.

The results of this review do not allow any conclusions regarding any possible link between improved knowledge and subjective feelings of security on the one hand and modifications of performance and reduced incidence rates of aggression on the other. Indeed, some studies reporting improved knowledge show an increase in aggression rates (Rice et al., 1985). This finding may accrue from the fact that participants are trained at the individual level, while effects are generally measured at the organizational level. In order to induce change at the organizational level, all individuals should have the same commitment and display a similar performance. Furthermore, coordination between trained participants is vital because interventions to handle aggressive situations usually involve more than one person. Arguing along these lines, it seems imperative that all members of the organization be equally committed and that the institutional structures are adapted to the intervention.

Another methodological difficulty, to which no answer can be offered here, is the time frame between the training course and the measurement of its effect. Short time frames, e.g., one week, may inflate positive findings, while long time frames, e.g., years, may neglect the influence of extraneous variables. Also, when using long time frames the initial effect of the training may diminish due, for example, to personnel turnover.

One of the most prominent difficulties is the way in which aggressive incidents and their effects are registered and enumerated. Some authors employ changes in reporting behavior (for example, Colenda & Hamer, 1991; Ore, 2002) which may on grounds of selective perception offer a distorted picture. Possibly the improved knowledge of aggression may incite persons trained in aggression management to report behavior they had not previously perceived as aggression. A study by Arnetz and Arnetz (2000) demonstrated a significantly higher willingness to report aggression. The training probably induces a higher sensitization to aggressive behavior and precursors thereof, which in effect is a desirable effect per se.

Better prevention of violence is dependent on employees' capacity to detect pending violent behavior. Research on this subject would pose serious methodological problems which could only be overcome by utilizing innovative empirical procedures. A possible but quite expensive solution in terms of time investment might consist of employing objective external observers participating in the study. This would be possible in pre–post measure designs as well as in control-group studies.

4 CONCLUSIONS

The international literature on evaluation studies as well as texts on evidence-based medicine conclude that social interventions, like training programs in aggression management, are particularly difficult to evaluate in terms of their efficiency (Petticrew, 2003). The more specific the social intervention examined, the higher the likelihood of detecting significant results. Interventions including training programs do, however, examine complex work and organizational environments involving multiple influencing variables. For an adequate evaluation of aggression management training programs it is most important, therefore, to include not only the quality of existing evidence in the field but also possible "non intervention" alternatives, e.g., the reluctance to introduce aggression management training in psychiatric wards. From an ethical point of view such evaluational research must be conducted before considerations on a training programs' cost effectiveness are made (Grades of Recommendation, 2004).

The results of this review demonstrate that staff knowledge and subjective feelings of security in handling aggressive incidents may be improved through training programs. It is, however, less evident as to what influence aggression management programs might have on the rate of aggressive incidents on wards. Some studies report an increase of postintervention aggression rates. But this might be due to a changed aggression perception of staff after a training program. It is extremely difficult to prove that aggression management training programs do actually reduce aggression rates. Based on the evidence of this review we can, however, conclude that at least no negative effects on aggression rates were observed.

These findings give rise to the following question: If we assume that aggression management training programs can augment subjective feelings of the security of staff but cannot reduce aggression rates, would this be sufficient to justify the introduction of aggression management programs? In our opinion the added value of an increase in security for handling aggressive situations should not be underestimated. In fact this may be one of the most important contributions in improving the management of aggressive situations on wards. Thus the introduction of comprehensive aggression management training in mental health and disability care institutions should therefore be recommended. Future empirical research will certainly need to examine the effects of aggression management programs in more robust studies with larger sample sizes. Evidence-based medicine adheres to the principle that "absence of evidence is not evidence of absence" (Alderson, 2004). This vantage point has also been adopted in the guidelines of the British *National Institute of Clinical Excellence* (NICE) for the short term management of aggression in psychiatric wards (NICE, 2005). Although the authors of these guidelines could not find any relevant evidence for the effectiveness of training programs to reduce aggression rates they are in favor of the introduction of training interventions including deescalation strategies, physical defense, and coercive measures. These recommendations were based on the best available clinical evidence and match the reported evidence from most of the primary studies reviewed in this article. Comprehensive aggression management programs should empower staff to adopt adequate management strategies for any type of aggressive patient behavior. Training programs should hence include deescalation strategies as well as training in physical defense techniques.

If, and only if, future empirical research produces significant evidence that aggression management training does cause more harm than benefit, should the above recommendations be reviewed.

REFERENCES

Alderson, P. (2004). Absence of evidence is not evidence of absence. *British Medical Journal, 328,* 476–477.

Allen, D. (2001). *Training careers in physical intervention: Research towards evidence-based practice.* Kidderminster: British Institute for Learning Disabilities.

Allen, D., McDonald, L., Dunn, C., & Doyle, T. (1997). Changing care staff approaches to the prevention and management of aggressive behavior in a residential treatment unit for persons with mental retardation and challenging behavior. *Reserch in Developmental Disabilities, 18,* 101–112.

Allen, D., & Tynan, H. (2000). Responding to aggressive behavior: Impact of training on staff members' knowledge and confidence. *Mental Retardation, 38,* 97–104.

Anke, M., Bojack, B., Krämer, G., & Seiaelberg, K. (2003). *Deeskalationsstrategien in der psychiatrischen Arbeit.* Bonn: Psychiatrie-Verlag.

Arnetz, J. E., & Arnetz, B. B. (2000). Implementation and evaluation of a practical intervention program for dealing with violence towards health care workers. *Journal of Advanced Nursing, 31,* 668–680.

Baker, P. A., & Bissmire, D. (2000). A pilot study of the use of physical intervention in the crisis management of people with intellectual disabilities who present challenging behavior. *Journal of Applied Reserch in Intellectual Disabilities, 13,* 38–45.

Calabro, K., Mackey, T. A., & Williams, S. (2002). Evaluation of training designed to prevent and manage patient violence. *Issues in Mental Health Nursing, 23,* 3–15.

Carmel, H., & Hunter, M. (1990). Compliance with training in managing assaultive behavior and injuries from inpatient violence. *Hospital and Community Psychiatry, 41,* 558–560.

Colenda, C. C., & Hamer, R. M. (1991). Antecedents and interventions for aggressive behavior of patients at a gero-psychiatric state hospital. *Hospital and Community Psychiatry, 42,* 287–292.

Fähndrich, E., & Ketelsen, R. (2004). Die medikamentöse Behandlung des psychiatrischen Notfalls. In Ketelsen, R., Schulz, M., & Zechert, C., (Eds.), *Seelische Krise und Aggressivität: Der Umgang mit Deeskalation und Zwang* (pp. 80–88). Bonn: Psychiatrie-Verlag.

Farrell, G., & Cubit, K. (2005). Nurses under threat: A comparison of content of 28 aggression management programs. *International Journal of Mental Health Nursing, 14,* 44–53.

Feldt, K. S., & Ryden, M. B. (1992). Aggressive behavior: Educating nursing assistants. *Journal of Gerontological Nursing, 18*(5), 3–12.

Fitzwater, E. L., & Gates, D. M. (2002). Testing an intervention to reduce assaults on nursing assistants in nursing homes: a pilot study. *Geriatric Nursing, 23,* 18–23.

Forster, P. L., Cavness, C., & Phelps, M. A. (1999). Staff training decreases use of seclusion and restraint in an acute psychiatric setting. *Archives of Psychiatric Nursing, 13,* 269–271.

Fuchs, J. M. (1998). Kontrollierter Umgang mit physischer Gewalt und Aggression in der Psychiatrie? Bericht über ein Praxisseminar. In: Sauter, D., & Richter, D. (Eds.), *Gewalt in der psychiatrischen Pflege* (pp. 59–72). Bern: Huber.

Gertz, B. (1980). Training for prevention of assaultive behavior in a psychiatric setting. *Hospital and Community Psychiatry, 31,* 628–630.

Grades of Recommendation, Development, and Evaluation (GRADE) Working Group, (2004). Grading quality of evidence and strength of recommendations. *British Medical Journal, 328,* 1490–1494.

Grube, M. (2001). Aggressivität bei psychiatrischen Patienten: Einflussmöglichkeiten durch ein Selbstschutztraining. *Der Nervenarzt, 72,* 867–871.

Hagan, B. F., & Sayers, D. (1995). When caring leaves bruises: The effects of staff education on resident aggression. *Journal of Gerontological Nursing, 21*(11), 7–16.

Hoeffer, B., Rader, J., McKenzie, D., Lavelle, M., & Stewart, B. (1997). Reducing aggressive behavior during bathing cognitively impaired nursing home residents. *Journal of Gerontological Nursing, 25*(5), 16–23.

Hurlebaus, A. E., & Link, S. (1997). The effects of an aggressive behavior management program on nurses' levels of knowledge, confidence and safety. *Journal for Nurses in Staff Development, 13,* 260–265.

Ilkiw-Lavalle, O., Grenyer, B. F. S., & Graham, L. (2002). Does prior training and staff occupation influence knowledge acquisition from an aggression management training program? *International Journal of Mental Health Nursing, 11,* 233–239.

Infantino, J. A., & Musingo, S.-Y. (1985). Assaults and injuries among staff with and without training in aggression control techniques. *Hospital and Community Psychiatry, 36,* 1312–1314.

Jambunathan, J., & Bellaire, K. (1996). Evaluating staff use if crisis prevention intervention techniques: A pilot study. *Issues in Mental Health Nursing, 17,* 541–558.

Lee, S., Gerberich, S. G., Waller, L. A., Anderson, A., & McGovern, P. (1999). Work-related assault injuries among nurses. *Epidemiology, 10,* 685–691.

Lehmann, L. S., Padilla, M., Clark, S., & Loucks, S. (1983). Training personnel on the prevention and management of violent behavior. *Hospital and Community Psychiatry, 34,* 40–43.

Martin, K. H. (1995). Improving staff safety through an aggression management program. *Archives of Psychiatric Nursing, 11,* 211–215.

Mason, T., & Chandley, M. (1999). *Managing violence and aggression: A manual for nurses and health care workers.* Edinburgh: Churchill Livingstone.

Maxfield, M. C., Lewis, R. E., & Cannon, S. (1996). Training staff to prevent aggressive behavior of cognitively-impaired elderly patients during bathing and grooming. *Journal of Gerontological Nursing, 22,* 37–43.

McDonnell, A. (1997). Training care staff to manage challenging behavior: An evaluation of a three day training course. *British Journal of Developmental Disabilities, 43,* 156–162.

McGowan, S., Wynaden, D., Harding, N., Yassine, A., & Parker, J. (1999). Staff confidence in dealing with aggressive patients: A benchmark exercise. *The Australian and New Zealand Journal of Mental Health Nursing, 8,* 104–108.

Mortimer, A. (1995). Reducing violence on a secure ward. *Psychiatric Bulletin, 19,* 605–608.

Needham, I., Abderhalden, C., Haug, H. J., Dassen, T., Halfens, R. J. G., & Fischer, J. E. (2004). The effect of a training course in aggression management on the prevalence of aggression and coercive measures in inpatient psychiatric settings: A randomized controlled trial. In: I. Needham (Ed.), *A nursing intervention to handle patient aggression: The effectiveness of a training course in the management of aggression (PhD-Thesis)* (pp. 109–124). Maastricht, NL: Universitaire Press Maastricht.

Needham, I., Abderhalden, C., Meer, R., Dassen, T., Haug, H. J., & Halfens, R. J. G. (2004). The effectiveness of two interventions in the management of patient violence in acute mental inpatient settings. *Journal of Psychiatric and Mental Health Nursing, 11,* 595–601.

NICE. (2005). *Clinical practice guidelines for violence: The short-term management of disturbed/violent behavior in psychiatric in-patient and emergency departments guideline.* National Institute for Clinical Excellence.

Nijman, H. L. I., Merckelbach, H. L. G. J., Allertz, W. F. F., & à Campo, J. M. L. G. (1997). Prevention of aggressive incidents on a closed ward. *Psychiatric Services, 48,* 694–698.

Ore, T. (2002). Workplace assault management training: An outcome evaluation. *Journal of Healthcare Protection Management, 18*(2), 61–93.

Parkes, J. (1996). Control and restraint training: A study of its effectiveness in a medium secure psychiatric unit. *Journal of Forensic Psychiatry, 7,* 525–534.

Paterson, B., Turnbull, J., & Aitken, I. (1992). An evaluation of a training course in the short-term management of violence. *Nurse Education Today, 12,* 368–375.

Perkins, J., & Leadbetter, D. (2002). An evaluation of aggression management training in a special educational setting. *Emotional and Behavioral Difficulties, 7,* 19–34.

Petticrew, M. (2003). Why certain systematic reviews reach uncertain conclusions. *British Medical Journal, 326,* 756–758.

Philips, D., & Rudestam, K. E. (1995). Effect of nonviolent self-defense training on male psychiatric staff members' aggression and fear. *Psychiatric Services, 46,* 164–168.

Poster, E. C. (1996). A multinational study of psychiatric nursing staff beliefs and concerns about work safety and patient assaults. *Archives of Psychiatric Nursing, 10,* 365–373.

Rice, M. F., Helzel, M. F., Varney, G. W., & Quinsey, V. I. (1985). Crisis prevention and intervention training for psychiatric hospital staff. *American Journal of Community Psychology, 13,* 289–304.

Richter, D., & Berger, K. (2001). Patientenübergriffe auf Mitarbeiter: Eine prospektive Untersuchung der Häufigkeit, Situationen und Folgen. *Der Nervenarzt, 72,* 693–699.

Richter, D., Fuchs, J. M., & Bergers, K.-H. (2001). *Konfliktmanagement in psychiatrischen Einrichtungen.* Münster/Düsseldorf: Gemeindeunfallversicherungsverband Westfalen-Lippe, Rheinischer Gemeindeunfallversicherungsverband, Landesunfallkasse Nordrhein-Westfalen.

van Rixtel, A. M. J., Nijman, H. L. I., & Jansen, A. (1997). Aggressie en psychiatrie: Heeft training effect? *Verpleegkunde, 12,* 111–119.

Robson, L. S., Shannon, H. S., Goldenhar, L. M., & Hale, A. R. (2001). *Guide to evaluating the effectiveness of strategies for preventing work injuries: How to show whether a safety intervention really works* (No. DHHS (NIOSH) Publication No. 2001–119). Cincinnati, USA: National Institute for Occupational Safety and Health.

Shah, A., & De, T. (1998). The effect of an educational intervention package about aggressive behavior directed at the nursing staff on a continuing care psycho-geriatric ward. *International Journal of Geriatric Psychiatry, 13,* 35–40.

Sjöström, N., Eder, D. N., Malm, U., & Beskow, J. (2001). Violence and its prediction at a psychiatric hospital. *European Psychiatry, 16,* 459–465.

Smooth, S. L., & Gonzales, J. L. (1995). Cost-effective communication skills training for state hospital employees. *Psychiatric Services, 46,* 819–822.

Steinert, T. (2004). Indikation von Zwangsmaßnahmen in psychiatrischen Kliniken. In: Ketelsen, R., Schulz, M., & Zechert, C. (Eds.), *Seelische Krise und Aggressivität* (pp. 44–52). Bonn: Psychiatrie-Verlag.

Steinert, T., Vogel, W. D., Beck, M., & Kehlmann, S. (1991). Aggressionen psychiatrischer Patienten in der Klinik. *Psychiatrische Praxis 25,* 221–226.

St. Thomas Psychiatric Hospital. (1976). A program for the prevention and management of disturbed behavior. *Hospital and Community Psychiatry, 27,* 724–727.

Thackrey, M. (1987). Clinician confidence in coping with patient aggression: Assessment and enhancement. *Professional Psychology, Research and Practice, 18,* 57–60.

UKCC. (2001). *The Recognition, prevention, and therapeutic management of violence in mental health care.* United Kingdom Central Council for Nursing, Midwifery and Health Visiting.

Weisman, R. L., & Lamberti, J. S. (2002). Violence prevention and safety training for case management services. *Community Mental Health Journal, 38,* 339–348.

Whittington, R., & Wykes, T. (1996). An evaluation of staff training in psychological techniques for the management of patient aggression. *Journal of Clinical Nursing, 5,* 257–261.

Wilkinson, C. L. (1999). An evaluation of an educational program on the management of assaultive behavior. *Journal of Gerontological Nursing, 25*(4), 6–11.

V

THE ORGANIZATIONAL CONTEXT

12

Locating Training Within a Strategic Organizational Response to Aggression and Violence

KEVIN J. MCKENNA AND BRODIE PATERSON

1 BACKGROUND

Work-related violence is a serious problem within healthcare that diminishes the quality of working life for staff, compromises organizational effectiveness, and ultimately impacts negatively on the provision of services to users. Recognition of the increased risk in mental health services imposes professional, statutory, and moral imperatives upon employers to provide staff with safe, clinically effective training in the management of work-related violence.

While increasing recognition of the problem has been a welcome development, this increased awareness has frequently resulted in responses in which the provision of training has been regarded as the predominant, if not only, requirement. This "training as singular solution" response has been identified to be potentially problematic in that, while it represents an organization's dawning recognition of the problem, the emphasis on the interpersonal dimensions of violence inherent in such approaches often neglect the wider structural dimensions at both societal (Swanson et al., 2002), and organizational levels (Colton, 2004).

Such over-emphasis on the role of training can foster the creation of organizational "reactive responses" in which crisis management takes precedence over crisis prevention, and meaningful opportunities for clinical and organizational learning are lost. At best, what is achieved is a partial response to the problem, while at worst the result may be the erroneous illusion that the problem has actually been addressed.

Paterson, McComish, and Bradley (1999) suggested that organizations have somewhat unfortunately tended to adopt one of two responses to the problem of workplace violence, neither of which is helpful. The first is "avoidance" i.e., simply to ignore the problem which, while quite obviously problematic was, until comparatively recently, a commonplace strategy in many areas of health and social care. The second is to acknowledge that a problem exists but to frame the problem either solely or largely as a problem of individual staff skill deficits which are remediable by "training." Leadbetter (2003) has described an incremental framework of stages through which organizations typically progress toward an eventual integration of training into an overall organizational response (See Figure 1). Such progress is not, however, inevitable and organizations can, and indeed do, regress.

The International Labor Organization (ILO, 2000), has urged caution in the utilization of over-simplistic solutions to the issue of workplace violence generally and particularly those which may be over-reliant on training. They advocate the adoption of what they have described as "high road" approaches characterized by the notion of the "smart organizations," i.e., those in which learning is a function of continuous reflection on current experiences which develops the organizations capacity to meet existing and future demands (Senge et al., 1999). Such learning requires detailed attention to the nature of the problem of violence in terms of both individual and organizational dimensions (Colton, 2004). It has been suggested that what is required is a "total organizational response" in which a partnership between the organization, employees, representative associations, and individual workers is necessary (Cox & Cox, 1993).

Despite potential limitations, the provision of training will continue to play a central role in most organizations efforts to manage aggression and violence. The provision of training, however, poses a unique challenge to both healthcare professionals and organizations. For professionals, the uniqueness of this challenge rests on the premise that understanding, managing, and responding to violence within healthcare must be situated within the context of the unique relationship that exists between the protagonist and victim. This contextual approach to the problem requires the consideration of the professional, legal, legislative, moral, and ethical parameters within which this care relationship exists. For organizations, the challenge is how, strategically, to locate training within an organizational framework which adequately and equally addresses the concerns of all involved, while meeting their statutory health and safety obligations and addressing their corporate risk management function.

For a variety of reasons, organizations have sometimes not fully appreciated the complexities involved in understanding aggression and violence as being embedded within a professional relationship, which has resulted in the provision of training in isolation from the context in which the problem occurs (Leadbetter and Paterson 2005).

- Denial: An "If you can't stand the heat get out the kitchen" blame culture. Staff who raise concerns are often seen as over anxious and/or incompetent. "Whistle blowers" and activists are often scapegoats. Violent incidents are seen as isolated events, predominantly caused by individual failure, or by chance. No agency policies exist. Responses are haphazard and ad hoc.
- Ignoring: The risks of service user violence is perceived but not addressed. This is often a result of unhelpful beliefs and ideologies and/or fear of exposing the problem. Recording and reporting are not encouraged and active measures to suppress the debate may be imposed. High absenteeism/sickness absence. Focus on crisis management, rather than strategic service delivery.
- Awakening: Risks are acknowledged, but within an "it's part of the job" culture. Resistance to formal action and a fragmented agency response. Causal connections are not perceived. No overall management responsibility. The problem is "owned" by front-line staff and often the agency training section. Victims can share experiences and "whistle blowers" can speak out. Support systems are criticized. Consultants become involved. Policies are developed. These are often vague, unrealistic, and focus on what staff cannot do, rather than the specification of acceptable responses. "Reductionist" training is introduced. Training "gurus" are given credibility. Lack of routine post-incident "debriefing" limits agency and individual learning.
- Breakthrough: Management studies the costs and consequences and concludes that a different approach is required. One coordinating manager assumes responsibility. Policies are developed but remain fragmented. A more rational approach to the problem is adopted. Diversification of training, holistic training. Training "gurus" lose credibility. Outcomes assume importance.
- Management: Practices and procedures are amended. Integration of different policies. Attention is given to warnings and causes and increased understanding of causal chains. Senior Management assumed responsibility.
- Integration: Safety is integrated in all activities. Pro-active approach at all levels. Aggression is seen as directly related to work tasks, rather than individual staff qualities. Effective liaison with service users. A total organizational response model is implemented.

Source: Leadbetter (2003).

Figure 1. Organisational consciousness in responding to violence.

While other chapters have addressed the need for attention to the problem of aggression and violence at an individual level, this chapter will focus on the problem from an organizational perspective. In practice however, these approaches must be complementary. While it must be stressed that the provision of training is only one component of any total organizational response, this chapter will specifically address the problem of how to locate training within such wider integrated responses. An enabling framework is presented which describes how organizations can embed training in a strategic approach that addresses the concerns of key stakeholders, including those from clinical practice, health and safety, risk management, and organizational policy perspectives.

2 TRAINING

The Council of Europe recommendations *Concerning the Protection of the Human Rights and Dignity of Persons with Mental Disorder* (2004), binds member states that provide training to staff working with persons with mental disorder with training in:

- Protecting the dignity, human rights, and fundamental freedoms of persons with mental disorder
- Understanding, prevention, and control of violence
- Measures to avoid the use of restraint or seclusion
- The limited circumstances in which different methods of restraint or seclusion may be justified, taking into account the benefits and risks entailed, and the correct application of such measures

The extent to which these recommendations have been translated into practice varies greatly between, and within, healthcare organizations. One reason may be that it is widely acknowledged that the research base in support of such training continues to be inadequate. Despite positive indications from some key studies of significant potential benefits (Richter & Needham, 2005), other studies have suggested that training can have negative impacts. On balance, however, current professional opinion offers qualified support for training (Royal College of Psychiatrists, 1998).

A further reason, however, for this apparent failure in many settings, is that organizations have had to struggle with the lack of clarity surrounding the structures, processes, and content of training programs, and how to integrate these into a cohesive organizational strategy.

The lack of established training structures and the absence of formal regulations governing the provision of training have been highlighted as concerns by reports from both professional bodies and public enquiries (Blofeld, 2003; United Kingdom Central Council, 2002). Estimates suggest that in the UK alone there are now more than 700 training providers and more than 100 different systems of training (National Institute of Clinical Excellence, 2005; Tucker, 2005). This diversity of training providers and approaches is further complicated by the absence of systematically collected evidence regarding the content of training or the background and qualifications of providers (UKCC, 2002). Subsequently, organizations face the dilemma of how to reconcile the urgent need to provide training, with the controversy and lack of consensus as to what constitutes safe, effective, and acceptable practice. This is especially apparent in the organization's struggle to select physical intervention training as Paterson et al. (1999, p. 46), cautioned: "while some programs are excellent, others are of extremely dubious quality."

In addition to structural issues there are also procedural concerns. A recent UK report, while acknowledging improvements in some services resulting from isolated instances of good practice, expressed concern at the huge variation which exists within and between trusts in the procedural organization of training. These concerns included the lack of standardization of content and the considerable variation with which staff were required to attend training. Furthermore the provision of "off the shelf" approaches to training, in the absence of any structured analysis of needs, has resulted in staff receiving training in which the content reflected the "experience and preference of the trainers rather than a rational analysis" of their training needs (National Audit Office, 2003, p. 24).

While the difficulties with training have received most attention within the UK (NAO, 2003; UKCC, 2002), their experience is not unique. A review within Irish healthcare concluded that training provision is currently unregulated, inconsistent, and often delivered without reference to staff practice settings. This has resulted in considerable financial, and human, resources being invested in some unproven methods of training which may not only be ineffectual from clinical and safety perspectives, but difficult to defend legally, professionally, or morally (McKenna, 2004).

Professional and organizational dissatisfaction have fueled considerable effort and significant advances in addressing these difficulties. Following the recommendations of the Bennett Inquiry (Blofeld, 2003) that a standardized national approach to training be established as a matter of urgency, the National Institute for Mental Health in England (NIMHE), undertook a major review of training within the UK and are now establishing an accreditation scheme for trainers (NICE, 2005). Other UK initiatives in the standardization of training content and the development of a service specific curriculum for mental health and disability services in particular, are major achievements which might address many of the current deficits and impact on training provision far beyond the geographical scope of their mandate.

While these initiatives are hugely encouraging in addressing some of the structural inadequacies, there has been less attention paid to the processes involved in providing training at organizational level. This is unfortunate in that, while accreditation may monitor the quality of providers and standardization ensures the quality of content, the challenge for organizations remains how to effectively translate these innovations into practice.

At national level, effectively addressing the provision of training requires the achievement of a collective and collaborative effort between employers, employees, professional, and statutory bodies (ILO, 2002). Within organizations, the integration of training requires clear and determined leadership (Colton, 2004), and the adaptation of a strategic approach (Leadbetter, 2003). While the rationale for a clearly-led, unified approach seems intuitively obvious, achieving such cohesion within organizations seems to have been difficult to accomplish in practice. Cameron (2001) suggests that public sector organizations achieve only limited success in genuine joint-working as a function of individual units being focused on singular rather than unified agendas, particularly when singular agendas are overlaid with professional boundaries and different statutory responsibilities.

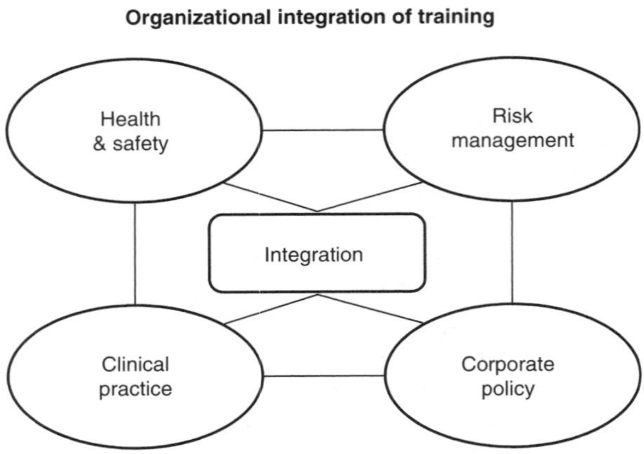

Organizational integration of training

Figure 2. Organizational integration of training (McKenna, 2005).

An alternative strategy in an organization's quest for a unified response is the adaptation of the balanced scorecard approach developed by Kaplan and Norton (1996), for the purpose of increasing organizational performance. Essentially the balanced scorecard is a management technique which improves systems approaches to problems by identifying the critical success factors necessary to achieve goals, and addressing these through balanced attention to each perspective (Hepworth, 1998). While originating in the business world, this approach has been successfully adapted to public services (De Waal, 2003), within the health services (Moulin, 2004), and to the design and provision of training (McKenna, 2005).

Effective organizational training strategies must balance the provision of safe, professional, and clinically skilful management of the violent client with the safety needs of the staff, and the organizations' statutory health and safety, and corporate risk management obligations. Subsequently, the critical success factors necessary for the organizational integration of training requires that it adequately and equally meets the needs of these key stakeholders, including those from clinical practice, health and safety, risk management, and corporate policy perspectives. The Matrix of Organizational Training Effectiveness (McKenna, 2005) describes an enabling framework which can structure organizations' efforts to effectively embed training within a governance framework by recognizing the central role of each of these perspectives (Figure 2).

3   HEALTH, SAFETY, AND WELFARE PERSPECTIVE

Employers have a statutory obligation to provide a safe workplace for their employees, and others. The indisputable risks associated with aggression and violence within healthcare, and within mental health services in particular, pose a clear organizational health and safety obligation which must be addressed within any integrated response.

Two critical considerations for healthcare organizations from a health and safety perspective are the magnitude of the problem, and the service-specific nature of the associated risks. It has been reported that US healthcare workers are at a greatly increased risk of nonfatal assault (NIOSH, 1996), with hospital workers risk of assault more than four times that of staff in private sector industries (BLS, 1999). Similarly, the Australian health service has the highest rate of occupational workplace violence (Zinn, 2001), while in Sweden, 60% of all occupational injuries resulting from work-related violence reported to the relevant statutory agency, occurred within the health and social services sector (Menckel & Viitasara, 2002). Within the Irish health services, assault is the third leading cause of accidents for staff, accounting for 14.9% of all occupational injuries reported in 2000 (Advisory Committee on Health Services Sector, 2001). In England, 95,501 assaults were reported on healthcare staff in 2002 (NAO, 2003), with a nurse's occupational risk of physical assault second only to security and protective services personnel (Budd, 2001).

Inherent in this recognition of the problem as a service-specific hazard is the legislative mandate that organizations evaluate the associated risks, provide staff with the necessary training to mitigate against identified risks, and to provide staff who are exposed to aggression and violence with the necessary support.

European Health and Safety legislation has evolved from a collection of statutory instruments specific to hazardous materials, to the adaptation of broader principles which were enshrined in the adaptation of the 1989 European Framework directive on safety and health (Byrne, 2001). While the issue of work-related violence is not specifically mentioned within this framework, or within the legislation of individual countries, there are highly relevant obligations implied under the general duty clause of the legislation. This clause obligates employers to exercise all due care in assessing risks to safety and health within the place of work which are likely to result in accident or injury, and to put in place all reasonably practicable protective and preventive measures to minimize identified risks.

This duty to assess risks has been made explicit in many countries in the obligation to conduct a written assessment of risks to employees which should be subject to periodic review, both as a matter of routine, and in response to significant changes in the workplace. From this assessment, employers must then produce a safety statement which highlights the identified risks, outlines the preventive and protective measures in place, and the procedures for any related emergency circumstances (Safety, Health, and Welfare at Work Act, 2005).

One clearly explicit preventive strategy is the obligation of employers, in so far as is reasonably practical, to provide staff with the information and training necessary to ensure their safety which should, similarly, be subject to periodic review as a matter of routine, and adapted to take account of new or changed risk situations. Where employers seek assistance in providing such training they must ensure that those engaged for this purpose possess the relevant knowledge, experience, and competence to do so. The "reasonably practicable" duty requires that employers undertake all measures up to the point at which any further measures would be grossly disproportionate in regard to the unusual, unforeseeable, and exceptional nature of any other circumstance or occurrence (Safety, Health, and Welfare at Work Act, 2005).

While failure to comply with available guidelines on the management of aggression and violence may not, in itself, be a statutory offence, health and safety authorities have pointed to their reliance on the general duty clause for enforcement authority (Occupational Safety and Health Administration, 2004). Employers may be cited under this clause for failing to institute measures to prevent, or mitigate against, recognized hazards. Subsequently, prudent healthcare organizations must ensure that the provision of training in the management of aggression and violence satisfies the prevailing statutory obligations imposed by the relevant local legislation.

4   RISK MANAGEMENT PERSPECTIVE

Risk management initiatives within healthcare originated in response to the progressively escalating costs associated with litigation. Clinical risk management has evolved from these initiatives into a broader, clinical governance effort, which also encompasses patient and staff safety, and quality improvement efforts in service delivery (McElhinney & Heffernan, 2003). Clinical risk management strategies have incorporated successful initiatives from other high-risk industries including the practices of blame-free reporting and root cause analysis. The ultimate objective is to identify and analyze risks associated with the provision of services, and to put in place control measures, against which these mitigate, in order to ensure the safety of patients and staff, and the protection of the assets and reputation of the organization (McElhinney & Heffernan). This requires that organizations monitor the frequency and magnitude of actual occurrences in addition to near misses, i.e., potential adverse events in which the avoidance of harm was a function of chance rather than the effective utilization of control measures. Successfully managing risk requires that this effort is continuous, proactive, and systematic. The very significant risks to patients, staff, and organizations inherent in the management of aggression and violence have firmly placed this issue on the organizational risk management agenda.

There has been universal identification of the risks to staff. While there is consensus that minor injuries are frequent and major injuries are rare (McKenna, 2004), these result in high levels of absenteeism (Nijman, Bowers, Oud, & Jansen, 2005). For the few who suffer major injuries the personal, professional, and risk management consequences can be profound. An Irish study reported that 39 psychiatric nurses had retired prematurely between 1993 and 2001, and a further 35 nurses were on extended sick leave resulting directly from injuries sustained from work-related aggression and violence (Psychiatric Nurses Association, 2002). In rare cases there have been even more catastrophic consequences, as highlighted in the media coverage of fatalities of psychiatric nurses in both the UK and France.

In addition to the risks posed to staff, the management of aggression and violence may also pose serious risks to service users. A report to the US Senate reported 24 deaths, in the 1998 fiscal year, related to the use of restraint and seclusion within care settings, and speculated that in all likelihood many more deaths had occurred as few states maintained systematic records of such fatalities (General Accounting Office, 1999). Similar reviews within the UK (Paterson et al., 2003), reported 12 deaths related to physical restraint within the health and social care services, while the publication of the inquiry into the death of a patient within a UK acute psychiatric setting highlighted the associated risks, and the need for cohesive staff training (Blofeld, 2003).

In addition to the risk of physical injury, there is increasing evidence that aggression and violence is also a source of significant psychological distress for both patients and staff. Staff may experience a range of emotional, social, biophysiological, and cognitive reactions subsequent to occurrences of aggression and violence (Lanza, 1992), while patients have reported psychological distress, including reenactments of distressing memories, while being restrained and have experienced isolation, fear, and shame in the aftermath (Bonner, Lowe, Rawcliffe, & Wellman, 2002).

Apart from the serious physical and psychological risks, working continuously in an atmosphere of normative abuse and threat may be profoundly damaging to the confidence and morale of staff. This may impact on the quality of professional care in the future through the loss of expertise related to those individuals who either terminate employment or change clinical specialty subsequent to such exposure (Badger & Mullan, 2004).

From an organizational perspective there are also significant financial implications. The UK National Audit Office estimated that the direct cost of work-related violence to the NHS is likely to be at least £69 million per annum which, they point out, does not include human costs such as physical and psychological pain, increased stress levels, or the impact on staff confidence and retention (NAO, 2003). McKenna (2004) noted the absence of robust actuarial measures of the cost of the problem as remarkable but estimated the cost to be in millions of Euro on an annualized basis. While these reports have highlighted direct costs, others have described indirect costs, including the recruitment and orientation of new staff following resignations or disabilities, the extra burden placed on staff during absences, and lowered staff morale (Dawson, Johnson, Kehiayan, Kyanko, & Martinez, 1988). It has been argued that other cost factors should also be considered, such as the increasing number of successfully contested litigations challenging employers over their failure to provide a safe place of work, and for failing to protect third parties from injury (Blair & New, 1991).

Considering that many of these potentially serious risks are foreseeable, organizations may be challenged to demonstrate that all reasonable, practicable, control measures were put in place to satisfy the duty of care owed to patients and staff. While this duty includes multiple measures, one explicit control measure is the duty to ensure that staff are provided with the necessary knowledge and skills to ensure their competence to safely, and effectively, manage such occurrences. Consequently, from a risk management perspective, it is critical that the provision of training considers and addresses the inherent risks from the perspectives of the service user, the staff, and the organization.

5   THE PRACTICE PERSPECTIVE

The management of aggression and violence should not, however, be considered solely in the context of statutory obligations or organizational mandate. From a professional perspective, what is also demanded is the compassionate and skilful care of those involved which requires that staff are competent to recognize, assess, and intervene with individuals experiencing difficulty in controlling their behavior. More than twenty years ago Edwards and Reid (1983, p. 68), cautioned that to accept all violence by patients within mental settings as being inevitable is "fatalistic and nihilistic" and contended that violent behaviors are symptoms "crying out for treatment." Lion (1987, p. 883), suggested that the "compassionate and intelligent care" of patients experiencing difficulty in controlling their behavior demands that staff "be fully competent and skilled in the management" of such behaviors. These propositions raise two fundamental questions: what are the skills required, and how can such skills be taught to, or learned by, staff?

While manifestations of aggression and violence vary greatly between, and within, service settings, these can be functionally categorized as "verbal abuse," "threats," and "physical assaults" (McKenna, 2004). As there is some evidence of a linear relationship between verbal and physical aggression (Maier, Stava, Morrow, Van Rybroek, & Baumaan, 1987), staff need to be able to recognize, assess, and skillfully intervene to de-escalate verbal aggression and threats. While verbal aggression is by far the most commonly encountered manifestation of aggression within health care, some staff are also susceptible to the risk of physical assault (McKenna). These members of staff need to be competent in patient, and situation-specific, risk assessment, and risk management strategies. In addition, staff need to be able to manage their own personal safety, and to effectively free themselves from potential or actual assaults. There are a number of settings within mental health care in which staff are not only authorized, but required, to physically contain individuals when this is the only clinically correct option. Such staff, in addition to the skills above, need to be able, safely and effectively, to contain others in a manner which acknowledges and manages the inherent risks to all involved while preserving the therapeutic relationship.

While the mandate for clinicians to be competent in the management of aggression and violence has been advocated for some time, recent guidelines have focused on the repertoire of knowledge and skills required by staff to develop such competence (British Institute of Learning Disability, 2001; National Institute for Mental Health in England, 2004; NICE, 2005; UKCC, 2002). While central themes of content have been consistently identified, later guidelines have placed much greater emphasis on the requirement that training content be determined by needs assessment (NICE), an aspiration that is also explicit in the most recent code of practice on workplace violence agreed by the International Labor Organization (ILO, 2003).

The implementation of this shift from prescriptive to needs-assessed training content may challenge the prevailing reliance on proprietary training providers whom Leadbetter and Paterson (2005) argues adopt "reductionist" approaches to training, and the practice of providing "one size fits all" systems of training which have increasingly been called into question (NAO, 2003).

While this chapter proposes no commentary on the quality of individual training providers or programs, what is suggested is the need to examine fundamental difficulties in the existing relationship between proprietary providers and professional practice. The provision of systems approaches to training, in which the compilation of course content is divorced from the practice context, is inherently problematic in that such approaches assume that professional practice be framed around the training, rather than vice versa. While the interventions included in such programs may be appropriate or effective within a particular setting, this is a function of chance rather than design in the absence of a service-specific needs analysis. More significantly, there is no mechanism whereby interventions which might be inappropriate are filtered out, causing potential difficulties in translating training to practice.

From a professional practice perspective, training must be informed by, and respond to, the various manifestations of aggression and violence encountered, and the challenges which staff are required to manage within their practice. Training which is effectively functionally aligned to practice promotes the refocusing of interventions from the treatment of aggression and violence, as a distinct entity to one which manages such behaviors within the context of professional care.

6   THE POLICY PERSPECTIVE

Policies, procedures, and practices reflect how actions are guided and performed within organizations. Policy can be defined as a guideline which has been formalized by administrative authority to direct action to some purpose, while procedures detail the operational specifics as to how the organization wishes these policies to be carried out. Practices, conversely, are more vague in both origin and execution, and while they may include behaviors created by policy, they may also include those that originate from habit, tradition, or general problem-solving efforts (Stevens, 1995).

The function of policy is to provide staff with the information necessary to guide their decision making and inform their actions. In effect, they provide the boundary structure for the individual's decision-making scope. In this way, employee actions within the established rule structures are protected from later reprimand. Clarity of rule structures guide employees as to what course of action they may take, and protect them from the precarious position of having to make decisions in circumstances of uncertainty (Perrow, 1988).

The need for policies which support and guide the management of aggression and violence has been identified by professional and regulatory bodies (BILD, 2001; ILO, 2003; NIMHE, 2004). The UKCC (2002) called for practices and procedures to be supported by accessible comprehensive policies which are subject to regular review. The Irish nursing board requires all clinical areas to have "well-defined and rationally structured" policies, and nurses to be thoroughly familiar with the specific legal provisions governing any utilized interventions (An Bord Altranais, 1997). NIMHE positive practice standards require that frameworks which guide staff should be subject an annual review which incorporates evidence from local audits, occurrences, inquiries, and positive practice initiatives. Despite these calls, policies have been found lacking in a number of important areas, including guidance on the use of physical interventions (UKCC), while others (NAO, 2003), have voiced concern that staff were often not adequately involved in formulating policies, and that the majority of policies had not been subject to legal review.

One major concern, resulting from the absence of clear policies, is that staff must rely on practice as their primary guide. While some practices may be excellent, their lack of critical appraisal and formal authorization creates organizational ambiguity, and places staff in a state of uncertainty as to the expectations and authorization of interventions employed to manage aggression and violence encountered in their practice. Reliance on practice rather than policy also complicates the design and delivery of training as the content must, in all instances, comply with the legislative, professional, and policy frameworks within which services are delivered. While not all situations in practice can be anticipated, the central values and guiding principles of the organization can, and should, inform and be communicated in training. The potential for this communication within training is hindered if the shared understanding between the provider of training and the organization, which is necessary to ensure that training congruence with the organizational frameworks which support and guide staff, is absent or ambiguous in the first instance.

7 NEED FOR INTEGRATION

The effective provision of training requires that these four critical success perspectives are adequately and equally addressed. These perspectives should not be considered as mutually exclusive, in that all individuals within the health care organization are essentially agents of each perspective, the difference being one of degree. Assignment and commitment of clear leadership at a senior level of the organization is crucial (Colton, 2004) to achieve and maintain a balance between perspectives and avoid singular approaches which mitigate against the development of "integration" (Leadbetter & Paterson, 2005).

Some organizations have, however, tended to approach the issue of training by assigning responsibility to either individual persons or departments within the organization. These have included clinicians with a particular interest or expertise in the area, or the alignment of responsibility to budgetary allocation with those who hold the budget charged with selecting the training response. While, in some instances, individual clinicians and departments have accomplished very impressive results, the lack of unified focus has inherent fundamental weaknesses. In some instances, the administrative rather than clinical selection of training, while perfectly well intentioned, has failed to appreciate the multidimensional complexity of the problem. Similarly, responses driven primarily from risk management, or health and safety perspectives, run the risk of the "tick box" phenomenon of organizations being in a position to demonstrate compliance with the statutory mandates to provide training which, in reality, have neither enhanced staff clinical competence or patient care.

Adapting a balanced scorecard approach helps to ensure that all critical perspectives are considered, and provides a methodology for the organization and the training provider to structure the design and provision of training. The provider can methodically evaluate training needs by collaboratively exploring practice and safety concerns related to aggression and violence with staff and service managers, and by reviewing health and safety audits, risk management data, and the legislative and policy frameworks specific to each service.

From this critical appraisal, the provider must be competent in selecting a range of verbal intervention techniques, disengagement skills, and therapeutic holding skills which address the concerns of staff and are congruent with professional, legislative, and policy frameworks within which services are provided.

The Matrix of Organizational Analysis of Training (MOAT) (McKenna, 2005), describes this effort as a five-stage process of training analysis, from which service-specific training is designed that:

- Responds to the safety and practice concerns of staff
- Addresses statutory health and safety obligations
- Addresses corporate risk management concerns
- Includes only interventions which are professionally, legally, and organizationally permissible
- Is congruent with organizational philosophy and policy.

The MOAT was developed in response to concerns related to the provision of training, which were highlighted in a large scale study within one Irish health authority (McKenna, 2004). Following a critical review, a radical reorganization of training provision, utilizing the MOAT framework, has been initiated. While initial results indicate that the approach both informs and challenges practice, the effectiveness of the framework as a core structure for training provision is now being systematically evaluated (Figure 3).

8   STEP ONE: WORK-SETTING TASK ANALYSIS

The primary evaluation of training needs analysis requires the development of a clear understanding of the care provided and tasks undertaken by staff within a particular work setting. This is fundamental as the potential manifestations of

Matrix of organizational analysis of training

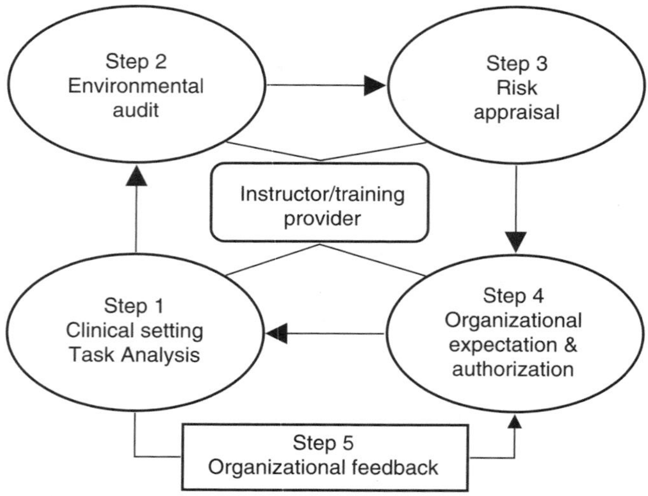

Figure 3. Matrix of organizational analysis of training (McKenna, 2005).

aggression and violence are embedded within the tasks associated with provision of care (McKenna, 2004). For example, there will be considerable variance between what might be anticipated on an acute admission unit, in which staff are required to involuntarily detain and administer treatments, to acutely ill individuals and residential units, in which supportive care is provided to individuals with more stabilized enduring illnesses.

As the source of this information is practice based, this evaluation is ideally done on site and should include unit-based staff and leadership. One useful template to guide this analysis is Poyner and Warne's (1988) framework, which describes the potential for violence as an interactive process between patient, staff, interactional, and environmental variables. The critical output from this evaluation is that the training provider develops an understanding of the practice and safety concerns of staff which must inform the content of training.

This consultation process also facilitates the exploration of other key issues with staff, including the accuracy and completeness of reporting patterns, and including any under-reporting of verbal abuse, threats, and less serious assaults. The expectations of staff from training should also be explored so that necessary information and skills are included. It is equally important to determine that staff have realistic expectations of training, both in terms of clarity and scope. Requests for training can reveal issues for which training is an incomplete, inadequate, or inappropriate response. Both staff and unit leadership need to appreciate the limitations of training and that, irrespective of the quality of the training, it cannot compensate for systems problems or questionable practice. This clarification of expectations avoids the frustration which is inevitable when training is employed in response to either a system or practice issue which, invariably, remains only partially, or totally, unresolved.

9   STEP TWO: ENVIRONMENTAL AUDIT

Having developed an understanding of the care context, the next assessment seeks to identify potential hazards for staff which are inherent in either the tasks undertaken or the environment of care. This consultation should be incorporated into the risk assessment framework being employed to satisfy the organizations health and safety mandate. This evaluation should be conducted in liaison with those responsible for health and safety within the unit of service, and might include the review of environmental audits, in addition to reviewing the structures, practices, and systems of working in relation to the management of aggression and violence. While remediation of environmental factors such as crowding, acuity, and aesthetics are beyond the scope of the training provider, a comprehension of these can help inform the context of the training provided while simultaneously ensuring that the limitations of training responses are understood by all. The critical output from this understanding is that training is informed by, and addresses, the potential hazards in the environment in which staff work, including those which are a function of high risk populations which might be served.

10   STEP THREE: RISK APPRAISAL

The next phase of the assessment progresses from the understanding of the care context and associated hazards, to the development of a clear understanding of the risks, including near misses, which have been encountered by staff within the work area. This review should be conducted in liaison with those responsible for risk management within the unit and should review the frequency of recorded incidents, the severity of recorded occurrences, the site, location, and time of occurrences, and the occupation, grade, and role of staff involved and/or injured. In analyzing formal records, it is important to be aware of their limited reliability due to under reporting of work-related violence by staff. Formal records should be considered in conjunction with the information about reporting behaviors elicited from staff during the previously conducted consultations (Step one). The purpose of this evaluation is to identify the potential risks to patients, staff, and the organization actually encountered in the practice setting. The critical output from this understanding is that training is informed by, and responds to, the risk concerns of staff in addition to addressing high risk, high frequency, and problem-prone challenges, which staff actually encounter.

11 STEP FOUR: ORGANIZATIONAL EXPECTATION AND AUTHORIZATION

While all staff in care settings share the fundamental values existing within professional relationships, there is great variation in the legal, legislative, professional, and organizational structures within which this care is provided. Having developed an understanding of the care context, and the inherent hazards and risks, this phase of the assessment seeks to establish clarity as to how the organization expects and authorizes staff to manage occurrences of aggression and violence. This assessment should be conducted in liaison with those who are organizationally, and professionally, accountable and responsible for the development and enforcement of policies and procedures within the service, usually the service manager. This review involves the critical appraisal of the range of interventions deemed necessary from the previous stages of the assessment process, and ensuring that proposed interventions are legally, professionally, and organizationally permissible. While at the extremes many of these decisions are clear, there are frequently areas of ambiguity. One example is the use of physical disengagement interventions, which range from simple attempts to effect releases, to those which may be more functionally effective but are aversive to the protagonist. The decision as to which techniques are included in the training needs to be explored and, while informed by risk analysis and unit-based values, must be authorized by the manager and supported with clear operational policy and procedures. A second, increasingly encountered, issue is the employment of security staff in services, sometimes with a lack of clarity as to their exact role expectation. Such situations place all staff, and the organization, in a highly precarious position of uncertainty as to what such staff are expected, or authorized, to do and, equally importantly, what they are not. The removal of ambiguities in relation to the scope and role of all staff can lower the inherent stress in managing occurrences of aggression and violence and reduce the potential for miscommunication or error. The critical output from this assessment is that training is informed by, and is fully congruent with, the legal, professional, and policy parameters which prevail within the service, and that the content is aligned with the responsibilities of those staff receiving training. Staff frequently have to make very difficult decisions in haste, often under extreme circumstances. It is critical therefore, that the opportunity exists for staff to explore and consider the frameworks governing and supporting their decision-making in such circumstances. While training presents an ideal forum to incorporate such exploration, what is absolutely crucial is that the training provided is informed by, and consistent with, the policies and values of the organization.

The completion of the first four steps of assessment informs the preparation of a draft program of training which is then returned for review by the service manager. This process of approval provides clarity for the training provider and the organization as to the exact content and duration of training. Following approval, organizational aspects of training delivery are finalized, including venue, equipment, and communication with staff. The delivery of training is outside the scope of this chapter but should be delivered within best practice as described elsewhere (see BILD, 2001; NICE, 2005; NIMHE, 2004; UKCC, 2002).

12   STEP FIVE: ORGANIZATIONAL FEEDBACK

Following the delivery of training, the opportunity should exist for the provision of feedback. The structure and focus of this feedback should, ideally, be agreed with the service manager prior to the delivery of training. This review may include systems issues such as attendance records, course evaluation by participants, and evaluation of venue and equipment. Other significant organizational issues include the validation that the agreed course content was actually delivered and the level of staff performance, competence, and mastery of the course material. In addition, issues or practices of concern which have emerged during the training should be discussed. While it is difficult to be prescriptive in the actual content of this review, what is critical is that the opportunity exists for the exploration of concerns providing a completion of the organizational training provider loop.

Organizations vary in how responsibilities for service delivery, health and safety, risk management, and corporate policy are delegated. While some have individual persons or departments assigned to each of the components, others rely on individuals or departments for more than one of these responsibilities. The MOAT framework should be considered, therefore, as a functional, rather than departmental, assessment of training needs which translates organizational consideration of critical perspectives into practice by methodically incorporating these considerations in the provision of training.

13   PROACTIVE AND REACTIVE TRAINING

The process described above structures the organization's effort to proactively provide training which aims to ensure safety, and enhance the clinical effectiveness of staff while meeting their obligation to institute control measures which mitigate against identified hazards and foreseeable risks. While such proactive responses are the penultimate goal, there are circumstances in which immediate reactive training is appropriate. Examples of such circumstances might include a change in the patient population being served by a particular unit, or in response to an individual patient who poses a particular behavioral management difficulty. In either event, what is significant is that the problem being encountered in the practice setting is either outside the scope of the proactively provided training, or challenges staff coping skills in the management of particular behaviors. In such circumstances, situation-specific or patient-specific training should be available to staff as a matter of urgency. The assessment of such reactive training can be approached using the same considerations and framework, the essential difference is that the impetus for training might originate from a safety perspective; hence the need to deliver training is more emergent.

The assessment process which informed the provision of all proactive and reactive training should be accurately recorded. These records demonstrate the attempts of the organization to take all reasonable measures in their duty to protect others by engaging in a structured consultation process to identify and address safety concerns. These cumulative records of unit-based training form a compendium of planned proactive training efforts supported by a series of solution-focused specific training responses. Together these represent a developmental process, not only for the practice staff involved, but also for other related departments and for the organization. This developmental process which embeds training into a governance framework goes some way toward actualizing the "high road" approach typical of "smart organizations" by consistently and continuously reflecting upon, and learning from, experiences in a way that develops the capabilities of both the organization and the individuals within it (Senge et al., 1999).

14 CONCLUSION

Long-standing tendencies to explain workplace violence in healthcare, with reference to the actions of the protagonists, and a deficit of evidence of sufficient quality to guide best practice in the prevention and management of violence, have proved an invidious combination. The causes of aggression and violence are multifactorial and may constitute acute or chronic manifestations of a range of medical and psychological conditions. These behaviors require skillful clinical assessment and a range of interventions which may range from supportive reassurance to the management of an actual, or impending, medical or safety emergency (McKenna, 2004). The causes of the crises which can give rise to aggression are, however, often embedded in the structural arrangements of care, and the culture of services, rather than solely consumer pathology (Fisher, 2003).

The reality of these events within healthcare settings, and within mental health settings in particular, requires that staff are provided with the training necessary to safely and effectively manage such occurrences. Effective provision of such training requires the implementation of a strategic systematic approach to ensure that the needs of service users, staff, and the organization are adequately, and equally, addressed in a balanced and comprehensive manner. The provision of training is, however, a complex task which reflects the multidimensional etiology and various theoretical understandings of the problem.

Attempts to provide training have encountered difficulties with structures, processes, and content which have been highlighted in the professional and regulatory reports. The absence of regulation has resulted in a proliferation of proprietary training programs which are often heavily marketed to organizations who, in many instances, continue to lack understanding of the integrated approach necessary, and their organization's specific training needs. The fundamental concern with such approaches is that professional practice becomes subordinate to the content of proprietary programs rather than such programs being subordinate to the needs of professional practice. The inherent weakness in such approaches is simply the application of a product solution to a process problem.

While the complexity of providing training has become increasingly clear to organizations, there has been less attention to providing strategies as to how to address this complex issue. Rather than simply challenging the current reliance on proprietary training, what needs to be challenged are the assumptions that underpin this reliance. Most fundamental among these is the consideration of the management of aggression and violence as distinct from the patient care. What is required is to refocus our efforts on the skilful management of patient care rather than the skilful management of aggression and violence.

Despite, or perhaps because of, these problems, very real advances have been made in the professional attention to the issue, which offers new opportunities for the contribution of training to patient care to be fully realized. The actualization of this potential, however, will require that more attention is paid to the professional and organizational processes of training, and returning the management of aggression and violence to the domain of professional practice, rather than aggressive marketing or budgetary authority. The MOAT framework describes one such effort by outlining an approach which places clinical practice as the central determinant of training, while adequately and equally considering and meeting the needs of the organization.

REFERENCES

Advisory Committee on Health Services Sector (2001). *Report of the advisory committee on health services sector*. Dublin: National Authority for Occupational Safety and Health.

An Bord Altranais (1997). *Guidance to nurses and midwives on the management of violence/challenging behavior*. Dublin: An Bord Altranais.

Badger, F., & Mullan, B. (2004). Aggressive and violent incidents: Perceptions of training and support among staff caring for older people and people with head injury. *Journal of Clinical Nursing, 13*(4), 526–533.

Blair, D. T., & New, S. A. (1991). Assaultive behavior: Know the risks. *Journal of Psychosocial Nursing, 29*(11), 25–31.

Blofeld, J. (2003). *An independent inquiry set up under HSG(94)27 into the death of David "Rocky" Bennett*. Cambridge: Norfolk, Suffolk, and Cambridgeshire Strategic Health Authority.

Bonner, G., Lowe, T., Rawcliffe, D., & Wellman, M. (2002). Trauma for all: A pilot study of the subjective experience of physical restraint for mental health patients and staff in the UK. *Journal of Psychiatric and Mental Health Nursing, 9*, 465–473.

British Institute of Learning Disabilities (2001). *Code of practice for trainers in the use of physical interventions*. Kidderminster: British Institute of Learning Disabilities.

Budd, T. (2001). *Violence at work, findings from the British Crime Survey*. London: Home Office.

Bureau of Labor Statistics (1999). *Non-fatal assaults at work*. Washington, DC: United States Department of Labor.

Byrne, R. (2001). *Safety, health and welfare at work law in Ireland: A guide*. Dublin: Nifast.

Cameron, A. (2001). *The art of partnership: A practical guide*. Kidderminster: British Institute of Learning Disabilities.

Colton, D. (2004). *Checklist for assessing your organization's readiness for reducing seclusion and restraint*. Virginia: Commonwealth Centre for Children and Adolescence Staunton.

Council of Europe (2004). *Council of Europe Committee of Ministers Recommendation (2004)10 of the Committee of Ministers to member states concerning the protection of the human rights and dignity of persons with mental disorder*. Available at https://wcd.coe.int/ViewDoc.jsp?id=775685&Lang=en

Cox, T., & Cox, S. (1993). *Psychosocial and organizational hazards: Control and monitoring*. Occupational Health Series, 5. Copenhagen: World Health Organization.

Dawson, J., Johnson, M., Kehiayan, N., Kyanko, S., & Martinez, R. (1988). Response to patient assault: A peer support program for nurses. *Journal of Psychosocial Nursing, 26*(2), 8–15.

De Waal, A. (2003). The future of the balanced scorecard: An interview with Professor Robert S. Kaplan. *Measuring Business Excellence, 7*(1), 30–35.

Edwards, J., & Reid, W. (1983). Violence in psychiatric facilities in Europe and the United States. In: J. Lion & W. Reid (Eds.), *Assaults within psychiatric facilities* (pp. 61–70). Philadelphia: W. B. Saunders and Company.

Fisher, J. (2003). Curtailing the use of restraint in psychiatric settings. *Journal of Humanistic Psychology, 43*(2), 69–95.

General Accounting Office of the United States (1999). *Report to congressional requesters: Mental health: Improper restraint or seclusion places people at risk.* Washington, DC: United States General Accounting Office.

Government of Ireland (2005). *Safety, health, and welfare at work act.* Dublin: Government Publications Office.

Hepworth, P. (1998). Weighing it up–a literature review for the balanced scorecard. *Journal of Management Development, 17*(8), 559–563.

International Labor Office, International Council of Nurses, World Health Organization, Public Services International (2002). *Framework guidelines for addressing workplace violence in the health sector.* Geneva: International Labor Office.

International Labor Organization (2000). *Violence at work.* Geneva: International Labor Organization.

International Labor Organization (2003). *Code of practice on workplace violence in services sectors and measures to combat this phenomenon.* Geneva: International Labor Organization.

Kaplan, R. S., & Norton, D. P. (1996). Using the balanced scorecard as a strategic management system. *Harvard Business Review*, Jan–Feb***, 75–85.

Lanza, M. (1992). Nurses as patient assault victims: An update, synthesis, and recommendations. *Archives of Psychiatric Nursing, 6*(3), 163–171.

Leadbetter, D. (2003). *CALM training services instructors manual.* Menstrie: CALM Training services.

Leadbetter, D., & Paterson, B. (2005). *From moral panic to moral action.* Paper presented at the Child Welfare League of America/Cornell University/Stirling University Joint symposium on high risk interventions in human services. New York: Cornell University.

Lion, J. (1987). Training for battle: thoughts on managing aggressive patients. *Hospital and Community Psychiatry, 38*, 882–884.

Maier, G., Stava, L., Morrow, B., Van Rybroek, G., & Baumaan, K. (1987). A model for understanding and managing cycles of aggression among psychiatric inpatients. *Hospital and Community Psychiatry, 38*(5), 520–524.

McElhinney, J., & Heffernan, O. (2003). Using clinical risk management as a means of enhancing patient safety: The Irish experience. *International Journal of Health Care Quality Assurance, 16*(2), 90–98.

McKenna, K. (2004). *Study of work-related violence.* Kells, County Meath, Ireland: North Eastern Health Board.

McKenna, K. (2005). Locating training within a comprehensive organizational strategy to manage aggression and violence in health and social care. In: T. Palmstierna H. Nijman & N. Oud (Eds.), *Proceedings of the 4th European Congress on Violence in Clinical Psychiatry.* Amsterdam, Netherlands: Oud Consultancy.

Menckel, E., & Viitasara, E. (2002). Threats and violence in Swedish care and welfare: Magnitude of the problem and impact on municipal personnel. *Scandinavian Journal of Caring Sciences, 16*, 376–385.

Moulin, M. (2004). Eight essentials of performance measurement. *International Journal of Health Care Quality Assurance, 17*(3), 110–112.

National Audit Office (2003). *A safer place to work: Protecting NHS hospital and ambulance staff from violence and aggression. Report HC 527 Session 2002–2003.* London: The Stationery Office.

National Institute of Clinical Excellence (2005). *Violence: The short-term management of disturbed/violent behavior in psychiatric in-patient settings and emergency departments.* London: National Institute of Clinical Excellence.

National Institute for Mental Health in England (2004). *Mental health policy implementation guide developing positive practice to support the safe and therapeutic management of aggression and violence in mental health in-patient settings.* Worcestershire: National Institute for Mental Health in England.

Nijman, H., Bowers, L., Oud, N., & Jansen, G. (2005). Psychiatric nurses' experience with inpatient aggression. *Aggressive Behavior, 31,* 217–227.

NIOSH (1996). *Violence in the workplace. Risk factors and prevention strategies.* Washington, DC: Government Printing Office Publication: National Institute for Occupational Safety and Health.

Occupational Safety and Health Administration (2004). *Guidelines for preventing workplace violence for health care and social service workers.* Washington, DC: US Department of Labor, Occupational Safety and Health Administration.

Paterson, B., Bradley, P., Stark, C., Saddler, D., Leadbetter, D., & Allen, D. (2003). Restraint-related deaths in health and social care in the UK: Learning the lessons. *Mental Health Practice, 6*(9), 10–17.

Paterson, B., McComish, S., & Bradley, P. (1999). Violence at work. *Nursing Standard, 13*(21), 43–46.

Perrow, C. (1988). *Complex organizations: A critical essay* (3rd ed.). New York: Random House.

Poyner, B., & Warne, C. (1988). *Preventing violence to staff.* London: HMSO Publications.

Psychiatric Nurses Association (2002). *Assault on nurses: PNA launch campaign for compensation.* Dublin: Psychiatric Nurses Association.

Richter, D., & Needham, I. (2005). Effectiveness of training interventions in the management of violence in health care: A systematic review. In: T. Palmstierna H. Nijman & N. Oud (Eds.), *Proceedings of the 4th European Congress on Violence in Clinical Psychiatry.* Amsterdam, Netherlands: Oud Consultancy.

Royal College of Psychiatrists (1998). *The management of imminent violence: Clinical practice guideline to support mental health services.* London: Royal College of Psychiatrists.

Senge, P., Kleiner, A., Roberts, C., Ross, R., Roth, G., & Smith, B. (1999). *The dance of change: The challenges of sustaining momentum in learning organizations.* New York: Doubleday.

Stevens, B. (1995). *The nurse as executive* (3rd ed.). Maryland: Aspen Publications.

Swanson, J. W., Swartz, M. S., Essock, S. M., Osher, F. C., Wagner, H. R., Goodman, L. A., et al. (2002). The social-environmental context of violent behavior in persons treated for severe mental illness. *American Journal of Public Health, 92*(9), 1523–1531.

Tucker, R. (2005). *Social Care Risk Assessment.* Guardian, 19 October 2005. Available at http://society.guardian.co. uk/socialcare/story/0,,1595039,00.html

United Kingdom Central Council (2002). *The recognition, prevention, and therapeutic management of violence in mental health care.* London: United Kingdom Central Council for Nursing Midwifery and Health Visiting.

Zinn, C. (2001). Health service ranked as the most violent industry in Australia. *British Medical Journal, 323,* 1386–1387.

13

Safety and Security in Psychiatric Clinical Environments

SEAMUS COWMAN

1 INTRODUCTION

In mental health services, violent and assault behavior is manifested in many different directions including patient violence and assault on staff; patient violence and assault on other more vulnerable patients; violence and assault from outsiders; patient violence toward visitors and the public generally. Violent death by suicide is also occurring with increasing frequency and within the hospital setting. The resulting situation is one where environmental dangers must be reduced and this must be accompanied by arrangements for increased safety and security precautions to protect staff and patients of the mental health services.

The literature investigating violence has consistently highlighted the patient/client as the perpetrator of violence. However, there is a growing recognition that work-related violence in health care is also attributed to relatives, friends, and members of the public. The challenge of maintaining safe, secure, and therapeutic clinical environments for staff and patients in mental health is complicated by the increased frequency in the number of relatives and visitors as a source of work-related violence. What is also very clear from the literature is that the experience of staff assault transcends professional boundaries and international frontiers and is a pervasive and persistent problem.

The increased concern among employees, employers, and professional organizations over the escalation in violence and aggression has created an urgent requirement for proactive national and international strategies in safety and security across mental health services. Despite improved initiatives in areas such as risk assessment and staff training, there remains a paucity of readily available data regarding the safety of mental health services. The coordination and establishment of a minimum data set across mental health services must be a priority as this will allow for the identification of where and how changes should be made in order to improve safety and security.

Despite the concerns of the Health and Safety Authorities about violence and assault in health care, in many countries there is an alarming lack of clarity on matters of procedure and policy pertaining to ward safety and security in hospitals. Across the psychiatric services there is a bewildering array of practices ranging from an open door policy, to locked wards and doors, and confiscation of patients clothing and personal property, some of which borders on the infringement of human rights, liberty, and the rights and choices of patients.

This chapter will review important issues directly and indirectly related to safety and security in psychiatric services. The content of the chapter will explore the core concepts underpinning safety and security; examine the concerns of formal bodies such as health and safety authorities. The importance of organizational culture and issues of direct importance to health service practitioners will also be reviewed. Controversial issues such as prosecution, the involvement of police, and the role dilemma for health professions created through the opposing roles of security and caring are significantly influential factors. The final section of the chapter outlines a case study on safety and security with the results highlighting variation and a lack of overall policy, procedure, or agreement on best practice in safety and security. The case for similar studies in safety and security in other jurisdictions is made in order to allow comparison and the creation of a minimum data set which ultimately will contribute to international standards on safety and security.

2   DEFINITIONS OF SAFETY AND SECURITY

Definitions of safety and security in mental health services often rely on descriptions of services currently available so that a given level is often defined by default. There is wide variation between services regarding levels of physical security, inappropriate placement, and patient mix. Kennedy (2002) discussed safety and security and defined it in three main contexts; environmental; relational, and procedural (Figure 1).

2.1   Environmental Safety and Security

Environmental safety and security refers to constructional and hardware issues, which are often introduced at high capital cost. Such measures include building access, door and window types, CCTV, general and personal alarms, mobile phones. High standards of maintenance and decoration are also significant environmental factors.

Environmental Safety and security	Design and maintenance of estate and fittings, building access. CCTV, Alarms, Mobile Phones
Relational Safety and security	Quantitative: staff–patient ratios Qualitative: quality of care, therapeutic regimes
Procedural Safety and security	Policy and procedure Patient level: systems and routines for checking and searching System levels: arrangements for risk management, professional governance, audit, training

Figure 1. Definitions and concepts in safety and security (Kennedy, 2002; Kinsley, 1998).

2.2 Relational Safety and Security

Relational safety and security refers to the quality of care, patient/staff ratios, treatment, recreational regimes, and therapeutic rapport.

2.3 Procedural Safety and Security

Procedural safety and security is the focus of much attention at operation level. It includes policy and procedures related to checking, searching, and imposed restrictions on patients/clients of the mental health care system. Management of violent incidents, control and restraint, deescalation, breakaway techniques, risk assessment, and seclusion are also features of procedural safety and security. Many organizational efforts such as audit and training are focused on this area of safety and security.

3 HEALTH SERVICE BODIES

The extensive range of international literature and data from health service bodies and related agencies has described the exposure of health care staff to patient violence in the workplace with some of them attempting to provide direction. The US Department of Labor (1998) reported that more assaults occur among health care and social services workers than in any other sector. It is also worth noting that almost two-thirds of the nonfatal assaults occurred in nursing homes and other establishments providing residential care and other social services. A great concern expressed in many reports, for example the US Department of Labor and the Irish North Eastern Health Board (2004), is the likely underreporting of violence and a persistent perception within the health sector that assaults are part of the job for employees of mental health services.

The need for comprehensive plans and systems aimed at maintaining safety and security in the workplace requires immediate action. Many unconventional approaches to improving safety and security are recommended. For example, in the US psychiatric setting, Qadir (1982) raises the issue of the practice of using airport-style metal detectors and full body searches for patients entering and leaving wards. In Ireland, for example, the Health and Safety Authority (2001) has suggested that organizations in the health sector: review work practices and procedures and what precautions are in place; evaluate the type of security presence to provide a deterrent and protection for staff; evaluate the requirements for devices such as alarms (personal and general) surveillance (CCTV); mobile phones, two way radios, and panic buttons.

Gould (2000) highlighted that according to the UKs Health and Safety Executive, nursing is Britain's most dangerous occupation. The Department of Health in the UK (2000a) produced a report on safety in high-security hospitals and suggested that patients be locked in their rooms at night because of lapses in security and the wide availability of pornography and illicit drugs.

The variance across the world in approaches to maintain safe and secure environments in mental health care settings is noteworthy. For example the US, in contrast to the European Union, has initiated very specific proactive measures to combat violence and promote safety and security. In some states of the US, Mental Health Security Technicians are employed to promote safer environments for care. The duties and responsibilities of the Security Technician encompass elements of safety and security including: behavior management; observing patients for potential violence or socially destructive behavior with intervention as required: security monitoring and control; emergency response coordination; transportation of patients. In contrast the EU, in the absence of key security posts such as a Mental Health Security Technician, requires mental health professionals to take on more confrontational approaches with patients and clients. The responsibility for security monitoring and control also lies with mental health care staff.

More recently the National Institute of Clinical Excellence (NICE, 2005) produced guidelines for effective prevention and short-term management of violence in adult psychiatric inpatient settings and emergency departments. The recommendations contained in the NICE guidelines, as best practice, are based on the best available evidence and can make a significant contribution toward ensuring safe and secure environments in mental health services. Whereas the guidelines do not comprehensively focus on safety and security in a specific sense it does provide direction in key areas central to safety and security such as: environment and alarm systems; prediction including warning signs, risk assessment, and searching.

4 ZERO TOLERANCE

Zero tolerance to workplace violence and aggression has emerged in contemporary health service policy and mental health discourse. It has gained widespread support as its emphasis and stance is acceptable. It is interesting to note that discussion on zero tolerance has taken place at all levels including governmental, political, societal, and professional. An obvious omission from much of the discussion is the requirement for a broad organizational approach which ensures the necessary human and physical resources required to implement and maintain a zero tolerance approach.

Whittington (2002) reviews the concept of zero tolerance and identifies a number of inherent problems. There is a lack of clarity in defining the problem behavior of violence. It may also be the case that implementing a zero tolerance approach in mental health services may disturb the subtle balance which needs to be struck in deciding what is acceptable staff and patient behavior in any health care interaction. In mental health services a sudden move, from what has traditionally been a lax attitude (violence accepted as part of the job), to one of zero tolerance may raise serious tensions and hostilities that lead to further confrontation. This may have further serious implication for mental health care staff in observing a zero tolerance approach and also maintaining an environment of trust with a therapeutic regime.

Clements, DeRanieri, Clark, Manno, and Kuhn (2005) attributes the concept of zero tolerance to mainstream media which report and sensationalize extremely violent incidents in health care; for example concentrating only on the "gunman" or "knife attack" type of violence. Another factor driving the zero tolerance agenda is the influence of powerful organisations such as the American Nurses Association which published a Bill of Rights for Registered Nurses. The Bill of Rights which was published in 2001 states that nurses have a right to work in an enviornment that is safe (Wiseman 2001). There is also an increasing number of mandates from significant bodies highlighting the duty of employers to provide safe environments (ILO, 2002; US Department of Labor, 1998). The National Institute of Occupational Safety and Health (NIOSH) (2003) argues there is a requirement for a zero tolerance assessment team consisting of interdisciplinary members which would be responsible for continuous review of reported workplace violence as well as any recommendations that would lead to the prevention of any further violent incidents.

There is general agreement within the literature among those that strongly advocate a zero tolerance approach that the essential requirements include the development of an identification system for potential violence, a system of response to threats or violent events, and constructive support procedures after the event.

5 CLINICAL ENVIRONMENT CONCERNS

Sanders, Milner, Brown, and Bell (2000) investigated aggression among psychiatric admissions ($n = 199$) and identified that almost a quarter of patients admitted, reported thoughts of violence directed at specific individuals. Nearly one in ten patients owned a weapon and one in twenty admitted to carrying them. It is the case that owning and carrying weapons are recognized risks of violence (Ferris, Sandercock, Hoffman, Silverman, & Carlisle, 1997). Ryrie and McGowan (1998) highlighted the illicit use of drugs among psychiatric inpatients as a major security issue.

Concerns about ward safety and security in a London-wide survey is reported by Bowers et al. (2002), which demonstrated wide-scale variation in safety measures and security features across acute admission wards. Bowers et al. through a correlation matrix of data demonstrated two independently varying clusters of security type.

One type of security represented an emphasis on the protection of the patient from himself or herself, and the second type of security emphasized the protection of staff and patients from other patients.

Cowman and Walsh (2004) reported on a population study of acute admission psychiatric wards in the Republic of Ireland. The study identified great variation between hospitals with no overall policy or agreement on what is best practice in terms of safety and security. There were not only differences between hospitals, but also between male and female wards in the same hospital. The study by Cowman and Walsh also reported on a lack of standardized security measures at the entrance to hospital wards, and the limited access to security guards suggested that nurses were expected to adopt more confrontational roles during episodes of violence.

In 2002, in response to the high level, and serious nature of assaults, the Minister for Health and Children in Ireland established a task force to examine incidences of assaults on psychiatric nurses and to investigate reasons for such assaults with a view to the determining effective preventative measures. A further objective of the task force was to put in place a compensation scheme to be applied to nurses in incidences of serious physical and psychological injury. The task force was established in response to a survey undertaken by the Psychiatric Nurses Association of Ireland. The Psychiatric Nurses Association (2002) survey highlighted a high level of physical assaults on staff, which resulted in absence from work through sick leave and stress. The task force concluded that the environment is a major factor in the cause of incidences of violence and that workplace evaluation should be instituted in all facilities to identify existing hazards (Department of Health and Children, 2003).

In some jurisdictions, the increased concerns over safety and security have given rise to publications from prominent mental health professional bodies. For example, the Royal College of Psychiatrists in the UK (2000), in recognizing that the clinical environment may be a factor that influences the development of violent incidents, developed guidelines on appropriate general layout and structure of the clinical environment. The guidelines provided direction on a number of elements in the clinical environment that serve to influence and trigger the development of violent incidents. The guidelines from the Royal College of Psychiatrists proposed that, in managing and providing care to psychiatric patients, the following areas should be considered:

- Access to privacy (telephones, toilets, showers, privacy for conversations with visitors and friends)
- Access to spacious facilities (confrontations may result from cramped conditions)
- Access to open spaces and fresh air (patients being able to leave ward)
- Making the clinical setting more "homely" (access to television, having a wardrobe/locker, access to private telephones)

Other important environmental factors identified were boredom, lack of therapy, and social groups. The infrastructure was highly significant in ensuring a safe environment, for example entrances and exits in sight of staff, accessible exit doors, moveable objects being of a safe weight, size, and construction. The Royal College of Psychiatrists (2000) concluded that the prevailing therapeutic environment of a clinical area influences the type of security arrangements and the level of workplace violence.

6 ORGANIZATIONAL CULTURE

In a context of change in the Australian mental health care system, Wilson et al. (1995) argued that approaches to improving safety must be systematic, ongoing, and include a commitment to resources and leadership. The Department of Health (UK) (2000b) summarized features of an organization's culture that promoted safety. Such features included:

- People are prepared to report problems, errors, and "near misses."
- There is an atmosphere of trust.
- There is respect for skills and abilities of frontline staff.
- There is an ability and willingness to learn and to implement improvements.

The National Patient Safety Agency (NPSA) which was established in the UK in 2001 has introduced a national reporting and learning system for adverse events across the NHS in England and Wales. The electronic reporting system collects structured and unstructured data about patient safety incidents and has now been incorporated into local risk management systems. There are positive reports on the introduction of the reporting system in particular its effects in reducing a culture of blame which has permeated mental health services. Over the years, inquiry after inquiry into mental health services, particularly in the area of suicide/homicide most often reported on system failure and the process of investigation was most often perceived as adversarial with staff feeling culpable.

There is sufficient evidence available to suggest that the culture of the clinical environment of care can influence the development of violent incidents. Skills in supervision have always been central to ensuring effective models of clinical governance in the acute psychiatric setting (Rogers & Topping-Morris, 1997). In reflecting on some of the early work on the culture of psychiatric clinical environments it could be argued that some elements may be evident in today's acute psychiatric services. A study by Mason (1993) in a high-security mental health setting identified small groups of negative and positive staff and a large group of "toggle staff" who would switch allegiances to whoever was in charge at the time. If a negative person was in charge then the "toggle staff" would be negative, and if a positive person was the ward leader then they would become positive. In a study on culture, Morrison (1990) identified different types of staff. One type was the "superman" which referred to the strongest and toughest nurse on the ward who is known for their ability to handle any patient that steps out of line.

The Royal College of Psychiatrists (1999) provided advice and guidelines to individual staff and trainees on establishing a culture of personal safety in clinical

practice. The advice and guidelines included a number of useful practical suggestions such as preserving personal privacy through not divulging home address, tele-
phone number, or personal information to patients; personal appearance engenders
confidence and trust; expensive, flamboyant, or sexually provocative clothing may
be misinterpreted by a patient; clothing should not be tight in case the staff member
has to move quickly; a scarf, long hair, and loose items of clothing should be
avoided; isolation should always be avoided; familiarity with the emergency alarm
system is essential; at night staff should avoid walking in poorly lit isolated areas
either inside or outside buildings. Staff should not be expected to make assessments
alone in an emergency situation or at night, always assess the level of security and
avoid situations which compromise safety; a personal alarm should be worn and care
should also be taken when conducting an interview and, where possible, other members of staff should be present; if the staff cannot control a disturbance the police
should be called without delay.

7   PROSECUTION OF PATIENTS

The amount of interest and the number of publications on the prediction and management of violence is not matched by a similar emphasis on systematically reporting assaults to the police or assault being followed by prosecution of the assailant
(Coyne, 2002). Over many decades there is evidence of widespread workplace violence toward all health care staff groupings: nurses (Paterson, McCornish, & Bradley,
1999), social workers (McCurry, 1999), district nurses (Finney, 1988), general practitioners (Tolhurst et al., 2003), doctors (Zahid, Al-Sahlawi, Shahid, Awadh, & Abu-
Shammah, 1999), and psychotherapists (Bernstein, 1981). A recent study (NEHB,
2004), conducted in a large geographical health care setting in Ireland, identified
widespread systematic assaultive behavior as a pervasive problem across health care
settings and against all health care staff: ambulance personnel, care attendants, child
care workers, community welfare officers, management/administration staff, med-
ical/dental staff, nursing, paramedical, support e.g., domestic, staff.

The emerging pattern in health services is one of high levels of assault in a
working environment that may be considered to be unsafe. It has been suggested
(Turnbull, 1999) that the public have learned that assaulting doctors, nurses, and
other health care staff brings few punishments or sanctions unlike, for example,
assaulting a member of the police. Therefore, safety and security in mental health
services is further undermined by creating the false impression that if a patient's
crimes are ignored then these patients are justified in learning that their conduct is
acceptable. It has also been reported (Convit, Isay, Otis, & Volavka, 1990) that a
small proportion of patients are responsible for a large percentage of the violence
that occurs. It is therefore likely that a policy of prosecuting this offending group is
likely to have a dramatic effect in increasing safety and security in the environs of
mental health services. Unfortunately, there is a strongly held view among health
care professionals that violence is an occupational hazard in mental health care and

that staff in this field should expect to be assaulted. There is the additional view that patients in receipt of mental health care are to some extent not responsible for their acts in times of severe illness (NEHB, 2004).

Formally the health services have responded to perpetrators in one form or another, albeit inadequate. For example, in the event of assaultive behavior, institutions have taken action against perpetrators including discharge to more secure and restricted care environments; increased medication or changed treatment regimes; more punitive measures such as seclusion or removal of privileges such as leave. Nork, Zonana, and Phillips (1992), argues that prosecution may encourage responsibility and is therefore a therapeutic intervention. The prospect of prosecution may also represent a form of reality orientation in the form of limit setting (Miller & Maier, 1987) and therefore may serve as a force against further acts of violent behavior. The disadvantages of a policy of prosecution for assaultive behavior is that such a policy may alienate patients and clients from the mental health services and may lead to further acts of violence being carried out in the community.

If mental health care institutions are to pursue an active policy of prosecution of patients for violent and assaultive behavior it is extremely important that robust procedures and protocols are put in place. Nork et al. (1992), suggests some key actions in this regard including:

- Clearly presenting and explaining to patients their rights and responsibilities on admission
- Developing criteria for pursuing prosecution as a matter of hospital policy
- Violent incidents should be reviewed by clinician(s) not involved with the treatment of the perpetrator of the violent act
- Findings of the screening evaluation should be reviewed by hospital administration and the Clinical Director
- In the event of a decision to proceed with the prosecution, treatment staff should not be responsible for filing the complaint

8 THE ROLE OF THE POLICE

In recent years, the involvement of the police and law enforcement agencies has played an increasingly important role in the management of people with mental illness. This in the major part has arisen from a policy of deinstitutionalization in the care and management of persons with a mental illness and a policy of normalization, integration, and community care. The primary purpose of police intervention in the lives of persons with a mental illness most often arises from the power and authority of the police to protect the safety and welfare of the community. The initial role of the police can be to transport persons for psychiatric evaluation and treatment where the individual may be a danger to themselves or others. A violent act or the likelihood of violence underlines the majority of psychiatric emergencies involving the police.

It is suggested (Lamb, Weinberger, & DeCuir, 2002) that from the standpoint of the police it is clear that police officers need, and want, assistance from mental health professionals when they are called upon to deal with complex situations involving mentally ill people. Similarly mental health professionals who become involved in psychiatric emergencies without police support may feel less competent to handle certain situations of violence and aggression. Therefore, it may be concluded that, in cases of mental health emergencies incorporating violence, neither the police nor the mental health care system alone can serve effectively and it is essential both systems work closely together (Zealberg, Santos, & Pucket, 1996). What is also notable is that there is more likely to be police and mental health services cooperation in the community care area rather than the institution. Yet it is the case that the acute inpatient psychiatric service is often the location where mentally ill people are at their most volatile, thus leaving staff in their most vulnerable position. Any future proposals for police and mental health services collaboration must, ideally, represent an integrated approach across community and hospital services. Such cooperation across state services could serve as a powerful means of reducing the threats and incidents of violence perpetrated against mental health care staff.

Prediction and, at the very least, anticipation of psychiatric patients who are likely to be violent must be a central working philosophy of any acute psychiatric service (Blumenthel & Lavender, 2000). Risk assessment is, therefore, an essential activity in ensuring safe environments for staff and patients. The creation of safe and secure environments is heavily dependent upon mental health professionals having well-developed skills in clinical reasoning and decision-making. In mental health the process of decision-making is determined as being enormously complex, requiring rapid decision-making in stressful clinical circumstances. It is important to note that expert nurses rely extensively on their personal knowledge and experience and the better that nurses felt that they knew the patient, the lower the level of subjective risk reported (Trenoweth, 2003).

It has been reported that skillful clinical management training will reduce the number of assaults toward staff and diminish the severity of any injuries subsequent to such assaults (Carmel & Hunter, 1990). Authoritative bodies, such as the National Audit Office (2003), recommend that each employer conduct a training needs analysis, and that training should be relevant to the risk management and clinical concerns of those being trained. Similarly in Ireland, the Health and Safety Authority (2001), in promoting staff safety and security concluded that there is a clear need for the availability of authoritative advice on best practice in training staff to deal with aggression and violence, and recommend an interagency collaborative effort to develop guidelines as a priority.

9 PROFESSIONAL ROLE DILEMMA: SECURITY VERSUS CARING

Across the European Union (EU) mental health services generally, the role of security rests predominantly with the health professionals mainly nurses. This may be quite different to the USA and Canada where acute psychiatric and forensic services employ security guards. The health professions, in providing care for unstable patients, also have a duty to ensure a safe and secure environment and they may be required to use procedures such as physical restraint and seclusion. The contradictory roles of carer and enforcer of rules for safety and security has the potential to create role tensions and a dilemma for health care professionals by impacting on the central tenets of trust and professional caring (Burrows, 1991).

Traditionally, the large asylum/psychiatric hospital was built with a primary objective of using security to keep the mentally ill away from society and provide an internal structure and environment which was safe and secure. The large outer perimeter wall around the hospital, barred windows, locked doors, and institutional routines during the early period of the mental health care were created for reasons of safety and security. In recent years, mental health policy has moved from a predominant model of institutional care to a more open and integrated model of community care. It would appear that the more open approach to the delivery of mental health care has been accompanied by an escalation in workplace violence. However, the relationship between the two has not been described to any great extent in the literature.

The changing health policy has also impacted on the role of mental health care professionals. For example, the traditional role of the psychiatric nurses is moving from one of custodian to therapist (Cowman, Farrelly, & Gilheaney, 2001). There are considerable role tensions in operationalizing security procedures in psychiatric nursing (Mason, 2002) and the impact of the security role on the professionalization of psychiatric nursing remains unclear at this point in time.

10   CASE STUDY IN SAFETY AND SECURITY

A population study was undertaken involving all acute admission psychiatric wards in the Republic of Ireland (Cowman & Walsh, 2004). The results of this study provide important insights into current practices in safety and security and additionally will serve as a useful benchmark for other, similar, studies. A descriptive research survey design was adopted with the use of a questionnaire for data collection. The aim of the study was to describe safety and security procedures on acute admission psychiatric wards and to report on patterns and trends. In adhering to ethical requirements, each director of nursing was approached and permission to undertake the study was obtained.

A questionnaire and accompanying letter was sent to directors of nursing of each psychiatric institution with an admission ward ($n = 37$, which included a total of 43 acute psychiatric wards). The type of admission facility ranged from a ward in the traditional large psychiatric hospital to a more modern unit in a general hospital. The accompanying letter provided information about the study and requested the director's permission, and also cooperation, with the study. The nurse in charge of each ward completed the questionnaire.

10.1   Instrument for Reporting on Safety and Security

An identified deficiency in mental health services is the lack of an appropriate instrument which can be used practically and easily by clinical practitioners to report on safety and security in clinical services. There are strong arguments to suggest that regular reporting on safety and security by clinical practitioners should be standardized across clinical areas. Such an approach could provide valuable data and insights into existing practices and how improvements can be made. An appropriate survey instrument (Ward Safety and Security Rules Survey questionnaire) to examine safety and security in psychiatric clinical environments has been used by Bowers et al. (2002), in a London-wide survey of psychiatric services. The questionnaire was subsequently modified and used by Cowman and Walsh (2004) in an Irish-based study on safety and security. Some of the main findings from the survey of acute psychiatric wards in the Republic of Ireland are reported in this case study.

The Ward Safety and Security Rules Survey instrument essentially sets out to incorporate content based around actions and procedures which traditionally, and presently, serve to provide a safe and secure environment. The Instrument contains five distinct sections and obtains data related to:

- A profile of each ward including the number of beds, ratio of qualified to unqualified staff, access to a psychiatric ICU, and the presence of a seclusion room.
- A survey of items which, through custom and practice and for security reasons, are banned from wards. Respondents were asked to identify by tick boxes which items were always, sometimes, and never banned. The respondents were also given the opportunity to report on additional items banned on wards.
- Practices related to searching of patients, visitors, and property.
- Current practices in areas such as locking of bathroom door, removal of plugs from baths, testing for alcohol or illegal drugs.
- The presence or absence of security features such as security desk and access to security guards, swipe cards, intercom, CCTV, panic alarms. Frequency of door-locking over the previous six months on a seven point scale ranging from never to always. The Advisory Committee of the Health and Safety Authority in Ireland (2001), as far back as 2001, suggested that all organizations evaluate the requirements for devices such as personal alarms, surveillance, CCTV.
- An additional space is provided on the instrument for other comments on ward safety and security.

10.2   Results

The Ward Safety and Security Rules Survey instrument was administered to all acute psychiatric wards in the Republic of Ireland. A response rate of 86% was obtained and this included 37 acute admission wards (1,033 beds) from the total of 43 in the Republic of Ireland. The mean number of beds per ward was 29, ranging from 13 to 50 beds.

In terms of clinical facilities, only 55% of wards had an intensive care unit and 49% had access to a seclusion room. It is noteworthy that 28.5% of acute wards had access to both an ICU and seclusion room and 20% had neither access to an ICU or seclusion room.

A summary of results is contained in Table 1. There was great variation in the nature of banned items across different wards. The results indicate that items always banned in one hospital are only sometimes, or never, banned in another. Items that one might expect to be always banned are not. For example, scissors were always banned in only 68% of wards. Solvents such as glue and lighter fluid were always banned in only 70% of wards.

Table 1. Summary of Banned Items in Acute Admission Wards

Banned Items			
Alcoholic drinks	37(100%)	–	–
Batteries	1(3%)	10(27%)	26(70%)
Disposable razors	15(41%)	16(43%)	6(16%)
Flexes and cables	7(19%)	20(54%)	27(27%)
Illegal drugs	36(97%)	–	1(3%)
Lighters and matches	31(84%)	6(16%)	–
Medications and tablets	35(94%)	1(3%)	1(3%)
Nail files	8(22%)	23(62%)	6(16%)
Pencils and pens	2(5%)	13(35%)	22(60%)
Penknives	35(95%)	2(5%)	–
Perfume and aftershave	3(8%)	18(49%)	16(43%)
Plastic bags	5(13%)	21(57%)	11(30%)
Razor blades	29(78%)	8(22%)	–
Scissors	25(67%)	11(30%)	1(3%)
Solvents, e.g., glue	26(70%)	11(30%)	–
Weapons, e.g., hunting knife	37(100%)	–	–

	Always/Yes	Sometimes	Never/No
Searches			
Bag search	30(81%)	7(19%)	–
Pockets search	23(62%)	14(38%)	–
Rub-down search	5(14%)	32(86%)	–
Strip search	1(3%)	8(21%)	28(76%)
Return from leave search	4(11%)	26(70%)	7(19%)
Bed space search	1(3%)	32(86%)	4(11%)
Visitors searched	3(8%)	34(92%)	–

	Always/Yes	Sometimes	Never/No
Restrictions			
Bathrooms locked	31(84%)	4(11%)	5(5%)
Taps/plugs removed	1(3%)	6(16%)	30(81%)
Plastic cutlery	20(54%)	17(46%)	–

(Continued)

Table 1. Summary of Banned Items in Acute Admission Wards—Cont'd

	Always/Yes	Sometimes	Never/No
Locked cleaning cupboard	36(97%)	1(3%)	–
Access to boiling water	16(43%)	12(33%)	24(24%)
Urine or blood test for illegal drugs on admission	6(16%)	29(78%)	2(6%)
Report to police if drug discovered	15(41%)	9(24%)	12(32%)
Urine/blood test for illegal drugs on return from leave	33(89%)	4(11%)	–
Breath/blood test for alcohol on return from leave	25(68%)	12(32%)	–
Door security and alarms			
Swipe card at ward entrance		6(16%)	31(84%)
Key pad at ward entrance		4(11%)	33(89%)
Intercom system at ward entrance		14(38%)	23(62%)
Personal panic alarm for staff		34(92%)	3(8%)
Panic alarm in office only		4(11%)	33(89%)
Emergency response telephone extension		12(32%)	25(68%)
CCTV on ward		11(30%)	26(70%)
Security desk at unit entrance		4(11%)	33(89%)
Access to security guards at all times		18(49%)	19(51%)
Rapid response team on call at all times to respond to violent crises		15(40%)	22(60%)
Patients made to pay for damage to hospital property		5(14%)	31(84%)
Patients prosecuted for violent assaults		6(16%)	31(84%)
Problem visitors refused entry		27(73%)	10(27%)

Historically, in mental health care, searching of patients and property was a major activity for staff working in psychiatric services. In this study 81% of wards always conducted a bag search on admission. Pocket searching was sometimes conducted on 38% of wards and bed spaces were always searched in only 3% of wards. Bathrooms are a frequent location for patient self harm and it is, therefore, important to note that 84% of bathroom doors are always kept locked when not in use and 81% of wards never remove plugs from baths when not in use. Plastic cutlery is never used in 54% of wards and in 78% of wards cutlery is never counted after use.

There were varied practices reported by respondents when dealing with illegal drugs, only 16% of wards always conducted a urine or blood test for illegal drugs on admission. If drugs are discovered, 32% of wards never report it to the police. Random urine or blood tests on patients for illegal drugs were never conducted in 19% of wards.

Measures aimed at ensuring staff security were lacking and the results indicate that 84% of wards do not have a swipe-card system at the ward entrance. Only 11% have a keypad system and 38% have an intercom system at ward entrance. An interesting finding is that only 3% of wards reported that all rooms have a panic alarm and CCTV was available on 30% of wards. Only 11% of wards reported the presence of a security desk at the unit's entrance and 49% of wards had access to security guards at all times. It should also be noted that only 40% of wards had a rapid response team on call at all times to respond to violent crises.

Damage to property is frequently a feature of violent outbursts and 84% of wards do not require patients to pay for damage to hospital property nor do they prosecute patients for violent assaults.

The issue of locked doors in psychiatric hospitals has been a frequent source of controversy over the years. In this study 27% of wards always had the door locked and 16% of wards never locked the door. An interesting pattern is that the doors are more likely to be locked in wards with a small number of beds than wards with a large number of beds.

10.3 Discussion of Case Study Results

One of the most striking features of the results was the variation in results with a clear lack of overall policy, procedure or agreement on what is best practice in terms of safety and security.

Clinical facilities and infrastructure appear to be factors influencing and determining approaches to support best practice. The fact that 20% of wards had neither access to an ICU or seclusion room must be a concern given the fact that seclusion is used as a measure to combat violent and assaultive patient behavior. The literature supports the need for intensive observation of some groups of patients and, within psychiatric wards as a whole, it is well documented that a small number of patients are involved in a high percentage of the violent incidents that occur (Mortimer, 1995).

Locking of ward doors in managing inpatients may be considered a controversial practice and has been considered within the code of ethics and debated as illegal detention of voluntary patients (Bowers et al., 2002). In this study there appears to be a lack of protocol and rationale in the practice of locking ward doors, as 27% of wards always had the door locked and 16% of wards never had the door locked. Any discussion on locked doors is complex. On the one hand, it raises issues of morality, ethics, and legality, while on the other there are service issues relating to the requirement to secure patients with a propensity to abscond, and to prevent access to the ward by outsiders on an open basis.

The use of alcohol and illegal substances is currently a major problem in society and poses new and varied challenges for nurses working in clinical psychiatry. In this study, patient-searching practices and testing for illegal drugs, and alcohol, on admission, and when returning from weekend leave, are not entirely consistent with the scale of the problem in society. Based on the results, it may be argued that nurses and health service employers are very tolerant of violent behavior given the fact that in 32% of wards the discovery of illegal drugs is never reported to the police. Also a majority of wards do not require patients to pay for damage to hospital property and do not prosecute patients for violent assaults.

The lack of standardized security measures at the entrance to hospital wards requires further examination. Keypad systems and swipe-cards are in limited use across wards. The limited number of wards with a security desk and access to security guards may suggest that nurses are expected to adopt more confrontational roles during episodes of violence. The lack of such security measures places frontline clinical mental health care staff in a vulnerable position and employers and managers alike must regularize practices in the interest of safety and security.

The results of the case study demonstrate a lack of overall coherent policy and procedure in safety and security measures across acute admission wards in one country. A critical point arising from the study is the extent to which similar results may be obtained from mental health services in other countries. A key question is, to what extent do the disparate practices revealed in the results of this study account for the escalation in violent episodes and assaultive behavior in psychiatric services in recent years?

It is important to note the wide range of similarities in safety and security between this case study and a similar study undertaken in London by Bowers et al. (2002). The similarity in findings is interesting given the fact that mental health services in Ireland and the UK are provided under distinctively different types of mental health legislation. The mental health legislation governing Irish services dates back to 1945 and in the UK, to 1983.

There are, however, distinctive differences in key areas between the results of the Irish study (Cowman & Walsh, 2004) and the London study (Bowers et al., 2002). When compared to the UK, a psychiatric patient admitted to the mental health service in Ireland is likely to enter a more restrictive environment through the range of items banned in the ward environment and the practice of routinely searching the patient and their belongings. Acute admission wards in London have a much smaller number of beds and it would appear that elements of security are geared toward combating the drugs culture, for example when compared to Ireland, CCTV is more prominent in communal places, probably in an attempt to control drug deals. The stronger emphasis on staff personal security in Ireland through the provision of personal alarms and the banning of items may be a reflection of a stronger nursing union culture in psychiatric nursing. Such a culture ensures that workers' rights to safe environments are upheld, and appropriate interventions developed or equipment provided.

One of the fundamental questions relates to the relationship between safety and security measures, and violence. Specifically, does an increase in safety and security lead to a proportionate increase in violence and assault? There is little available evidence to support this contention and it would appear that the therapeutic milieu and staff–patient relationship are significant factors influencing the type and level of security. James, Fineberg, Shah, and Priest (1990) reported more violent incidents on a locked psychiatric intensive care unit when nursing shifts included a higher proportion of agency or bank staff. The results of the study by James et al. indicates that human interaction and familiar relationships have a role to play in ensuring maintaining a safe environment.

Although not every incident of violence can be prevented, the adoption of practical measures as outlined in this case study may help to lessen the incidences of violence and assault, and may reduce the severity of injuries to employees. Some of the characteristic features of the traditional mental hospital were the strong emphasis on security, restrictive practices, and physical measures in combating violent and assaultive behavior. However, the policy direction of recent years has resulted in the location of services away from the large hospital and toward smaller units located in general hospitals and community care. The new locations for care require a different type, and level, of safety and security and, in the planning and design of new psychiatric units, planners must pay particular attention to safety and security features.

10.4   Looking to the Future

The results of the case study highlights a less than satisfactory situation in meeting safety and security requirements, and this is worrying given the trend of increased violence in mental health services. There is an urgent requirement for similar studies in other countries to allow for comparison and the establishment of a minimum data set.

Given the increased concerns among employers, employees, and professional organizations over the escalation in workplace violence, there is an urgent requirement for the establishment of agendas on safety and security in mental health services across all areas of mental health services delivery. Standards and best practice must be promulgated from within each country and this will require political commitment in order to strengthen the agenda of safety and security in mental health services. The consolidation and regularization of safety and security procedures is essential to the creation of stable mental health care settings that are safe and secure for patients and staff, and espouse a therapeutic milieu. In progressing and strengthening the safety and security agenda a number of actions are required including:

- Undertaking regular audits/surveys similar to that outlined in the case study reported here in order to determine and regularize safety and security measures across countries.
- The publication of position papers and guidelines on safety and security from within individual countries which will inform and direct employers and appropriate professional bodies.
- Each country must establish a forum, which includes stakeholders, to develop, agree, and publish best practice guidelines and policy for safety and security in psychiatric acute admission wards.
- Establishment of national directives on risk assessment and staff training in the management of workplace violence.
- The availability of specific funding initiatives for research is essential to the establishment of credible and robust approaches to safety and security.

REFERENCES

Bernstein, H. A. (1981). Survey of threats and assaults directed towards psychotherapists. *American Journal of Psychotherapy, 35*(4), 542–549.

Blumenthel, S., & Lavender, T. (2000). *Violence and mental disorder: A critical aid to the assessment and management of risk*. New York: Jessica Kingsley.

Bowers, L., Crowhurst, N., Alexander, J., Callaghan, P., Eales, S., Guy, S., et al. (2002). Safety and security policies on psychiatric acute admission wards: Results from a London-wide survey. *Journal of Psychiatric and Mental Health Nursing, 9*, 427–433.

Burrows, S. (1991). The special hospital nurse and the dilemma of therapeutic custody. *Journal of Advances in Health and Nursing Care, 1*(3), 21–38.

Carmel, H., & Hunter, M. (1990). Compliance with training in managing assaultive behavior and injuries from inpatient violence. *Hospital and Community Psychiatry, 41*(5), 558–560.

Clements, P. T., DeRanieri, J. T., Clark, K., Manno, M. S., & Kuhn, D. W. (2005). Workplace violence and corporate policy for health care settings. *Nursing Economics, 23*(3), 119–124.

Convit, A., Isay, D., Otis, D., & Volavka, J. (1990). Characteristics of repeatedly assaultive psychiatric inpatients. *Hospital and Community Psychiatry, 41*, 1112–1115.

Cowman, S., & Walsh, J. (2004). Safety and security procedures in psychiatric acute admission wards. *Nursing Times Research, 9*(3), 185–193.

Cowman, S., Farrelly, M., & Gilheaney, P. (2001). An examination of the role and function of the psychiatric nurse in clinical practice. *Journal of Advanced Nursing, 34*(6), 745–743.

Coyne, A. (2002). Should patients who assault staff be prosecuted? *Journal of Psychiatric and Mental Health Nursing, 9*, 139–145.

Department of Health (2000a). *Report of the review of security at the high security hospitals*. London: HMSO.

Department of Health (2000b). *An organization with a memory*. London: Department of Health www.doh.gov.uk/cmo.orgmen.

Department of Health and Children (2003). *Report of the task force on assault on psychiatric nurses*. Dublin: Department of Health and Children, (Unpublished).

Department of Labor (1998). *Guidelines for preventing workplace violence for health care service workers*. US Dept of Labor, Occupational Safety and Health Administration, OSHA 348, Washington, DC: Department of Labor.

Ferris, L., Sandercock, J., Hoffman, B., Silverman, M., & Carlisle, J. (1997). Risk assessments for acute violence to third parties: A review of the literature. *The Canadian Journal of Psychiatry, 42*, 1051–1060.

Finney, G. (1988). One false move. *Community Outlook*, April: 8–9.

Gould, D. (2000). Security alert. *Nursing Times, 96*, 26–28.

Health and Safety Authority (2001). *Report of the advisory committee on health services sector to the health and safety authority*. Dublin: Health and Safety Authority.

Health Services Advisory Committee (1987). *Violence to staff in the health services*. Sheffield: UK Health and Safety Executive.

International Labor Organization (2002). *Framework guidelines for addressing workplace violence in the health sector*. Geneva: International Labor Organization.

James, D. V., Fineberg, N. A., Shah, A. K., & Priest, R. G. (1990). An increase in violence on an acute psychiatric ward. A study of associated factors. *The British Journal of Psychiatry, 156*, 846–852.

Kennedy, H. G. (2002). Therapeutic uses of security: Mapping forensic mental health services by stratifying risk. *Advances in Psychiatric Treatment, 8*, 433–443.

Kinsley, J. (1998). Security and therapy. In: C. Kaye & A. Franey (Eds.), *Managing high security psychiatric care*. London: Jessica Kingsley.

Lamb, H. R., Weinberger, L. E., & DeCuir, W. J. (2002). The police and mental health. *Psychiatric Services, 53*(10), 1266–1271.

Mason, T. (1993). Seclusion as a cultural practice in a special hospital. *Educational Action Research, 1*(3), 411–423.

Mason, T. (2002). Forensic psychiatric nursing: A literature review and thematic analysis of role tensions. *Journal of Psychiatric and Mental Health Nursing, 9*(5), 511–520.

McCurry, P. (1999). Aggressive intent. *Community Care*, Nov/Dec:22–24.

Miller, R. D., & Maier, G. J. (1987). Factors affecting the decision to prosecute mental patients for crim-inal behavior. *Hospital and Community Psychiatry, 34*, 99–123.

Morrison, E. (1990). The tradition of toughness: A study of non professional nursing care in psychiatric settings. *Image: Journal of Nursing Scholarship, 22*(1), 32–38.

Mortimer, A. (1995). Reducing violence on secure wards. *Psychiatric Bulletin, 19*(10), 605–608.

National Audit Office (2003). *A safer place to work: Protecting NHS hospital and ambulance staff from violent aggression.* London: The National Audit Office.

National Institute of Clinical Excellence (NICE) (2005). *Violence: The short-term management of disturbed/violent behavior in in-patient psychiatric settings and emergency departments. Clinical Guideline 25.* London: NICE.

National Institute of Occupational Safety and Health (2003). *Developing and implementing a workplace violence prevention program and policy.* http://www.cdc.gov/niosh/ Accessed 31.01.06.

Nork, M. M. A., Zonana, H. V., & Phillips, R. T. (1992). Prosecuting assaultive psychiatric patients. *Journal of Forensic Sciences, 37*, 923–931.

North Eastern Health Board (2004). *Study of work-related violence. Committee on Workplace Violence.* Kells, Ireland: North Eastern Health Board.

Paterson, B., McCornish, A., & Bradley, P. (1999). Violence at work. *Nursing Standard, 13*, 43–46.

Psychiatric Nurses Association of Ireland (2002). *Assault Survey.* Psychiatric Nurses Association, 2 Gardiner Place, Dublin. Dublin: Psychiatric Nurses Association of Ireland.

Qadir, G. (1982). Violence in an open psychiatric unit. *Journal of Psychiatric Treatment and Evaluation, 41*, 409–413.

Rogers, P., & Topping-Morris, B. (1997). Clinical supervision for forensic mental health nurses. *Nursing Management, 4*(5), 13–15.

Royal College of Psychiatrists (1999). *Report of the collegiate trainee's committee working party on the safety of trainees. Council report CR78.* London: Royal College of Psychiatrists.

Royal College of Psychiatrists (2000). *National audit of management of violence in mental health settings.* London: Royal College of Psychiatrists.

Ryrie, I., & McGowan, J. (1998). Staff perceptions of substance use among psychiatric in-patients. *Journal of Psychiatric and Mental Health Nursing, 5*, 137–142.

Sanders, J., Milner, S., Brown, P., & Bell, A., J. (2000). Assessment of aggression in psychiatric admis-sions: Semi-structured interview and case note survey. *British Medical Journal, 320*(72420), 1112.

Tolhurst, H., Baker, L., Murray, G., Bell, P., Sutton, A., & Dean, S. (2003). Rural general practitioner experience of work-related violence in Australia. *Australian Journal of Rural Health, 11*(5), 231–236.

Trenoweth, S. (2003). Perceiving risk in dangerous situations: Risks of violence among mental health inpatients. *Journal of Advanced Nursing, 42*(3), 278–287.

Turnbull, J. (1999). Theoretical approaches to violence and aggression. In: J. Turnbull & B. Paterson (Eds.), *Aggression and violence: Approaches to effective management* (pp. 31–51). London: McMillan Press.

Whittington, R. (2002). Attitudes towards patient aggression amongst mental health nurses in the "zero tolerance" era: Associations with burnout and length of experience. *Journal of Clinical Nursing, 11*, 819–825.

Wilson, R. M., Runciman, W. B., Gibberd, R. W., Harrison B. T., Newby L., & Hamilton, J. D. (1995). The quality in Australian health care study. *The Medical Journal of Australia, 163*, 458–471.

Wiseman, R. (2001). The ANA develops Bill of Rights for Registered Nurses: know your rights in the work place. *American Journal of Nursing, 101*(11), 55–56.

Zahid, M. A., Al-Sahlawi, K. S., Shahid, A. A., Awadh, J. A., & Abu-Shammah, H. (1999). Violence against doctors: 2. Effects of violence on doctors working in accident and emergency departments. *European Journal of Emergency Medicine, 6*(4), 305–309.

Zealberg, J. J., Santos, A. B., & Pucket, J. A. (1996). *Comprehensive emergency mental health: Protocol for collaboration with the police department.* New York: Norton.

14

Ward Culture and Atmosphere

Joy A. Duxbury, Anna Björkdahl, and
Sheena Johnson

1   INTRODUCTION

Violence and aggression in the inpatient psychiatric setting has long been a major
cause for concern in the UK, and continues to be the subject of a considerable
amount of research, official reports, and policy documents (Lowe, Wellman, &
Taylor, 2003). This is also true of Switzerland and a number of other European countries, in particular Sweden, Finland, Norway, and, to some extent, Italy, where an
increasing amount of attention has been given to this subject (Bowers et al., 1999).
In contrast, a great deal of work has been conducted in America and the work of
Morrison (1998) has been significant in this field of research but more from an organizational and cultural perspective.

   The literature concerning aggression and violence in psychiatry from a broader
perspective is extensive and indicative of concerns surrounding a problem which has
been investigated from a number of angles. While this has commonly involved the
characteristics of staff and patients, a range of other factors external to the two parties or associated with their relationships and interactions has also been examined
(Secker et al., 2004). The influence of the ward atmosphere on the incidence of
aggression, for example, is one area that has been acknowledged for some time, particularly since the reported negative impact of the institution. Despite the processes
of deinstitutionalization however, the hospital setting remains the hub of mental
health services in many countries.

Nijman, a Campo, Ravelli, and Merckelbach (1999) have suggested that three models explaining the potential causes of patient aggression exist within the healthcare literature. The first two models are in stark opposition and focus upon "internal factors" as precursors to aggression, or "external factors." In other words, is an aggressive patient response the result of factors such as frustration, illness, fear, age, gender, ethnicity and so forth, or the result of external factors such as the environment? The external model highlights a number of environmental influences that can contribute to patient aggression rather than individual patient factors (Duxbury, 2002). Shepherd and Lavender (1999) suggest that violent incidents are, in fact, more likely to be preceded by external environmental and interpersonal antecedents of this nature than internal, symptom related ones. The "interactional–situational model" is the third identified view and focuses upon the interplay between patient and staff interaction and the situation that presents. For the purpose of this chapter a review of the ward atmosphere will incorporate elements associated with the external and situational/interactional models as both apply in different ways.

Environmental factors that contribute to the overall atmosphere of the ward and that can lead to aggression have been reported in a variety of studies (Jansen, Dansen, & Jebbnik, 2005; Nijman, 2002). Issues that have been explored range from design deficits, hospital census figures, patterns of assaults, ward turmoil commonly underpinned by poor staffing levels and the use of temporary staff, a lack of privacy and freedom, inadequate organization, vague ward polices, poor staff–patient interactions, and ineffective communication (Jansen et al.). Various aspects of the physical environment are also indicative (Nijman et al., 1999) as are factors pertaining to the ward milieu, power, rules, and limit setting. Situations and/or interactions which may precipitate patient aggression are clearly important and contribute to the overall atmosphere and underpinning culture of any ward.

Before a discussion of the literature specifically relating to ward culture, atmosphere, and aggression, a review of general organizational culture theory and the relationships identified between organizational culture and work outcomes is provided. This overview sets the scene for the ward-specific research introduced later in the chapter and establishes the benefits of a consideration of culture as a key factor in the experience of ward life, both for employees and patients.

2   ORGANIZATIONAL CULTURE

Harrison (1972) defined organizational culture in terms of the beliefs and values of the organization, which act as prescriptions for the way in which organizational members should work. Similarly Smircich (1983) stated that "culture serves as a sense-making device that can guide and shape behavior" (Smircich, p. 346). The study of organizational culture is, therefore, about understanding people's perceptions of the organizations in which they work, and how these perceptions influence their attitudes and behavior toward, and within, their work environment.

The general concept of culture has been around for many years with intellectual influences from both anthropology and sociology (Ouchi & Wilkins, 1985). However, the study and application of culture within an organizational context predominately dates from the 1970s and, in a reflection of its utility as a tool with which to gain insight into organizations, remains a large and growing area of organizational research. A similar concept to culture, primarily based within social and organizational contexts, is evident in "climate" literature and research. In brief, culture is typically viewed as a deeper, more stable phenomenon than climate, which is temporal and less resistant to change. The study of organizational climate preceded that of organizational culture and climate has been conceptualized as a "snapshot" of organizational culture (Mearns, Flin, Gordon, & Fleming, 1998) and is typically viewed as a component of culture, that is, information about the climate of an organization can provide insight into its culture. Although there is some disagreement between researchers as to the definitions, and appropriate measurement methods, of the culture and climate concepts (and indeed the terms are often used interchangeably, see Glisson and James (2002), Rousseau's (1988) description of climate demonstrates the close relationship the concepts of climate and culture have in practice. She, along with others, considered climate as consisting of shared perceptions and beliefs, making it similar to Schein's middle level of culture, detailed below. Having acknowledged the confusion that often exists between the two terms, the term culture is used throughout this section in an effort to ease comprehension for the reader.

A number of theorists have described culture. One of the most influential of these, Schein (1992), believed culture existed across three main levels: artifacts, e.g., organizational rules, procedures, and observable behaviors of employees, espoused values (which serve to determine employee beliefs about how things ought to be and what is important in the organization), and basic assumptions (unconscious assumptions about appropriate behavior and reactions in any given situation). Schein defined culture as:

> "A pattern of shared basic assumptions that the group learned as it solved its problems of external adaptation and internal integration that has worked well enough to be considered valid and, therefore, to be taught to new members as the correct way to perceive, think, and feel in relation to those problems." (Schein, 1992, p. 12)

It is widely accepted that organizations do not operate one overall culture, rather they are comprised of subcultures. Martin, Sitkin, and Boehm (1985) detailed how it is more realistic to study organizational culture as an umbrella under which multiple subcultures exist, and Jansen (1994), suggested a number of different subcultures that may exist within an organization, i.e., corporate, departmental, divisional, geographical location, issue-related, and professional. Attention of culture at the ward level, as opposed to the broader organizational, e.g., hospital level is therefore appropriate.

Both qualitative and quantitative research techniques are employed to research culture, for example interviews with employees which enable detailed discussion, and attitude questionnaire studies which typically measure Schein's middle level of organizational culture (and are often used within climate research).

Culture is widely promoted as a tool for gaining insight into the workings of an organization. Researchers have discussed culture as the key to understand what makes some organizations more successful than others (Martin, 1992; Peters & Waterman, 1982). Others have looked at the impact that culture has on the well-being and performance of organizations (Denison, 1996; Wilkins & Ouchi, 1983). Additionally, specific elements of culture, for example safety culture (Flin, Mearns, O'Connor, & Bryden, 2000; Guldenmund, 2000), have been examined, and culture shown to be related to the experience of accidents within the workplace. Moreover, it has been demonstrated that accident rates can be reduced through attention to, and improvement of, an organization's safety culture. Enquiries following safety incidents repeatedly identify cultural factors which significantly contributed to the chain of events preceding an incident for example Piper Alpha oil rig fire, (Cullen, 1990); Ladbroke Grove rail crash, (Cullen, 2001). The relevance of culture within a ward environment and its influence on employee and patient attitudes and behavior in relation to violent incidents is therefore clearly indicated.

A number of researchers have looked at culture in a healthcare context (Peck, Towell, & Gulliver, 2001; Scott, Mannion, Marshall, & Davies, 2003; Smith, 2002). Scott et al. reviewed the evidence between organizational culture and healthcare performance and concluded that there was sufficient evidence to suggest a relationship does exist they discussed the potential importance of patient involvement in the production of culture. Within mental health care, poor communication between staff and management, staffing levels, stress, and high workloads have been identified as responsible for low employee morale, which can be expected to influence the culture of the organization (Commission for Health Improvement, 2004). The importance of issues such as these is further indicated later in the chapter when discussing specific research relating to patient violence and aggression.

3   PATTERNS OF ASSAULT

Variants known to affect the probability of violence include not only the ward's physical environment and culture, as discussed, but also patterns of therapeutic activity, staff ratios which may affect levels of interaction, and, to a limited extent, seasonal variation (Flannery, Hanson, & Penk, 1994). Each impact upon, or is affected by, the nature of the ward organization. For example, the timing of assaults appears significant and often relates to location and levels of staff–patient interaction (Aquilina, 1991). For instance, Vanderslott (1998) demonstrated that aggressive incidents occurred more frequently in the daytime between 10:00 and 13:59 hours. Whittington and Wykes (1994a), showed some variability in their findings reporting that staff availability increased from 30% in the morning to over 70% between 18:00 and 19:00 hours. Rates of talking and listening also varied, with peaks of staff–patient interaction at lunchtime and between 16:00 and 17:00 hours. This, to some extent, supports the view that the nonavailability of staff can lead to peaks of violent behavior which has been noted in previous research. Grassi, Peron, Marangoni, Zanchi, and Vanni (2001) have reported in their more recent study that most violent episodes occurred during the day (150 episodes between 08:00 and 13:00, 45.6%), followed by afternoon/evening (35.9%), and then night (18.5%). This could reflect the organization of the ward where the admission of new patients occurs in the morning with a resulting increase in the level of turmoil in the ward atmosphere. Duxbury (2002) found that a number of incidents occurred during the evening/early night shift when staff numbers were reduced.

To some extent, days of the week have been identified as a feature of patient aggression (Aquilina, 1991; Hanson & Balk, 1992). Carmel and Hunter (1993) found, in a five-year study, that when compared to the rest of the week, Mondays and Tuesdays accounted for more staff injuries. Distribution throughout the week, while reported to be uniform by Grassi et al. (2001), also demonstrated that half of the incidents occurred within the first week of admission, many within the first two days. Flannery et al. (1994) similarly found that most staff assaults occurred on Tuesdays. The increase in activity that often occurs at the start of the week was suggested for this result. Carmel and Hunter argued that diminished patient contact may be contributory and that this is often the result of organizational patterns and routines when staff are busy attending to patients' medication, treatment, handover periods, or at mealtimes (Vanderslott, 1998).

In addition to time hot-spots, changes in the patterns of ward census can have a significant impact upon aggressive behavior. Overcrowding and staffing levels have been noted to be problematic. Invasions of personal space related to over-crowding have been reported by Ryden, Bossenmaier, and McLachlan (1991). Palmstierna et al. (1991) found that psychiatric patients, and those with schizophrenia in particular, were significantly more aggressive on days when the unit census was elevated. Grassi et al. (2001) reported that 53.1% of incidents in their five-year Italian study were registered when the number of patients in the unit was higher than allowed. On a crowded psychiatric unit, the patient may be exposed to over-stimulation (Krakowski & Czobar, 1994). This may be particularly problematic on admission when several environmental stressors come into play (Nijman et al., 1999). The National Institute for Clinical Excellence (NICE) in the UK recommends that bed occupancy should be decided at local level and that this should not be exceeded because overcrowding leads to tension, frustration, and overstretched staff. They also suggest that there should be a stable and consistent inpatient team, as high staff turnover, and overuse of short term bank, locum, and agency staff, may create an unsafe and potentially volatile environment. Grassi et al. (2001) in contrast, suggest this can have the opposite effect whereby the resulting high number of staff may lead to better patient interaction and monitoring that can reduce violence. They further argue that fluctuations in the daily population and the different characteristics of space organization among wards in different studies represent significant variables that can bias the evaluation of the consequences of overcrowding, and suggest more research is necessary to explore this area (Kumar, Ng, & Robinson, 1999).

Inactivity has also been found to be a problem with over one-third of service users (of a total 1,459) reporting dissatisfaction with the choice of therapies/activities offered during the day (Healthcare Commission, 2005). Nijman (2002), infact argues that exposure to demanding therapies may result in frustration, anger, and violence. Patterns of care and associated periods of time in the life of the ward therefore can invariably contribute to an overall ward atmosphere dependent upon how the combination is matched and catered for.

4 THE CONCEPT OF WARD ATMOSPHERE

Definitions of what constitutes a ward atmosphere are difficult to find. This is hardly surprising given the complexity of factors involved. A lack of distinction between a plethora of terms such as "ward and social atmosphere" (Jansson & Eklund, 2002), social ecology (Moos, 1974), ward culture, ward milieu, ward environment, and ward climate further complicates the issue. Edvardsson (2005) uses the term "atmosphere" to "include the understanding and description of a tone or mood in care settings or . . . of what is contained 'within the walls' of that setting" (Edvardsson, p. 8). He sees the concepts of atmosphere and climate as interchangeable metaphors describing the psychological conditions of a social region. Schalast and Redies (2005), in a similar fashion suggest that "the interaction of aspects of the material, social, and emotional conditions of a ward, which may—over time—influence the mood, behavior, and self concept of the persons involved" are indicative of a "ward atmosphere".

The term "ward atmosphere" in particular seems to be most commonly adopted in studies that focus upon psychiatric settings. Moos (1974) may have been influential in this trend, devising what soon became known as the Ward Atmosphere Scale (WAS). This was developed in the 1960s in an attempt to describe and measure the therapeutic atmosphere in psychiatric and drug treatment settings. The WAS consists of a 100-item questionnaire that measures views about the actual real ward, preferences about the ideal ward, and individual expectations about the ward in general. It comprises three dimensions that highlight relationships, personal growth, and system maintenance, each of which is reflected in 10 subscales.

This tool has been regarded as the most widely used to measure ward atmosphere in inpatient settings (Rossberg & Friis, 2003a). Still, it has been criticized for being dated, lacking content validity, its extensive size, and limited psychometric properties. However, the fact it is still used today indicates that the dimensions and subscales identified continue to be recognized and the scale comprehensive to use.

Rossberg and Friis (2003a) have endeavored to defend criticisms of the WAS. They argue that the anger and aggression, and the spontaneity subscales, measuring behavior and attitudes, both cover two distinctly different dimensions, yet include items closely related to each other. Changes have also meant that some of the original items have been eliminated to improve levels of intercorrelation. The authors found that by reducing a total of sixteen items to ten, and then to eight,

Table 1. The Dimensions and Subscales of the Ward Atmosphere Scale (Moos, 1974)

Relationship Dimension	Personal Growth Dimension	System Maintenance Dimension
Involvement	Autonomy	Order and organization
Support	Practical orientation	Program clarity
Spontaneity	Personal problems orientation	Staff control
	Anger and aggression	

psychometric properties were improved and the content made more contemporary (Rossberg & Friis, 2003b).

By using the WAS, Friis (1986) has suggested that patients with different psychiatric diagnoses may need different things from a ward. Psychotic patients for instance seem, according to Friis, to benefit most from a ward atmosphere which emphasizes support with less interaction, practical orientation, order, and organization. In contrast, nonpsychotic patients benefit from a high level on all the WAS subscales, except for staff control which should be low. Johansson and Eklund (2004) found that patients stress the importance of a supportive ward atmosphere but one which also has a comprehensive treatment program as well as general ward stability and spontaneity. These factors, it is argued, could be seen as parallels to theoretical frames of psychotherapeutic relationships between the therapist and the patient.

The impact of the ward atmosphere upon patient aggression and violence, albeit a complex phenomenon that affects, and is affected by, the approach adopted by staff, can be viewed broadly as an interplay between three different but commonly interrelated areas:

- Ward culture
- Structural environment
- Patterns of assaultive behavior

The first of which, the less tangible aspect, is ward culture and its associated organizational and individual relationships and styles. The second and third components are more tangible and include the structural environment and patterns of assaultive behavior that may contribute to the overall atmosphere and stability of the ward. To some extent this reflects the view of Middleboe, Schjodt, Byrsting, and Gjerris (2001) that the ward atmosphere comprises the psychological, social, and physical climate of the psychiatric ward, commonly also referred to as the ward milieu. Quirk and Lelliott (2001) have reported that research conducted in the UK supports the view that organizational pressures and a decline in nurse–patient relationships are having a negative impact upon the quality of care. They have summarized UK research from the 1990s which suggests that contact is limited, wards are perceived as boring and unsafe, and general conditions are thus criticized. Different aspects of the ward milieu and how this has affected therapeutic outcomes and patient satis-faction has been a focus (Middleboe et al. 2001). Little is known about how patients perceive their treatment environment and no recent studies exist that "directly" examine the patients' perception of the "atmosphere" of the ward and its impact upon aggression and violence. However, since we know from existing organizational culture studies that employee perceptions of organizational culture affect both employee behavior and negative work incidents, for example through its influence on unsafe working practices and accident rates, it is reasonable to assume that patient perceptions of ward culture (in conjunction with other factors such as ward structure) will affect patient behavior.

5   WARD CULTURE

Gesler and Kearns (2002), defined culture as:

> "The complex of socially produced values, rules, beliefs, literature, arts, media, penal codes, laws, political ideas, and other such diversions by which a society, or any social group, represents its view of the world as its members (or at least the members in charge) believe it is." (p. 12)

More specifically, according to Huxley (2002), culture can also comprise material objects (artifacts), social relations (sociofacts), and ideas (mentifacts), and thus staff–patient interaction and the rules of the ward are of particular importance in the healthcare setting.

The ward culture is significantly shaped by the organization of, and the philos-ophy and nursing style adopted in, each care setting. According to Cortis (2003), it is "within this reality, or world view, an individual's purpose in life is defined, and appropriate, sanctioned behavior within the social group is prescribed" (Cortis, p. 55). Kagawa-Singer and Chung (1994) argue that:

> "Culture therefore furnishes the beliefs and values that give individuals a sense of identity, self-worth, and belonging, as well as providing the rules for behav-ior. This enables the group to survive and provide for the welfare and support of its members." (Cortis, 2003)

This is of significant importance in an environment that is potentially dangerous.

Bowers (2002) has endeavored to establish what underpins a good ward culture, suggesting six underlying mechanisms, including the following: A *psychiatric phi-losophy*, a belief in the importance of *psychosocial factors*, *moral commitments* and choices such as bravery, honesty, and equality, *cognitive-emotional self-management, technical mastery* using interpersonal skills such as solving conflicts, *teamwork skills* to share the burden of care and maintain consistency in relation to rules and, finally, *organizational support*. Bowers found the latter to be crucial requiring policy clarity and stability, specialist training, clinical supervision, and a management that is present on the ward and integrated into clinical care. In his study, five positive outcomes were reported. *Positive staff attitudes* and a sense of purpose and enthusiasm, a *positive impact* whereby *therapy* levels increased, an increase in the amount of time spent with patients, and finally, less *conflict* and limited *containment* as a consequence.

The ward culture can also be influenced by what patients bring with them when admitted to the ward. Morrison et al. (2002) described the importance of understanding the "street nature" on three forensic maximum security wards. Due to the high level of violence and aggression on the wards, guards with protective outfits were installed preferably to protect staff. This resulted in less violence and lower staff injury rates, and promoted greater therapeutic activity. According to Morrison (1998), this was an example of how the ward's culture had to be adapted in response to a patient's background.

6   RULES AND POWER

From a more social perspective, the use of ward rules can be instrumental in the development and maintenance of the positive, or negative, culture of a ward. Studies have shown for example, that there is a negative relationship between fixed rules and patient aggression (Roper & Anderson, 1991). Assaults can also be triggered by the denial of services and impingements upon liberty. Subsequently there may be a relationship between the flexibility/inflexibility of ward nursing regimes and patient outcomes (Alexander & Bowers, 2004). From the client perspective, powerlessness is a closely related and predominant theme (Breeze & Repper, 1998; Goodwin, Holmes, Newnes, & Waltho, 1999). The picture that emerges is one of an intolerable environment (i.e., one that possesses a negative culture indicating that employee and patient attitudes toward their environment are negative) within which aggressive acts are seen as both justified and as a brief period of self empowerment albeit negatively communicated (Secker et al., 2004). The concept of power is complex and the literature fails to produce a single uniform definition, particularly pertaining to social power. Hokanson Hawks (1991) suggests that the best one can do is to make two broad distinctions dependent upon the context, that of power over and power to, the latter implying a degree of empowerment and autonomy. This, argue Breeze and Repper, require nursing staff to return some control to the patient, and offer care and support which is recognized by the patient as skillful and therapeutic. From their study using interviews, Alexander and Bowers found that the most commonly reported antecedents to incidents revolved around power struggles between staff and patients and an inability by staff to empathize with the clients' point of view, often resulting in rigid procedural ward rules. It is commonly forgotten that patient behavior may be the result of fear and distress whereby reassurance would have been of value. Rigidity may reflect the status of ward systems and their inability to facilitate individualized care (Pilgrim & Rogers, 1999). Roper and Anderson found that patient violence was associated with nurses' attitudes toward control, and that staff used ward structure to deny patients' requests.

Critchon (1997) examined nurses' responses to rule-breaking, which sometimes resulted in containment and moral judgments about patients. This may result in blame placement, a feature reported by Duxbury (1999) in her survey of nurses using critical incidents.

By reviewing eyewitness accounts of 921 incidents of aggression, Powell, Caan, and Crowe (1994) demonstrated that a range of antecedents could be identified. The most common factors reported involved hospital regimes and interactions with others. In contrast however, Bensley, Nelson, Kaufman, Silverstein, and Walker Shields (1995) found that patients identified a lack of rule clarity as a primary factor influencing assaults. Aubrey, Bradley, Siddique, and LeBlanc (1996) used the Ward Atmosphere Scale to measure the impact of environmental changes on staff and patients which included greater rule clarity, the instigation of fewer searches, and more flexibility pertaining to care. As a result patients reported an improved social climate.

Further studies have also shown the value of restriction when comparing alternative therapeutic models as it can be that inconsistencies with social and therapeutic rules can lead to violent and aggressive behavior. Katz and Kirkland (1990), for example, found that violence was more frequent on disorganized wards where leadership was absent and staff–patient interaction unpredictable. Inconsistency in limit-setting regimes appears to act as an additional communication stressor (Nijman, 2002; Nijman et al., 1999).

Parallels between cultural studies on safety are evident in that good leadership (as demonstrated through positive management attitudes toward safety) is accepted as a key component of ensuring that a positive safety culture is in place in an organization (Flin et al., 2000). Good leadership within a ward context, for example through the setting of clear rules, ensuring these rules are consistently interpreted by employees, and ensuring good communication methods are in place, is therefore likely to impact upon employee (and subsequently patient) behavior and a positive ward culture.

Therefore it seems patterns in social organization and staff behavior can be attributed to reductions in the frequency and severity of violence. However, if rules are to be beneficial then therapeutic relationships must underpin their implementation. Alexander and Bowers (2004), on the subject of ward rules, highlight an association between nurse–patient interaction and rules. Arguments about rule clarity, clear communication, and consistency are indicative and the absence of these factors are reportedly linked to patient aggression. Mistral, Hall, and McKee (2002) examined the impact of therapeutic community principles in the management of a number of detained patients. These included the communication of the aims and clarity of ward rules pertaining to smoking, alcohol, the use of illegal substances, and communal responsibilities. The authors reported improved levels of communication and improvements in the physical environment.

To date, it is difficult to determine conclusively whether rigid or flexible environments are the most effective therapeutic ways of managing psychiatric wards. However, it seems that patients may view rules positively if they are underpinned by a communicated concern for welfare, while they are more likely to incite aggression if imposed in an insensitive and punitive manner (Alexander & Bowers, 2004). Many of these studies highlight a need to regulate institutional responses to patient aggression to avoid the inappropriate use of impositions, ward rules, and sanctions (Alexander & Bowers). A positive organizational culture then can be seen as:

> "A pattern of basic assumptions . . . developed by a given group . . . to cope with its problems . . . and taught to new members as a correct way to perceive, think, and feel in relation to those problems." (Schein, 1989)

Secker et al. (2004) suggest that previous research indicates that the organization of care can be hugely influential in levels of aggression and violence within the ward environment. This then forms the basis of a well-defined ward atmosphere. As problematic communication between staff and patients appears to be a consistent theme in the literature then it seems that, in order to prevent aggression, treatment goals and ward rules need to be explained carefully.

7   THE NURSE–PATIENT RELATIONSHIP

An increasing emphasis upon research into nurse–patient contact has emerged, particularly on how nurses relate to patients. This, invariably, will have an influence upon the overall atmosphere of any ward. Cheung, Schweitzer, Crowley, Yastrubetskaya, and Tuckwell (1997) reported that most assaults are triggered by staff–patient interactions, a view echoed by Abderhalden, Needham, Friedli, Poelmans, and Dansen (2002), who recognized that staff attitudes and behavior (which form a core part of the ward culture) may be two of the most important factors modulating aggressive behavior. Situational variables should be taken into account when assessing the risk of violent behavior as limit-setting, pertaining to parameters of activity and choice, and poor staff attitudes can be inflammatory (NICE, 2005).

Sheriden, Henrion, and Baxter (1990), on reviewing 73 incidents, found that patients commonly viewed conflicts with staff as contributory and thus may become frustrated and angry if they perceive that nursing staff are inaccessible (Whittington & Wykes, 1996). Powell et al. (1994) reported 5–10% of incidents to be the result of misinterpretation in communication. Whittington and Wykes (1994b) suggest that certain staff members are prone to being assaulted, indicating problematic rather than therapeutic relationships. Furthermore, limit-setting styles such as belittlement, the use of platitudes, and solutions without options are reported to be ineffective interpersonal strategies (Lancee, Gallop, McCay, & Toner, 1995). However, it is also argued that staff distancing due to previous assaults can preempt future assaults (Whittington & Wykes, 1994a). The proposal that staff withdraw from problematic relationships with clients is not new (Smith & Hart, 1994). It seems there is a fine line between strong leadership styles and authoritarian attitudes when examine levels of violence (James, Fineberg, Shah, & Priest, 1990).

Overall, it is clear that the impact of interactional factors can be substantial. The problem is in determining whether this impact is positive or negative and in controlling the numerous variables that interplay in the overall process. The Healthcare Commission has reported that a significant percentage of patients feel that they are unable to speak to staff, that staff "wind them up," and that their complaints are not taken seriously. Duxbury (2002) has reported findings of a similar nature when interviewing patients about the cause of aggression and violence in one mental health unit. Breeze and Repper (1998) found, in their study using unstructured interviews, that where nurses were perceived by patients to demonstrate respect, time, skilled care, and a willingness to give some patients control and a degree of choice over their care, feelings of anger were reduced. This has clear implications for the development of therapeutic relationships and systems to facilitate empowerment which then, in turn, may promote a positive and effective ward culture and subsequent positive ward atmosphere. Harris and Morrison (1995) suggest that, for a successful therapeutic environment, the avoidance of power struggles.

8   WARD STRUCTURE AND DESIGN

The physical environment of a unit can also be considered a molding factor in the risk of violence (Grassi et al., 2001). The design of a ward can contribute to its general atmosphere. In a recent one-year study by Vanderslott (1998), a number of external variables were noted to be influential, including the location of assaults, which commonly occurred in the lounge and bedroom areas (Ryden et al., 1991). There is growing empirical evidence that supports the positive impact of changes to the physical environment in psychiatry, particularly the lounge where patients spend much of their time. In contrast, Hunter and Love (1996) report that violence is often problematic in the dining room area, and by making changes to the environment and promoting increased therapeutic communication between staff and patients at mealtimes, aggressive dining room incidents were reduced by 40% over a two-year period. Using action research, Devlin (1992) demonstrated that the remodeling of two wards improved patient and staff satisfaction significantly, and the rate of violence decreased by almost 50%. Recommendations have since been made for the reorganization of key areas such as interviewing rooms (Lilywhite, Morgan, & Walter, 1995). Guidelines from the Royal College of Psychiatrists (1998) recommend that hospital environments should be comfortable, safe, private, and homely. More recently, both the National Institute for Mental Health in England (NIMHE) and the National Institute of Clinical Excellence (NICE) recommend that the environment in which care is delivered be scrutinized and planned for more effectively. NICE (2005), for example, suggested that the physical and therapeutic environment can have a strong, mitigating effect on the short term management of disturbed/violent behavior. They recommend that the internal design of the ward should accommodate service users' needs for engaging in activities and individual choice. More specifically, they argue there should be provisions for privacy when making phone calls, receiving guests, and when talking to a member of staff. Additional studies have indicated that lack of space is associated with violence (Rabeinowitz & Mark, 1999). However, controversy exists over this issue with some studies indicating (Palmstierna and Wistedt, 1995), and others not confirming, this relationship (Nijman & Rector, 1999).

It has been suggested that, since the components of risk are dynamic and may change according to circumstance, risk assessment of the environment should be ongoing. In addition, noxious environmental factors should be controlled as much as possible. An environmental audit of 265 mental health and learning disability wards/units revealed that temperature and ventilation were poorly controlled, quiet spaces for patients and staff inadequate, including private spaces for interactions, and the ward design and size of some wards poor (Healthcare Commission, 2005). Sufficient means for controlling light, temperature, and ventilation should therefore be made available. This was reflected in staff and patient responses to a survey, although interestingly, nursing staff were generally more likely than service users to express dissatisfaction with aspects of the physical environment which was viewed as cramped and oppressive with limited facilities (Healthcare Commission). Simple low-cost techniques such as making alterations to furniture arrangements have been found to have a positive impact upon a ward's psychosocial atmosphere. Conversely, environmental alterations have also been reported to increase aggression and violence, resulting in a greater need for interventions such as seclusion and restraint (Brooks, Gilead, & Daniels, 1994).

9 IMPLICATIONS

The impact of the ward atmosphere, albeit a somewhat tenuous term, on the incidence of patient aggression and violence is set to rise, given the increasing challenges facing changing models of inpatient care. The National Service Framework for Mental Health in England stipulates that the highest quality of health care should be provided for mental health users, and that incidents of violence and aggression mitigate against achieving this goal (Secker et al., 2004). Research has demonstrated that conditions to meet standards in inpatient settings are not always available, and that the quality of the therapeutic environment is both affected and precipitated by aggression.

There is evidence of continued interest in interactive factors and the role of adverse situations and perceptions of staff and patients about them. This then suggests a clear need to identify those that precipitate negative staff behavior, and to clarify the way in which staff make clinical judgments that are commonly elicited and reinforced by employing organizations (Lowe et al., 2003). It seems a lack of engagement may be widespread (Healthcare Commission, 2005). This, in turn, has implications for Zero Tolerance Campaigns which reflect a culture that may compound the situation (Secker et al., 2004; Whittington & Higgins, 2002). Rather than adopt a position of Zero Tolerance, for example, it seems that mechanisms for emotional support, critical reflection and learning, and the pursuit of therapeutic accountability might be a way forward. In order to promote recovery, opportunities need to be provided for patients who are aggressive to express their feelings without being judged (Secker et al. 2004).

Nijman et al. (1999) has argued that even in cases in which psychopathology is the primary antecedent to aggression, the contribution of environmental and communication stressors cannot be ruled out. Furthermore he suggests that the examination of the ward variables on inpatient aggression is a neglected area of research which may be hindered by cost. The UK Healthcare Commission (2005) suggests that we should use what we already know when designing safer environments and endeavor to improve ward-based activities and care packages. Structural and supportive factors in the inpatient ward environment are reportedly of particular value in inpatient treatment and thus further prospective studies are needed to explore this issue further (Middleboe et al., 2001).

In this chapter, a range of literature has been explored, some of which directly relates to ward atmosphere and aggression, but much of which has been applied given the limited research available. Implications for policy, particularly in terms of standardizing procedures are evident. With regards to organizational culture Scott et al. (2003) suggest that there should be an increase in the use of theoretical culture knowledge in empirical work, in addition to longitudinal and cross-sectional studies. Both quantitative and qualitative methods should therefore be used as complements to each other. Ultimately, the immediate and primary function of social science research should be to direct the process of change in psychiatric inpatient care and examine indiscriminate phenomenon such as the ward culture and atmosphere. The need to examine this at different levels and from different perspectives cannot, therefore, be underestimated, and larger scale studies are warranted. The National Institute for Clinical Excellence (2005) recommend that prospective cohort studies in particular are required to identify antecedents to aggressive/violent behavior in adult inpatient psychiatric settings.

Changes in behavior within institutions that impact upon the ward environment and atmosphere are rarely due to one factor alone. It is clear that a number of variables can contribute to an untherapeutic ward atmosphere, which can precipitate aggressive behavior. The design of many of our wards/units fails to meet the many basic safety standards. Therefore it is vital that systems to ensure staff and service users are fully involved in the design process for every new mental health setting are in place. It seems clinically meaningful to allow patients to evaluate their own environment, particularly pertaining to design, milieu and rules, intervention priorities and regimes, and the nature of relationships. Information on patient perceptions of their environment can serve to inform us of the ward culture and aid the identification of negative cultures that may be having an impact on the occurrence of violent incidences. Furthermore, real efforts should be made to upgrade and improve existing wards. Client mix and overcrowding leads to "fire fighting" and, for many inpatient services faced with high bed occupancy figures and inadequate staffing, the delivery of a therapeutic service can become impossible. Action is required for both commissioners and managers to address this. High levels of boredom lead to an unstructured and untherapeutic system of care and, as boredom has been linked to violence, this warrants greater investigation. It is vital that the status of inpatient care is raised if time, resources, funding, and training is to be targeted to remedy a number of these issues (Healthcare Commission, 2005). The National Institute of Mental Health in England (2004) suggests that in order to minimize the risk of violence that effective organizational, environmental, clinical, and management approaches and mechanisms need to be in place and supported at various levels. Environmental safety and the promotion of a positive ward atmosphere is everyone's business! Furthermore, while professionals may be unable to resist the greater legal responsibilities of their present "gate-keeping" role, they should be encouraged to use their power responsibly and rediscover a partnership role rather than rely upon their authority. This will significantly impact upon the culture of the inpatient ward.

Useful guidance to services when considering, commissioning new, or refurbishing, mental health facilities such as that provided by the Royal College of Psychiatrists (1998) is a positive way forward. But first the Healthcare Commission (2005) suggests that an environmental audit is required against a set of evidence-based standards and agreed ideas for improvement. It is essential that policies and procedures are reviewed every twelve months, taking into account emerging European research, local audit, recommendations, and lessons to be learnt from reports, investigations, inquiries, and positive practice initiatives (NIMHE, 2004). Drawing upon the information available as a result of research in other organizational settings in terms of the impact, and successful management, of ward culture is also likely to prove beneficial. Furthermore, while there will inevitably be some differences between care settings and systems in Europe, it seems the problems associated with maintaining a positive ward atmosphere are very similar, and much can be learnt from greater collaboration between countries.

The most fundamental issue to be addressed is to ascertain, and then dissect, the features that comprise the ward atmosphere. Only then can the necessary range of meaningful data be collected, communicated, and used to contribute to a greater understanding of its impact upon patient aggression and violence.

REFERENCES

Abderhalden, C., Needham, I., Friedli, T., Poelmans, J., & Dansen, T. (2002). Perceptions of aggression amongst psychiatric nurses in Switzerland. *Acta Psychiatrica Scandinavica, 106,* 110–117.

Alexander, J., & Bowers, L. (2004). Acute psychiatric ward rules: A review of the literature. *Journal of Psychiatric and Mental Health Nursing, 11,* 623–631.

Aquilina, C. (1991). Violence by psychiatric inpatients. *Medicine, Science, and the Law, 31*(4), 306–312.

Aubrey, T., Bradley, L., Siddique, C. M., & LeBlanc, A. (1996). Program development in an acute psychiatric unit. *Journal of Mental Health, 5,* 507–514.

Bensley, L., Nelson, N., Kaufman, J., Silverstein, B., & Walker Shields, J. (1995). Patient and staff views of factors influencing assaults on psychiatric hospital employees. *Issues in Mental Health Nursing, 16,* 433–446.

Bowers, L. (2002). *Dangerous and severe personality disorder. Reaction and role of the psychiatric team.* London: Routledge.

Bowers, L., Whittington, R., Almik, R., Bergman, B., Oud, N., & Savio, M. (1999). European perspective on psychiatric nursing and violent incidents, management, education and service organization. *International Journal of Nursing Studies, 36,* 217–222.

Breeze, J. A., & Repper, J. (1998). Struggling for control: The care experiences of 'difficult' patients in mental health services. *Journal of Advanced Nursing, 28,* 1301–1311.

Brooks, K. L., Gilead, M. P., & Daniels, B. S. (1994). Patient overcrowding in psychiatric hospital units: Effects on seclusion and restraint. *Administration and Policy in Mental Health, 22*(2), 133–144.

Carmel, H., & Hunter, M. (1993). Staff injuries from patient attack: Five years' data. *The Bulletin of the American Academy of Psychiatry and the Law, 21*(4), 485–493.

Cheung, P., Schweitzer, I., Crowley, K. C., Yastrubetskaya, O., & Tuckwell, V. (1996). Aggressive behavior and extrapyramidal side effects of neuroleptics in schizophrenia. *International Clinical Psychopharmacology, 11,* 237–240.

Commission for Health Improvement (2004). *What CHI has found in: mental health trusts.* http://www.wales.nhs.uk/documents/mental_health_report03.pdf Accessed 31.01.06.

Cortis, J. D. (2003). Culture, values, and racism: application to nursing. *International Nursing Review, 50*(1), 55–64.

Critchon, J. (1997). The response of nursing staff to psychiatric inpatient misdemeanor. *Journal of Forensic Psychiatry, 8,* 36–61.

Cullen, W. D. (1990). *The public inquiry into the Piper Alpha disaster* (Vols. 1 & 2). London: HMSO.

Cullen, W. D. (2001). *The Ladbroke Grove rail inquiry.* Health and Safety Commission. London: HSE Books.

Denison, D. R. (1996). What is the difference between organizational culture and organizational climate? A native's point of view on a decade of paradigm wars. *Academy of Management Review. Academy of Management, 21*(3), 619–654.

Devlin, A. S. (1992). Psychiatric ward renovation: Staff perception and patient behaviour. *Environment and Behavior, 24*(1), 66–84.

Duxbury, J. (1999). An exploratory account of registered nurses' experience of patient aggression in both mental health and general nursing settings. *Journal of Psychiatric and Mental Health Nursing, 6*(2), 107–114.

Duxbury, J. A. (2002). An evaluation of staff and patients' views of and strategies employed to manage patient aggression and violence on one mental health unit: A pluralistic design. *Journal of Psychiatric and Mental Health Nursing, 9,* 325–337.

Edvardsson, D. (2005). *Atmosphere in care settings: Towards a broader understanding of the phenomenon.* Department of nursing. Umeå, Sweden: Umeå university.

Flannery, R. B., Hanson, M. A., & Penk, W. E. (1994). Risk factors for psychiatric inpatient assaults on staff. *Journal of Mental Health Administration, 21*(1), 24–31.

Flin, R., Mearns, K., O'Connor, P., & Bryden, R. (2000). Measuring safety climate: Identifying the common features. *Safety Science, 34,* 177–192.

Friis, S. (1986). Characteristics of a good ward atmosphere. *Acta Psychiatrica Scandinavica, 74*(5), 469–473.

Gesler, W. M., & Kearns, R. (2002). *Culture/place/health.* London and New York: Routledge.

Glisson, C., & James, L. R. (2002). The cross level effects of culture and climate in human service teams. *Journal of Organizational Behavior, 23,* 767–794.

Goodwin, I., Holmes, G., Newnes, C., & Waltho, D. (1999). A qualitative analysis of the views of inpatient mental health service users. *The Journal of Mental Health, 8,* 43–54.

Grassi, L., Peron, L., Marangoni, C., Zanchi, P., & Vanni, A. (2001). Characteristics of violent behavior in acute psychiatric inpatients: A five-year Italian study. *Acta Psychiatrica Scandinavica, 104,* 273–279.

Guldenmund, F. W. (2000). The nature of safety culture: A review of theory and research. *Safety Science, 34,* 215–257.

Hanson, R. H., & Balk, J. A. (1992). A replication study of staff injuries in a state hospital. *Hospital and Community Psychiatry, 43*, 836–837.

Harris, D., & Morrison, E. (1995). Managing violence without coercion. *Archives of Psychiatric Nursing, 9*(4), 203–210.

Harrison, D. (1972). *Understanding your organization's character*. Harvard Business Review, May/June, 119–128.

Healthcare Commission. (2005). *National audit of violence*. London: RCP.

Hokanson Hawks, J. (1991). Power: a concept analysis, *Journal of Advanced Nursing, 16*, 754–762.

Hunter, M. E., & Love, C. C. (1996). Total quality management and the reduction of inpatient violence and costs in a forensic psychiatric hospital. *Psychiatric Services, 47*(7), 751–754.

James, D. V., Fineberg, N. A., Shah, A. K., & Priest, R. G. (1990). An increase in violence on an acute psychiatric ward. *The British Journal of Psychiatry, 156*, 846–852.

Jansen, G. (1994). Safety culture: A study of permanent way staff at British Rail. Amsterdam: Vrije Universiteit.

Jansen, G. J., Dansen, T. W. N., & Jebbnik, G. (2005). Staff attitudes towards aggression in health care: A review of the literature. *Journal of Psychiatric and Mental Health Nursing, 12*, 3–13.

Jansson, J. A., Eklund, M. (2002). How the inner world is reflected in relation to perceived ward atmosphere among patients with psychosis. *Social Psychiatry and Psychiatric Epidemiology, 37*(11), 519–526.

Johansson, H., & Eklund, M. (2004). Helping alliance and ward atmosphere in psychiatric inpatient care. *Psychology and Psychotherapy, 77*(4), 511–523.

Kagawa-Singer, M., & Chung, R. (1994). A paradigm of culturally-based care in ethnic minority populations. *Journal of Community Psychology, 22*, 192–208.

Katz, P., & Kirkland, F. R. (1990). Violence and social structure on mental hospital wards. *Psychiatry, 53*, 262–277.

Krakowski, M. I., & Czobar, P. (1994). Clinical symptoms, neurological impairment, and prediction of violence in psychiatric inpatients. *Hospital and Community Psychiatry, 45*(7), 700–705.

Kumar, S., Ng, M. P. B., & Robinson, E. (1999). The crowded ward. *Psychiatric Services, 50*, 1499.

Lancee, W. J., Gallop, R., McCay, E., & Toner, B. (1995). The relationship between nurses' limit setting styles and anger in psychiatric inpatients. *Psychiatric Services, 46*(6), 609–613.

Lilywhite, A., Morgan, N., & Walter, E. (1995). Reducing the risk of violence to junior psychiatrists. *Psychiatric Bulletin, 19*, 24–27.

Lowe, T., Wellman, N., & Taylor, R. (2003). Limit-setting and decision-making in the management of aggression. *Journal of Advanced Nursing, 41*, 154–161.

Martin, J. (1992). *Cultures in organizations: Three perspectives*. Oxford: Oxford University Press.

Martin, J., Sitkin, S., & Boehm, M. (1985). Founders and the elusiveness of a cultural legacy. In: J. Martin. (Ed.). *Organizational culture*. Beverly Hills, CA, USA: Sage.

Mearns, K., Flin, R., Gordon, R., & Fleming, M. (1998). Measuring safety climate on offshore installations. *Work and Stress, 12*(3), 238–254.

Middleboe, T., Schjodt, T., Byrsting, K., & Gjerris, A. (2001). Ward atmosphere in acute psychiatric inpatient care, patients' perceptions, ideals and satisfaction. *Acta Psychiatrica Scandinavica, 103*, 212–219.

Mistral, W., Hall, A., & McKee, P. (2002). Using therapeutic community principles to improve functioning of a high care psychiatric unit in the UK. *International Journal of Mental Health Nursing, 11*, 10–17.

Moos, R. (1974). *Evaluating treatment environments: A social ecological approach*. New York: Wiley.

Morrison, E. F. (1998). The culture of caregiving and aggression in psychiatric settings. *Archives of Psychiatric Nursing, 12*(1), 21–31.

Morrison, E., Morman, G., Bonner, G., Taylor, C., Abraham, I., & Lathan, L. (2002). Reducing staff injuries and violence in a forensic psychiatric setting. *Archives of Psychiatric Nursing, 16*(3), 108–117.

National Institute of Clinical Excellence (2005). *Disturbed (violent) behavior: The short-term management of disturbed (violent) behavior in inpatient psychiatric settings*. London: NICE.

National Institute for Mental Health in England (2004). *Mental health policy implementation guide: Developing positive practice to support the safe and therapeutic management of aggression ad violence in mental health inpatient settings.* Leeds: Department Of Health.

Nijman, H. L. I. (2002). A model of aggression in psychiatric hospitals. *Acta Psychiatrica Scandinavica, 106,* 142–143.

Nijman, H. L. I., a Campo, J. M. L. G., Ravelli, D. P., & Merckelbach, H. L. G. J. (1999). A tentative model of aggression on inpatient psychiatric wards. *Psychiatric Services, 50*(6), 832–834.

Nijman, H. L. I., & Rector, G. (1999). Crowding and aggression on inpatient psychiatric wards. *Psychiatric Services, 50,* 830–831.

Ouchi, W., & Wilkins, A. L. (1985). Organizational culture. *Annual Review of Sociology, 11,* 457–483.

Palmstierna, T., Huitfeldt, B. & Wistedt B. (1991). The relationship of overcrowding and aggressive behaviour on a phychiatric intensive care uniit, *Hospital and Community Psychiatry* 42, 1237–1240.

Palmstierna, T., & Wistedt, B. (1995). Changes in the pattern of aggressive behavior among inpatients with changes in ward organization. *Acta Psychiatrica Scandinavica, 91,* 32–35.

Peck, E., Towell, D., & Gulliver, P. (2001). The meanings of "culture" in health and social care: A case study of the combined Trust in Somerset. *Journal of Interprofessional Care, 15*(4), 319–327.

Peters, T. J., & Waterman, R. H. Jr. (1982). *In search of excellence. Lessons from America's best-run companies.* New York: Harper and Row.

Pilgrim, D., & Rogers, A. (1999). *A sociology of mental health and illness* (2nd ed.). Buckingham: Open University Press.

Powell, G., Caan, W., & Crowe, M. (1994). What events precede violent incidents in psychiatric hospitals? *The British Journal of Psychiatry, 165,* 107–112.

Quirk, A., & Lelliot, P. (2001). What do we know about life on acute psychiatric wards in the UK? A review of the research evidence. *Social Science and Medicine, 53,* 1565–1574.

Rabeinowitz, J., & Mark, M. (1999). Risk factors for violence among long stay psychiatric patients: National study. *Acta Psychiatrica Scandinavica, 99,* 341–347.

Roper, J., & Anderson, N. (1991). The interactional dynamics of violence, part one: An acute psychiatric ward. *Archives of Psychiatric Nursing, 4,* 209–215.

Rossberg, J. I., & Friis, S. (2003a). Do the spontaneity and anger and aggression subscales of the Ward Atmosphere Scale form homogeneous dimensions? A cross-sectional study of 54 wards for psychotic patients. *Acta Psychiatrica Scandinavica, 107*(2), 118–123.

Rossberg, J. I, & Friis, S. (2003b). A suggested revision of the Ward Atmosphere Scale. *Acta Psychiatrica Scandinavica, 108*(5), 374–380.

Rousseau, D. (1988). The construction of climate in organizational research. In: I. Roberston (Ed.). *International review of industrial and organizational research.* New York: Wiley.

Royal College of Psychiatrists (1998). *Management of imminent violence. Occasional paper OP41.* London: Royal College of Psychiatrists.

Ryden, M. B., Bossenmaier, M., & McLachlan, C. (1991). Aggressive behavior in cognitively impaired nursing home residents. *Research in Nursing and Health, 14,* 81–95.

Schalast, N., & Redies, M. (2005). *Development of an assessment questionnaire (handout).* The sixth Nordic symposium on forensic psychiatry. Finland: Vaasa.

Schein, E. H. (1992). *Organizational culture and leadership.* San Francisco: Jossey-Bass.

Scott, T., Mannion, R., Marshall, M., & Davies, H. (2003). Does organizational culture influence health care performance? A review of the evidence. *Journal of Health Services Research and Policy, 8*(2), 105–117.

Secker, J., Benson, A., Balfe, E., Lipsedge, M., Robinson, S., & Walker, J. (2004). Understanding the social context of violent and aggressive incidents on an inpatient unit. *Journal of Psychiatric and Mental Health Nursing, 11,* 172–178.

Shepherd, M., & Lavender, T. (1999). Putting aggression into context: An investigation into contextual factors influencing the rate of aggressive incidents in a psychiatric hospital. *Journal of Mental Health, 8*(2), 159–170.

Sheriden, M., Henrion, R., & Baxter, V. (1990). Precipitants of violence in a psychiatric inpatient setting. *Hospital and Community Psychiatry, 41,* 776–780.

Smircich, L. (1983). Concepts of culture and organizational analysis. *Administrative Science Quarterly,*
28, 339–358.

Smith, D. (2002). Management and medicine – issues in quality, risk, and culture. *Clinician in*
Management, 11, 1–6.

Smith, M. E., & Hart, G. (1994). Nurses' responses to patient anger: From disconnecting to connecting.
Journal of Advanced Nursing, 20, 643–651.

Vanderslott, J. (1998). A study of violence towards staff by patients in an NHS Trust hospital. *Journal of*
Psychiatric and Mental Health Nursing, 5, 291–298.

Whittington, R., & Higgins, L. (2002). More than zero tolerance? Burnout and tolerance for patient
aggression amongst mental health nurses in China and the UK. *Acta Psychiatrica Scandinavica, 106,*
37–40.

Whittington, R., & Wykes, T. (1994a). An observation study of associations between nurse behavior and
violence in psychiatric hospitals. *Journal of Psychiatric and Mental health Nursing, 1,* 85–92.

Whittington, R., & Wykes, T. (1994b). Going in strong, confrontative coping by staff following assault
by a patient. *Journal of Forensic Psychiatry, 5*(3), 609–614.

Whittington, R., & Wykes, T. (1996). Aversive stimulation by staff and violence by psychiatric patients.
The British Journal of Clinical Psychology, 35, 11–20.

Wilkins, A. L., & Ouchi, W. (1983). The culture audit: A tool for understanding organizations.
Organizational Dynamics, 12, 24–38.

VI

CONSEQUENCES: HANDLING THE AFTERMATH

15

Psychological Responses Following Exposure to Violence

IAN NEEDHAM

1   INTRODUCTION

The definition of violence or aggression varies considerably even within the scientific community. Some researchers apply the term assault solely to the physical dimension (Owen, Tarantello, Jones, & Tennant, 1998), but for others, verbal acts constitute assault (Chambers, 1998; Gates, Fitzwater, & Meyer, 1999; Vanderslott, 1998). Sometimes sexual harassment (Vanderslott) or unwanted sexual acts (Flannery, Hanson, & Penk, 1995) or contacts (Morgan & Porter, 1999) are used in conjunction with patient violence. Some authors refrain from defining violence and leave the definition of it to the victims (Hauck, 1993). Thus, differing operational definitions render data collection and the comparison of aggression rates difficult. For the purpose of this chapter, no standardized definition of violence is adopted and patient violence is used synonymously with patient aggression. The sole specification is that only patient aggression or violence toward carers—not horizontal violence or aggression (among patients or among staff) or from carers to patients—will be considered.

Parallel to the increase in societal aggression, health care facilities are becoming increasingly dangerous places (O'Connell, Young, Brooks, Hutchings, & Lofthouse, 2000). Mental health facilities have even been referred to as one of the "most hazardous work settings" (Caldwell, 1992, p. 837). In Australia, the health industry is the most violent of all industries (Jones & Lyneham, 2000) and the British Crime Study has shown that nursing is the occupation with the second highest risk of assault, second only to the security and protective services (Budd, 1999). Considerable variation of patient aggression exists even when using a standardized instrument for the registration of aggression. Nijman et al. (1999) found a range of 0.4–33.2 aggressive incidents (mean = 9.3) on acute admission wards in various countries when these were recorded employing the revised version of the Staff Observation of Aggression Scale. A recent Swiss study demonstrated a rate of 3.51 aggressive incidents per 100 hospitalization days (Needham et al., 2004) in acute psychiatry. In spite of such variation it is safe to say that patient aggression is most predominant in psychiatric and emergency health care settings.

Many health care professionals are exposed to patient aggression. In a German investigation in a psychiatric setting, 128 doctors, 50 psychologists and 55 social workers reported their exposure to violence by patients with 55% reporting a career prevalence of severe assault. Social workers had lower rates of exposure to violence than psychologists and physicians (Steinert, Beck, Vogel, & Wohlfahrt, 1995). A Canadian report demonstrated that 40.2% of psychiatrists (n = 136) had been assaulted at least once (Chaimowitz & Moscovitch, 1991) in their career. The one year incidence of self-reported violence toward 284 physicians was 30 violent incidents giving rise to a standardized incidence rate—taking the age and gender distribution of the Swedish working population into consideration—of 0.18 (Arnetz & Arnetz, 2001). However, nurses are the professional group most subjected to patient violence (Blow et al., 1999; Haller & Deluthy, 1988; Noble & Rodger, 1989; Tam, Engelsmann, & Fugere, 1996). In an American one year study, for example, nurses endured 120 of the 135 injuries inflicted on all staff (Carmel & Hunter, 1989). Nurses' spatial and temporal proximity to patients incur that they have the most contact with violent patients (Ernst, 1988) and thus are the most affected (Fottrell, 1980; Geser, 1999). Because nurses provide a 24-hour care service they are the professionals taking the brunt of such aggression (Vanderslott, 1998). For this reason, the investigation on psychological responses following exposure to violence concentrates mainly on the nursing profession.

Research on physical injuries inflicted on health care staff by patients is common (Bensley et al., 1997; Hanson & Balk, 1992; Lee, Gerberich, Waller, Anderson, & McGovern, 1999; Noble & Rodger, 1989) with rates for physical injury ranging from 2% (Noble & Rodger, 1989) to 16% (Carmel & Hunter, 1993). A recent study conducted in Germany revealed that 10% of healthcare workers (predominantly nurses) needed medical treatment after assault, and one nurse contracted life-threatening injuries (Richter & Berger, 2000). Another study revealed 35 assault-inflicted injuries per 100 employees per year with 73% of health carers reporting at least one minor injury during the past year (Bensley et al.). In a survey of 40 nurses who had been randomly assaulted by a patient, 21% of the respondents reported suffering life-endangering or multiple injuries, including fractures, lacerations, bruises, and loss of consciousness (Lanza, 1983). Fractures requiring surgery have also been reported (Chiang, 2005). In a study by Blow et al. (1999), 3024 patient-to-staff assaults were recorded averaging a rate of 2.28 assaults per patient and 87% were classified as battery without a weapon resulting in the necessity for 20% of staff to seek medical attention (Blow et al.).

Although serious injuries occur much more rarely than "minor" forms of violence resulting in little or no physical injury (Fottrell, 1980; Whittington & Wykes, 1992), psychological and emotional wounds may linger on and interfere with normal working and leisure lifestyles for months or years after the incident (Rippon, 2000). In a study of psychiatric patients' violence to staff, only 2% of the assaults led to major physical injuries as compared to 59% which induced no detectable injury (Noble & Rodger, 1989). Furthermore, psychological sequelae of violence have been deemed, by nurses themselves and by the literature, as petty and not worthy of serious research (Haller & Deluthy, 1988; Whittington & Wykes). Apparently physical consequences of patient aggression are often taken more seriously than other sequelae as illustrated by Rippon, who reports that, after a sexual assault one nurse received no support. After being punched by a patient, however, she was assisted. Richter reiterates this point by reporting that organizational response to workplace injuries—such as violence-induced injury—is mainly related to physical lesions only (Richter, 2005).

Psychological responses to patient violence often take longer for victims to come to terms with. In a study by Baxter, Hafner, and Holme (1992), 49% of nurses assaulted by psychiatric patients expressed the belief that it takes several months to recover emotionally from an assault. Another investigation (Richter & Berger, 2000) reports that 14% of assaulted staff suffer from some severe symptoms of post-traumatic stress disorder (PTSD). In a study on the short- and long-term effects of patient assault, the authors demonstrate that, one year following the aggression, some nurses suffer from moderate to severe PTSD (Ryan & Poster, 1989). On an organizational level, Richter notes that the effects of psychological sequelae for the organization cannot be estimated (Richter, 1998).

This chapter aims to identify and categorize predominant psychological responses following exposure to violence on health care workers, especially on nurses. An electronic search was conducted to identify articles on the subject. In addition to the electronic search, experts from the European Violence in Psychiatry Research Group (EViPRG) were consulted and crossreferencing of relevant articles was conducted. Published texts including at least two psychological responses from 1983 onward were considered. Due to the incidence of psychiatric disorder in many health care settings, texts from all available domains were utilized. In order to demonstrate the global nature of the problem of patient violence, the focus was widened to include reports on psychological sequelae from any country. Thus the search aimed at inclusiveness and sensitivity in order to discover the greatest possible variability of the subject.

The range of psychological responses reported here was extended to include biophysiological, emotional, cognitive, and social reactions according to the categorization of Lanza (1992). The four categories are conceptualized in the following manner:

- Biophysiological effects refer to nonvisible somatic responses in a physiologically involuntary fashion.
- Emotions are sentiments not associated with any kind of psychological or psychiatric pathology but rather, are common or "normal" feelings.

- Cognition is defined as a non-emotive mode of perceiving, including perception of self or referring to a person's system of beliefs or convictions.
- Social interaction refers to interpersonal exchange.

2 RESULTS

After application of the inclusion and exclusion criteria the electronic and hand search revealed 27 articles for inclusion in this review. Three unpublished studies (Chiang, 2005; Hauck, 1993; Vincent, Perlt, Sørensen, & Winther, 2000) were drawn to our attention by experts. The 27 articles are characterized and arranged in alphabetical order in the appendix. The most prominent psychological responses are presented according to the nursing domains (psychiatric, emergency, residential and gerontological, general and mixed settings) in Table 1. As most of the reports are available from the nursing literature there is an obvious bias toward this profession and it is therefore questionable whether the findings are transferable to other health care professions.

2.1 Biophysiological Effects

Anxiety or fear is the most frequently reported biophysiological effect. Anxiety may occur in a generalized form (Lanza, 1983; Ryan & Poster, 1989; Whittington & Wykes, 1992) and fear may relate, for example, to the workplace (Arnetz & Arnetz, 2001; Bin Abdullah, Khim, Wah, Bee, & Pushpam, 2000), or patients (Fernandes et al., 2002). Fear can be differentiated as fear of the perpetrator or of other patients (Hauck, 1993; Lanza; Whittington & Wykes), fear for oneself or one's family (Fry, O'Riordan, Turner, & Mills, 2002), fear of permanent side effects of the assault or of becoming physically dependent on others (Lanza), fear of retaliation toward the aggressor (Lanza; Ryan & Poster), fear of co-workers, or of the future (Hauck). The reported rates of fear range from 12.4% (Richter & Berger, 2000) to 49% (Arnetz & Arnetz) (n = 85 and 8,531, respectively).

Patient aggression may lead, in a minority of cases, to a fully established posttraumatic stress disorder (PTSD) or isolated symptoms of this. PTSD is a long-lasting anxiety response following a traumatic or catastrophic event, and consists of various symptoms in the following groups: persistent re-experience of the traumatic event, e.g., including images, thoughts, or perceptions, recurrent distressing dreams; persistent avoidance of trauma-associated stimuli, e.g., thoughts, feelings, or conversations, efforts to avoid activities, places, or people that arouse recollections of the trauma, inability to recall an important aspect of the trauma; and persistent symptoms of increased arousal such as difficulty falling or staying asleep (American Psychiatric Association, 1994). Isolated PTSD symptoms have been reported implicitly or explicitly by numerous authors (Table 1). Caldwell reports that 137 of 224 (56.1%) traumatized clinical staff in psychiatry contracted some PTSD symptoms but only 22 (9.8) suffered the full clinical PTSD (Caldwell, 1992). In one study of

Table 1. Synopsis of the Most Prominent Nonsomatic Symptoms (P = Psychiatric Setting, E = Accident & Emergency, R = Residential/Gerontological Setting, M = Mixed Settings, G = General)

			Biophysiological					PTSD				Cognitive		Emotional														Social			
	Domain	Country	Body Tension	Disquiet/Irritability	Headache	Sleep Disorder, Nightmares	Stress	Avoidance	Increased Arousal	Persistent Re-experience	Disbelief	Personal Integrity Threatened	Transformed Perception	Anger	Anxiety or Fear	Apathy, Indifference	Apprehension, Distress, Upset	Exhaustion, Fatigue, Strain	Frustration, Resignation	Guilt, Self-blame, Shame	Helplessness	Hurt, Insult, Disappointment	Powerlessness	Resentment, Annoyance	Sadness, Unhappiness	Shock, Surprise	Doubts on Job Appropriateness	Relationship to Patient Impaired	Professional Performance Impaired	Insecurity at Work
Adams and Whittington (1995)	P	UK						•		•	•																			
Arthur et al. (2003)	P	US				•																							•	
Caldwell (1992)	P	US				•		•	•	•	•			•	•		•													
Chiang (2005)	P	TW I				•			•	•					•		•													
Flannery et al. (1991)	P	US																	•	•						•		•		
Flannery et al. (1995)	P	US						•	•	•			•	•		•	•													•
Fry et al. (2002)	P	AUS				•																							•	
Hauck (1993)	P	CH	•				•	•	•	•		•	•	•			•	•			•			•	•	•	•		•	•

(Continued)

Table 1. Synopsis of the Most Prominent Nonsomatic Symptoms (P = Psychiatric Setting, E = Accident & Emergency, R = Residential/Gerontological Setting, M = Mixed Settings, G = General)—Cont'd

		Biophysiological					PTSD			Cognitive			Emotional													Social			
Domain	Country	Body Tension	Disquiet/Irritability	Headache	Sleep Disorder, Nightmares	Stress	Avoidance	Increased Arousal	Persistent Re-experience	Disbelief	Personal Integrity Threatened	Transformed Perception	Anger	Anxiety or Fear	Apathy, Indifference	Apprehension, Distress, Upset	Exhaustion, Fatigue, Strain	Frustration, Resignation	Guilt, Self-blame, Shame	Helplessness	Hurt, Insult, Disappointment	Powerlessness	Resentment, Annoyance	Sadness, Unhappiness	Shock, Surprise	Doubts on Job Appropriateness	Relationship to Patient Impaired	Professional Performance Impaired	Insecurity at Work
Lanza et al. (1991) — P	US					•					•	•				•										•		•	
Lanza (1983) — P	US	•	•	•	•					•			•	•	•			•	•	•				•	•				
Murray and Snyder (1991) — P	US			•															•					•	•				
Richter and Berger (2000) — P	D						•	•	•					•															
Richter (2005) — P	D																												
Ryan and Poster (1989) — P	US	•					•	•	•				•	•															
Whittington and Wykes (1992) — P	UK				•				•					•			•												

Study			N studies reporting effect
Bin Abdullah et al. (2000)	E	SGP	6
Fernandes et al. (2002)	E	CDN	3
Hislop and Melby (2002)	E	UK	6
Levin et al. (1998)	E	US	3
Suserud et al. (2002)	E	S	7
Åström et al. (2002)	R	S	10
Chambers (1998)	R	UK	10
Gates et al. (1999)	R	US	7
O'Connell et al. (2000)	G	AUS	5
Arnetz and Arnetz (2001)	M	S	4
May and Grubbs (2002)	M	US	18
Menckel and Viitsara (2002)	M	S	17
Vincent et al. (2000)	M	DK	3

aggression, victims in a German psychiatric setting, not a single person suffered from fully established PTSD (Richter & Berger, 2000), which demonstrates the need to differentiate between isolated symptoms and all three dimensions of PTSD. A recent German study employing a prospective design with assessment at the time of the assault and with two follow up points (two and six months) found eight participants (17%) suffering from fully fledged PTSD (Richter, 2005).

2.2 Cognitive Effects

Various threats to personal integrity or pride are reported, with some victims perceiving themselves as disrespected, unappreciated, violated, robbed of their rights (Gates et al., 1999), humiliated (Hauck, 1993; Lanza, Kayne, Hicks, & Milner, 1991), compromised (Chambers, 1998), or intimidated, harassed, and threatened (Fry et al., 2002). Others perceive themselves as being at the mercy of the perpetrator (Hauck), while yet others experience disbelief that the assault occurred (Adams & Whittington, 1995; Chambers; Hislop & Melby, 2003; May & Grubbs, 2002; Ryan & Poster, 1989). Denial or rationalization of the assault (Lanza, 1983) or disbelief at being involved in the incident (Chambers) may also occur. Some incidents can lead to a radical transformation of the conception of the world, with some victims stating that nothing will ever be the same again (Hauck), that the event has a disruptive meaning (Flannery et al., 1995), or that the world has become less predictable (Gates et al.; Hauck) or threatening (Hauck).

2.3 Emotional Effects

Emotional reactions constitute the greatest variety of symptoms, with anger being the most frequently reported. Anger may be directed toward the nurses themselves, superiors (Hauck, 1993) or the institution (Chambers, 1998; Hauck) or of a general nature (Arthur, Brende, & Quiroz, 2003). The range of the percentage of nurses experiencing anger is greatest in the emergency services, with rates from 14% (n = 763) (Fernandes et al., 2002) to 68.6% (n = 35) (Bin Abdullah et al., 2000). Two groups of authors report higher anger rates following verbal aggression than physical aggression (Fernandes et al.; O'Connell et al., 2000). Anger is a predominant response in most cultures excepting one Chinese study. In Taiwan persons are socialized—according to the mores of collectivism—to control their anger and to be polite even in taxing situations (Chiang, 2005).

Guilt, self-blame or shame is also a prominent reaction to aggression and was reported in a majority of the studies. Some nurses feel guilty for not handling the situation in a more appropriate way (Hauck, 1993). In the Chinese study, shame was most prominent when nurses were slapped in the face because, in Taiwan, this part of the body is associated with loss of face:

> "I was so humiliated when the patient slapped me on the face. I lost face."
> (Chiang, 2005).

Feelings of guilt and self-blame are sometimes reinforced by superiors placing the blame for assaults on the victims (Hauck, 1993). Guilt sometimes occurs in conjunction with shame (Åström, Bucht, Eisemann, Norberg, & Saveman, 2002) and may lead to impairments in self-confidence (Hauck). The other emotional effects are shown in Table 1.

2.4 Social Effects

Assaults can affect (Gates et al., 1999; Suserud, Blomquist, & Johansson, 2002) or undermine (Flannery et al., 1995) the nurse–patient relationship and lead to behavior such as less eagerness to spend time with residents, less willingness to answer residents' call lights (Gates et al.), avoiding patients (Flannery et al.; Levin, Hewitt, & Misner, 1998), or adopting a passive role (Chambers, 1998). Some nurses report becoming callous toward patients (Levin et al.).

Nurse perceptions of their job competency and security at, or satisfaction with, the workplace may be affected. Some of the assaulted nurses question the normalcy of a job in which workers are assaulted (Hauck, 1993), or even consider changing their job (Bin Abdullah et al., 2000; Lanza, 1983). Some actually change ward or employer (O'Connell et al., 2000). Many assault victims feel insecure at work (Bin Abdullah et al.; Hauck; May & Grubbs, 2002; Vincent et al., 2000), more vulnerable (Fry et al., 2002; Lanza) or less in control (Lanza et al., 1991).

Patient aggression and assault can lead to real or perceived impairments in professional performance, leading nurses to doubt the quality of their work (Bin Abdullah et al., 2000), their competency (Whittington & Wykes, 1992), or perceive themselves as having failed.

2.5 Other Effects

The following effects of aggression on nurses were reported fewer than three times in the 27 articles used in this review: biophysiological (decreased energy, hyper vigilance and hyper alertness), cognitive (impaired concentration, increased cautiousness), emotion (burn-out, feeling confused, crying, feeling sorry for the perpetrator, dependency, depression, distress, embarrassment, laughter, numbness, resignation, thoughts of suicide, vulnerability), and social (impaired expression of feelings, changed or impaired relationships to co-workers or family members, stigmatization of victims).

3 DISCUSSION OF PSYCHOLOGICAL RESPONSES

The psychological responses were derived from studies conducted in nine countries and four settings which demonstrate the global nature of the problem. The variability of nurse reaction, vocabulary in which nurses express their reactions and a lack of standardization of terms expressing reaction are three possible reasons for the great number of responses. Because of the semantic proximity of some effects, e.g., guilt, self-blame, and shame, we summarized some effects into categories in the synoptic table (Table 1). This procedure is a trade-off between semantic precision and a manageable number of effects.

The most frequently reported effects are anger, anxiety (fear), and guilt (self-blame, shame). The data in Table 1 suggest that these three primary reactions occur in all domains and in most countries. Anger and anxiety are considered relatively normal reactions and should not be confused with pathology. Guilt, self-blame, and shame may be linked to the dual role of the carer—maintaining one's own rights while offering the best quality of care—in dealing with aggressive patients. Chambers (1998) remarks that some nurses tend to blame themselves, to assume responsibility and often to set themselves unrealistically high standards when attempting to deal with violent patients. Murray and Snyder (1991) report on healthcare workers' high expectations of themselves. Such high moral standards, while being laudable, may lead to the ethical dilemma of endeavoring to fulfill professional moral standards while concurrently wishing to safeguard and maintain the nurse's own rights.

Powerlessness is reported in the articles from all nursing domains except psychiatry. This finding may be associated with the socialization and education of psychiatric nurses. The high rates of aggression in psychiatric nursing may indicate habituation to, or better personal and structural resources for the managing of, patient aggression.

Because of the focus of the review on adverse effects on assaulted nurses, no references to those on whom patient aggression and assault have little or no effect are included in this chapter. Certain nurses are apparently not affected (Lanza, 1983; Vincent et al., 2000) and it is conceivable that patient aggression may have a positive effect, e.g., strengthening of certain personality traits, on some. As Flannery notes, 65% of nurses saw some meaning in the assault (Flannery, Fulton, & Tausch, 1991) and one group of authors notes that 54% of nurses had never considered leaving their jobs because of the incidence of violence.

The 28 predominant effects found here are the result of a simple enumeration process and do not reflect any association with severity of suffering of the victims. The number and quality of nonsomatic effects also seems to be affected by the research question and study design. An illustration of this difficulty is the nonsomatic reactions of anxiety and fear: possible explanations for the differing rates of anxiety or fear, ranging from 2.7% (trainee nursing aides) to 40.0% experienced caring staff, are sampling (assaulted versus non-assaulted, convenience vs. randomized sample), status (trainee vs. experienced), age of participants, setting (high-level aggressions care settings such as psychiatry or accident and emergency), or definition of threat, aggression, violence, and attack. A similar caveat applies to anger as the most frequently reported effect: while anger is reported in accident and emergency and general and mixed nursing settings, it occurs only in some psychiatric settings. This finding can be explained by the fact that most authors not reporting anger in psychiatric nursing (Adams & Whittington, 1995; Caldwell, 1992; Flannery et al.,

1995; Richter, 2005; Richter & Berger, 2000; Whittington & Wykes, 1992) conducted studies placing the emphasis on PTSD or related concepts. It must also be stressed that the apparent concentration of PTSD symptoms in the domain of psychiatric nursing (Table 1) may possibly be a product of researchers' interest in this syndrome rather than an expression of real rates in this nursing domain.

4 THE DYNAMICS OF PSYCHOLOGICAL RESPONSES

Wykes and Whittington (1994) have described the dynamics of reactions to patient violence in their "response cycle" which includes the following stages:

- *Impact.* The response is predominantly physiological and may occur some hours after the incident. Symptoms include high levels of arousal, shock, numbness, confusion, disorientation, heightened feelings of fear, vulnerability, helplessness, dependency, anger, appetite change, sleep loss, fatigue, and avoidance of the reminders of the incident.
- *Recoil.* The breakdown of feelings of security accompanied by the search for the reasons of the victimization, e.g., why me? Events prior to the assault are reinterpreted as omens of the incident as the victim tries to make sense of the happening. Victim preoccupation with the incident is indicated by extensive talking on the matter. Concurrently the assaulted may deny emotions and cognitions related to the assault.
- *Reorganization.* This is the period in which victims regain control over their emotions. It is often accompanied by discussions on the meaning of the attack. Here again, considerable variability exits with some victims feeling stronger and more resilient to stress. Others, however, may still be prone to relapse.

Little is known on the development of victim response over time. Some victims may experience symptoms of PTSD immediately after being traumatized, whereas others contract symptoms at a later stage, with relapses possibly happening years later (Sonnenberg, 1988). In his prospective analysis of PTSD, Richter found that these diagnoses generally decreased after two months but little further reduction of the symptoms were found in the same persons at six months, with a minority of subjects still suffering beyond the six month mark (Richter, 2005). Reoccurrence of symptoms may be triggered by events not related to the original assault. O'Rourke, for example, was recovering from a malicious violent attack by a patient and experienced flashbacks and nightmares shortly after the attack on the twin towers in Manhattan (O'Rourke, 2002). Lanza (1983) detected some long-term effects on nurses including re-experiencing earlier cognitive reactions, denial, rationalization, self-blame, increased perception of vulnerability. According to Flannery, many victims had still not regained their sense of control regarding the assault (Flannery et al., 1991). A study by Wykes and Whittington demonstrated a reduction of anxiety in victims of aggression as measured by the Spielberger State Anxiety Scale, and a general decrease in the number of victims reporting denial and re-experiencing at three weeks after the incident (Wykes & Whittington, 1991). However, great individual variation was identified in victims' reactions (Wykes & Whittington) and it remains debatable if the above-mentioned issues are symptoms of coping strategies.

5 DEALING WITH THE AFTERMATH OF PATIENT VIOLENCE

Given the above-mentioned psychological responses to patient violence, the question remains as to possible ways of handling the aftermath. Postincident care is necessary for both perpetrators and victims of violence. However, in this chapter the focus will be solely on the victims.

A widely used approach for victims to cope with patient aggression is psychological debriefing which aims to reduce victims' feelings of helplessness and fear and to provide a supportive emotional atmosphere until the event can be effectively integrated (Erdos & Hughes, 2001). Debriefing is a technique employed after major disasters, unusual violent events, and other particularly difficult or stressful situations. The procedure at best should be employed shortly (one or two hours) after the traumatic incident and at the latest three days after (Erdos & Hughes). The phases of debriefing (Erdos & Hughes) consist of:

- *Introduction*: explanation of purpose and guarantee of confidentiality.
- *Fact phase*: general explanation of the incident.
- *Feeling phase*: discussion of feelings.
- *Symptom phase*: description of symptoms.
- *Teaching phase*: drawing attention to symptoms and discussion of stress response.
- *Re-entry phase*: assurance and answering of questions by the facilitator, reiteration of confidentiality, planning of follow-up or referral to therapy.

Although debriefing is one of the most widely used offers for victims to aggression (Deahl, 2000) it has recently been criticized on methodological terms. Critics have noted, for example, that many studies on the effectiveness of psychological debriefing have small sample sizes, lack baseline measurement and are not prospective. Furthermore, the technique is difficult to investigate using rigorous research methodology (randomized controlled trials) (Deahl). The few RCTs conducted on debriefing have failed to demonstrate any procedural benefits (Deahl). It has also been noted that psychological debriefing may have a short, but not a long-term, effect on the traumatized (Deahl). Thus, more research in this area is required (Erdos & Hughes, 2001).

A less psychological offer to victims of patient violence has been proposed by Dawson, Johnston, Kehiayan, Kyanko, and Martinez (1988). They propose a peer support group for victims which is based on two concepts: A set of assumptions about the world (the belief in personal invulnerability, the world as a meaningful and comprehensible place, a positive view of oneself) and perceived role conflict after enduring violence (the ambiguous role of caregiver and victim) (Dawson et al.). After exposure to violence, the victims are approached by the Assault Support Team who make immediate contact or organize a schedule. Follow-up meetings are arranged if necessary (Dawson et al.). Although many victims expressed satisfaction with the peer group support system, the actual impact of the procedure is difficult to determine (Dawson et al.).

The Assaulted Staff Action Program (ASAP) is another among the many procedures aimed at reducing the psychological trauma of victimization following violence (Flannery et al., 1991). The ASAP team provides a 24-hour call service for aggression victims. The team members on call are assisted by supervisors. Any calls for ASAP assistance are responded to immediately in the form of debriefing. Medical care is provided if necessary. The ASAP team member discerns the victims' needs and possibilities (continuation of work, capability of sharing the experience with others, cognitive appraisal of the event). PTSD symptoms are also assessed. The team member offers to revisit the victim after three days (Flannery et al.). Flannery reports a "sharp" reduction in the victim's symptoms 10 days after the assault. (Flannery Jr., 2001). However, no statistics are reported.

An extreme case of a patient attack is reported in a personal account of a nurse who suffered a particularly malicious violent attack by a psychiatric patient (O'Rourke, 2002). Eye Movement Desensitization Processing (EMDP) was employed and helped successful recovery.

In spite of such laudable programs to alleviate the sequelae of patient violence on victims there is a general paucity of robust scientific evidence on the benefits of some of the methods. However, it is important that health institutions provide the possibility of support to affected persons even if scientific proof is missing.

6 AREAS FOR FUTURE RESEARCH

A basic problem regarding psychological responses to patient violence is the under-reporting of violent incidents. This is particularly the case on negative sequelae. One possible explanation for under-reporting is shame, guilt, denial, or fear of repercussion with administration (Chaimowitz & Moscovitch, 1991, p. 839). Paradoxically, some of the sequelae experienced after violence, e.g., shame and guilt, may constitute barriers to reporting such incidents. It also seems that the myth of "good" carers' exemption from patient violence or the stigmatization of the assaulted (Hauck, 1993) may contribute to under-reporting. Alternatively, carers' socialization to stoicism may also support this trend. Yet another explanation may be the role tension (caregiver versus victim) after being exposed to patient violence.

Another problem is the multitude of formats to register psychological responses which render comparison, and the generation of large data bases on the subject, difficult. The materials used in this chapter are a good illustration of the heterogeneity of research work in this field. The use of a standardized instrument, e.g., the PTSD instrument or Ryan and Poster's Assault Response Questionnaire, or a battery of instruments across different countries and settings would probably pave the way to acquire results which could be integrated in a systematic review.

Given the psychological responses and the suffering inflicted on carers, more attention must be placed on their preparation to handle the aftermath of patient violence. In a recent small-scale qualitative study on psychiatric nurse experience of patient aggression, the respondents were wary to report their emotional responses (Allin, Stantzos, & Needham, 2005). However, after prompting they readily reported their psychological responses. This may be indicative that emotions are considered subsidiary by some caring professions. The preparation of caregivers should also include a reflection of cognitive appraisal mechanisms. While, of course, role play and simulation cannot guarantee complete protection against negative psychological responses, they may contribute to their alleviation. In all these cases, caregivers' preparation should be evaluated employing strong scientific research designs to ascertain their effectiveness and establish evidence.

More research is obviously needed on procedures aimed at alleviating the aftermath of violence, e.g., psychological debriefing. However, given the idiosyncratic responses and the individual variation of carers' reactions to violence and other traumatizing events, such research is quite demanding. Also, the role of victims' coping strategies is an important research area. Wykes and Whittington have demonstrated that some forms of coping which are regarded as positive strategies, e.g., problem solving, may actually incur more short-term stress to the victims (Wykes & Whittington, 1991). This may indicate that coping is a very individual matter and that preconceptions must be questioned and coping individualized.

Certainly the most important research area must be located in strategies to avoid patient aggression in the first place. Given the multifaceted nature of violence, this requirement demands the collaborative work of all professionals to address the different aspects of violence management. Avenues to be addressed are the use of psychotropic substances to prevent potential, or to treat manifest, violence, the prediction of aggressive behavior (Abderhalden et al., 2002; Almvik & Woods, 1998), designing health care settings to prevent violence (Nijman & Rector, 1999; Palmstierna, Huitfeldt, & Wistedt, 1991), or specific training courses for staff in the management of patient aggression (Lehmann, McCormick, & Kizer, 1999; Needham et al., 2004; Nolan, Dallender, Soares, Thomsen, & Arnetz, 1999; Vanderslott, 1998).

7 APPENDIX: ARTICLES USED IN THE SYSTEMATIC REVIEW

Author(s)	Setting, Subjects, Sample	Study Type, Aim, Definition	Instrument, Analysis	Main results Related to Psychological Sequelae
Adams and Whittington (1995)	68 psychiatric nursing staff, UK. c	Prospective survey on verbal abuse and threats: TV	IRF, RIES, descriptive statistics, testing	50 episodes of verbal aggression reported by 20 nurses evoked intrusion and avoidance symptoms resulting in a score of 30.9 on the RIES, while an earlier study produced a RIES score of 10.3 following physical aggression
Arnetz and Arnetz (2001)	8531 (rr 61–76%) general hospital staff, S, c	Action research on association between patient violence and care quality: T, no definition of violence	Quality of care instrument, descriptive statistics and testing	284 hospital staff (12%) had experienced violence in the preceding year with the most common reactions being anger, sadness, disappointment and fear. Other reactions were post-violence cautiousness, fear, less enjoyment working with patients. Workplace violence was significantly related to non somatic symptoms
Åström et al. (2002)	506 (rr 78%) nursing staff in residential settings, S, c	Cross-sectional survey on incidence of violence and staff's emotional reactions: no definition	Questionnaire, descriptive statistics	A considerable proportion of nurses report aggression consequences such as powerlessness (56%), unhappiness (51%) and anger (49%). Shame (11%) and guilt (15%) were also reported
Arthur et al. (2003)	1131 Mental health professionals (non-nurses) (rr 18%) USA, c	Survey on exposure to violence and PTSD symptoms	Questionnaire, descriptive statistics	90% of all psychological consequences of the 690 respondents were Anger, feeling violated, irritability, impaired sense of professional identity, emotional detachment, loss of esteem, incapacity to sleep. 126 respondents reported no effect
Bin Abdullah et al. (2000)	35 (rr 86%) emergency staff, SNG, c	Survey on prevalence and effects of patient violence, PV	Questionnaire, descriptive statistics	94% reported psychological effects following patient violence including anger and irritability (69%), feelings of insecurity (69%), depression (3%) and anxiety (9%)
Caldwell (1992)	224 (rr 45%) mental health staff, USA, c	Survey on violence, consequences and debriefing: no definition	Questionnaire, descriptive statistics	62% (n = 138) of staff gave accounts of critical violence incidents with 61% reporting PTSD symptoms. 10% (23) met the criteria for PTSD

(Continued)

Appendix—Cont'd

Author(s)	Setting, Subjects, Sample	Study Type, Aim, Definition	Instrument, Analysis	Main results Related to Psychological Sequelae
Chambers (1998)	5 assaulted gerontological nurses, UK, c	Phenomenological study on experiences with violence: no definition	In-depth interviews, Colaizzi analysis	An exhaustive description of the experience of managing violent patients is given which includes experiences of powerlessness, resentment, resignation, and anger by the nurses
Chaing-Kuei (2005)	13 assaulted psychiatric nurses, TW, c	Qualitative interviews to establish assaulted nurses' experiences on patient violence, no definition	Content analysis	The nurses reported effects in various categories: Emotional (shock, fear, anxiety, shame, guilt, resignation, and sadness), bio-physiological (sleep and musculo-skeletal problems, body tension), social (changed in relationships to patients), social (disbelief and negative self-image, blame, impairment of nurse-patient relationship,), and cognitive (disbelief, positive reappraisal, perceived loss of self esteem)
Fermandes et al. (1999)	106 (rr 65%) emergency department staff in CND, c	Survey on perceived incidence and consequences of violence: no definition	Questionnaire, descriptive statistics	Nurses reported consideration of job change (38%), short, medium and long term impaired job performance (25%, 24%, and 19% respectively), fear of patients (73%), and impaired job satisfaction (74%)
Fermandes et al. (2002)	667 (rr 84%) emergency department staff, CND, c	Prospective survey on the effects of violence management: PV	Questionnaire, descriptive statistics	Surveys were conducted at baseline and at 3 and 6 months post-training with nurses constituting 56%, 55%, and 66% of the samples respectively. The impacts of verbal and physical violence are feeling upset, blame, fear of being alone with patient, increased irritability, anger, and headache
Flannery et al. (1991)	62 assaults on healthcare workers in a mental hospital, USA, c	Prospective survey on effects of an intervention for the assaulted, VP	Interviews, description of effects	During interviews conducted as part of the "Assaulted Staff Action Program" (ASAP) the victims reported on experiencing fright, anger, apprehension, sleep disturbances, intrusive memories, recall of traumatic incidents, and hyper vigilance

Study	Sample	Focus/Design	Method	Findings
Flannery et al. (1995)	19 assaults on psychiatric staff, USA, c	Prospective survey on frequency and impact of threats on carers, T	PTSD monitoring, descriptive statistics	Some of the nurses involved in 19 cases of severe threat experienced PTSD-like symptoms ($n = 9$) and disruption in mastery and meaning ($n = 11$)
Fry et al. (2002)	Community mental health staff ($n = 92$, rr 77%), AUS, c	Survey on characteristics of aggressive incidents and staff experiences with aggression, PV	Questionnaire based on the OAS, descriptive statistics	Respondents of the cross sectional survey reported anxiety (44%), emotional distress (35%), feelings of vulnerability, violation of psychological integrity (9%) including intimidation, harassment, and threat) and fear. Other experiences were e.g. nightmares, thoughts about further attacks, or preoccupation with risk and safety. "Less common" reactions were e.g. surprise annoyance, shock, laughter, or burnout
Gates et al. (1999)	60 nursing home nurses, USA, c	Focus group on perceptions of violence: PTV	Structured questions, content analysis, descriptive depiction of effects	In focus groups the victims of patient aggression report on the following feelings: Hurt, anger, frustration, resentment, sadness, feelings of hurt and unpredictability, lack of respect, shock, madness fear, feeling ban, and ambivalence
Hauck (1993)	Seven assaulted psychiatric nurses, CH, c	Content analysis on the experience of assaulted nurses: no definition	Open interview, coding, categorizing procedures	Assaulted nurses reported anger, resentment, guilt/self-blame, numbness, exhaustion/fatigue, threats to personal integrity, transformed perception, impaired capacity to express feelings, stigmatisation, doubts on job appropriateness, and feelings of workplace insecurity impairment in professional performance
Hislop and Melby (2002)	Accident and emergency nurses ($n = 26$, rr = 95%), UK, c	Phenomenological inquiry into the lived experience of violence: PTV	Giorgi method of analysis	The core category "why me?" of the lived experience of A&E nurses includes frustration, powerlessness, incapacity to understand being the target of aggression, embarrassment, and anger. In the core category "sense of isolation" respondents report feeling being left totally alone (by management), and fear (of personal injury)

(Continued)

Appendix—Cont'd

Author(s)	Setting, Subjects, Sample	Study Type, Aim, Definition	Instrument, Analysis	Main results Related to Psychological Sequelae
Lanza et al. (1991)	21 (rr unclear) psychiatric nurses, USA, sampling unclear	Prospective survey on characteristics of assaulted nurses: no definition	VIS, NSCF, descriptive statistics	Of the seven assaulted nurses, 30% felt more apprehensive, 10% more vulnerable, 10% less in control, 10% intended job change, and 10% experienced strained family relationships
Lanza (1983)	40 assaulted nurses in psychiatry, US, c	Explorative survey summarizing reactions to assault	Questionnaire, descriptive statistics	After administration of a questionnaire with 108 possible response reactions numerous short and long term emotional, social, bio-physiological, and cognitive reactions were found (e.g. anger, helplessness, anxiety, or changes in relationships to others). Some nurses were not prone to reaction after assault
Levin et al. (1998)	22 emergency department nurses, USA, c	Focus groups on nurses' views on assaults: P	Coding procedures, descriptive depiction of effects	Victims reported long-term chronic pain, muscle tension, loss of sleep, nightmares, flashback, anger, withdrawal from patients, callousness, burnout, impairment of personal relationships
May and Grubbs (2002)	86 (rr 69%) general, emergency, ICU nurses, USA, c	Survey on patient assaults on nurses: PTV	HASN, descriptive statistics, ANOVA	Victims of patient violence experienced: Decreased job satisfaction (65%), anger (66%), anxiety (53%), fear (36%), emotional distress (36%), disbelief (34%), powerlessness (23%), and impaired job confidence (20%)
Menckel and Viitasara (2002)	2380 (rr 85%) care workers, S, stratified sampling	Survey on prevalence and consequences of threats and violence: no definition of violence	Questionnaire, descriptive depiction of effects	Of the 2380 subjects 696 were nurses. The care givers most common reactions of the violence were: anger (41%), irritation (38%), sadness (35%), helpless or insulted (~33%), or frustration
Murray and Snyder (1991)	19 (rr 54%) assaulted psychiatric staff, USA, c	Survey to assess stress at 6 weeks post-assault: P	Questionnaire, descriptive depiction of effects	83% of assaulted nurses reported reactions of frustration, anger, self-criticism, disbelief, and sadness

Study	Sample	Survey	Method	Findings
O'Connell et al. (2000)	209 (rr 52%) general nurses, AUS, r	Survey on the perception and experience of violence: no definition	Questionnaire, descriptive statistics	95% of the sample had experienced verbal or physical aggression in the past year. Reactions to verbal violence were: Anger (71%), anxiety (29%), embarrassment (31%), fear (22%), frustration (73%), guilt (9%), helplessness (36%), hurt (47%), resentment (42%), or feeling burnt out (58%). Nurses having experienced physical aggression reported lesser percentages on the above effects
Richter and Berger (2000)	85 (rr 50%) assaulted psychiatric workers in D, c	Prospective survey on patient assault and consequences: P	Interview, PTSD questionnaire, descriptive statistics	The 85 assaulted carers (all bar two nurses) experienced shock (44%), despondency (7%), fear (12%). PTSD symptoms were also experienced: 11% re-experience (11%), avoidance (1%), and increased irritability (4%). None of the assaulted fulfilled all three criteria constituting a complete clinical PTSD
Richter (2005)	46 (rr ?) assaulted staff in D, c	Prospective analysis of assaulted care workers: no definition	PCL-C, IES-R, interviews	Of the 46 assaulted staff in nine state mental health institutions (70% nurses) eight persons met the criteria for PTSD at baseline. Posttraumatic stress was associated with the severity of physical lesions. Non participants at follow up had significantly higher IES-R scores. Generally PTSD rates reclined significantly among participants ($n = 35$) at the 2 and six month follow up assessments with the rates of three workers remaining stable
Ryan and Poster (1989)	61 assaulted nursing staff, USA, c	Prospective longitudinal survey on assault effects: PT	ARQ, ATPAQ, Interview, inferential statistics	The following reactions to violence were found: Anger (40–50%), anxiousness, feeling sorry for the perpetrator, feelings of inadequacy in preventing the aggressive incident (30–40%), increased body tension and awareness (40–50%), with social and cognitive responses having been experienced at "a lower rate"

(Continued)

Appendix—Cont'd

Author(s)	Setting, Subjects, Sample	Study Type, Aim, Definition	Instrument, Analysis	Main results Related to Psychological Sequelae
Suserud et al. (2002)	66 (rr 92%) ambulance service nurses, S, c	Survey on experiences with threats and violence: T, no clear definition of violence	Questionnaire, descriptive depiction of effects	Ambulance nurses having experienced violence perceived impairment of performance, anger, feeling confounded, shock, impairment of nurse-patient relationship, and difficulty to concentrate
Vincent et al. (2000)	660 (rr 69%) health care trainees; DK, c	Survey on assault consequences: PTSV	Questionnaire, descriptive statistics	Trainees in social work (428), nursing (228) and nursing aides (184) participated. Of the 660 students 428 had experienced violence of threats of violence. The main experiences were: Body tension, anxiety/fear (4.8%), anger (17.1%), powerlessness, indifference, exhaustion/fatigue, feelings of workplace insecurity
Whittington and Wykes (1992)	23 assaulted nurses, one assaulted doctor, UK, c	Prospective longitudinal survey on post assault strain and support: P	SSEV, SQ, VSQ, inferential statistics	Victims of patient violence were interviewed three times (< 72 h, 7, and 14 days). The following non somatic responses varied individually in intensity across time: Sleep disorder, night mares, anxiety/fear, exhaustion, with fatigue and irritability being the most prominent reactions

Note: rr = response rate, c = convenience sample, P = physical, V = verbal, T = threat
Countries: AUS = Australia, CH = Switzerland, CDN = Canada, D = Germany, DK = Denmark, S = Sweden, SGP = Singapore, TW = Taiwan, UK = United Kingdom, US = United States of America

Legend of Abbreviated Instruments Employed in the Chapter

ARQ = assault response questionnaire
ATPAQ = attitudes toward patient physical assault questionnaire
HASN = Hospital Assault Survey for Nurses
IES-R = impact of events scale revised
IRF = incident report form
NSCF = nursing staff characteristics form
OAS = overt aggression scale
PCL-C = posttraumatic stress disorder checklist—civilian
PTSD-Interview = post-traumatic stress disorder interview, German version
RIES = revised impact of events scale
SQ = strain questionnaire
SSEV = Spielberger's self evaluation questionnaire
VIS = victim interview schedule
VSQ = victim support questionnaire

ACKNOWLEDGEMENT

This chapter is based on the following article: Needham, I., Abderhalden, C., Halfens, R. J., Fischer, J. E., and Dassen, T. (2005). Non-somatic effects of patient aggression on nurses: a systematic review. *J Adv Nurs* 49(3):283–296.

I would like to thank all co-authors for the important contribution they made to this research work.

REFERENCES

Abderhalden, C., Needham, I., Almvik, R., Miserez, B., Dassen, T., Haug, H., et al. (2002). Clinical Validation of the German version of the Brøset-Violence-Checklist. *Unpublished paper.*

Adams, J., & Whittington, R. (1995). Verbal aggression to psychiatric staff: Traumatic stressor or part of the job? *Perspectives in Psychiatric Care, 2*(2), 171–174.

Allin, A., Stantzos, A., & Needham, I. (2005). Aggression from the inside: A qualitative study to discover nurses' experiences regarding patient aggression in psychiatric in-patient settings. In: N. Oud, H. Nijman & T. Palmstierna (Eds.), *Conference proceedings from the 4th European Congress on Violence in Psychiatry: "Good clinical evidence based practice for understanding and managing aggressive and violent behavior"* (pp. 201–217). Amsterdam: Oud Consultancy and Conference Management.

Almvik, R., & Woods, P. (1998). The Broset Violence Checklist (BVC) and the prediction of inpatient violence: Some preliminary results. *Perspectives in Psychiatric Care, 5*(6), 208–211.

American Psychiatric Association. (1994). *Diagnostic and Statistical Manual of Mental Disorders.* (4th ed.). Washington DC: American Psychiatric Association.

Arnetz, J. E., & Arnetz, B. B. (2001). Violence towards health care staff and possible effects on the quality of patient care. *Social Science and Medicine, 52*(3), 417–427.

Arthur, G. L., Brende, J. O., & Quiroz, S. E. (2003). Violence: Incidence and frequency of physical and psychological assaults affecting mental heath providers in Georgia. *The Journal of General Psychology, 130*(1), 22–45.

Åström, S., Bucht, G., Eisemann, M., Norberg, A., & Saveman, B. I. (2002). Incidence of violence towards staff caring for the elderly. *Scandinavian Journal of Caring Sciences, 16*(1), 66–72.

Baxter, E., Hafner, R. J., & Holme, G. (1992). Assaults by patients: The experience and attitudes of psychiatric hospital nurses. *The Australian and New Zealand Journal of Psychiatry, 26*(4), 567–573.

Bensley, L., Nelson, N., Kaufman, J., Silverstein, B., Kalat, J., & Shields, J. (1997). Injuries due to assaults on psychiatric hospital employees in Washington State. *American Journal of Industrial Medicine, 1*(1), 92–99.

Bin Abdullah, A. M., Khim, L. Y. L., Wah, L. C., Bee, O. G., & Pushpam, S. (2000). A study of violence towards nursing staff in the emergency department. *Singapore Nursing Journal, 27*(3), 30–37.

Blow, F. C., Barry, K. L., Copeland, L. A., McCormick, R. A., Lehmann, L. S., & Ullman, E. (1999). Repeated assaults by patients in VA hospital and clinic settings. *Psychiatric Services, 50*(3), 390–394.

Budd, T. (1999). *Violence at work: Findings from the British Crime Survey*. London: Home Office.

Caldwell, M. F. (1992). Incidence of PTSD among staff victims of patient violence. *Hospital and Community Psychiatry, 43*(8), 838–839.

Carmel, H., & Hunter, M. (1989). Staff injuries from inpatient violence. *Hospital and Community Psychiatry, 40*(1), 41–46.

Carmel, H., & Hunter, M. (1993). Staff injuries from patient attack: Five years' data. *The Bulletin of the American Academy of Psychiatry and the Law, 21*(4), 485–493.

Chaimowitz, G. A., & Moscovitch, A. (1991). Patient assaults on psychiatric residents: The Canadian experience. *Canadian Journal of Psychiatry, 36*(2), 107–111.

Chambers, N. (1998). "We have to put up with it: Don't we?" The experience of being the registered nurse on duty, managing a violent incident involving an elderly patient: A phenomenological study. *Journal of Advanced Nursing, 27*(2), 429–436.

Chiang, C. (2005). *Psychiatric nurses' experiences of physical assault by patients in Taiwan*. Chungtai: Central Taiwan University of Science and Technology.

Dawson, J., Johnston, M., Kehiayan, N., Kyanko, S., & Martinez, R. (1988). Response to patient assault. A peer support program for nurses. *Journal of Psychosocial Nursing and Mental Health Services, 26*(2), 8–11,15.

Deahl, M. (2000). Psychological debriefing: Controversy and challenge. *The Australian and New Zealand Journal of Psychiatry, 34*(6), 929–939.

Erdos, B. Z., & Hughes, D. H. (2001). Emergency psychiatry: A review of assaults by patients against staff at psychiatric emergency centers. *Psychiatric Services, 52*(9), 1175–1177.

Ernst, K. (1998). Freiwilligkeit und Zwang in der psychiatrischen Behandlung. *Deutsches Ärzteblatt, 95*(47), 2990–2996.

Fernandes, C. M., Bouthillette, F., Raboud, J. M., Bullock, L., Moore, C. F., Christenson, J. M., et al. (1999). Violence in the emergency department: a survey of health care workers. *Canadian Medical Association Journal, 161*(10), 1245–1248.

Fernandes, C. M., Raboud, J. M., Christenson, J. M., Bouthillette, F., Bullock, L., Ouellet, L., et al. (2002). The effect of an education program on violence in the emergency department. *Annals of Emergency Medicine, 39*(1), 47–55.

Flannery, R. B., Jr. (2001). The Assaulted Staff Action Program (ASAP): Ten year empirical support for Critical Incident Stress Management (CISM). *International Journal of Emergency Mental Health, 3*(1), 5–10.

Flannery, R., Fulton, P., & Tausch, J. (1991). A program to help staff cope with psychological sequelae of assaults by patients. *Hospital and Community Psychiatry, 41*(9), 935–938.

Flannery, R., Hanson, M., & Penk, W. (1995). Patients' threats. Expanded definition of assault. *General Hospital Psychiatry, 17*(6), 451–453.

Fottrell, E. (1980). A study of violent behavior among patients in psychiatric hospitals. *British Journal of Psychiatry, 136*, 216–221.

Fry, A. J., O'Riordan, D., Turner, M., & Mills, K. L. (2002). Survey of aggressive incidents experienced by community mental health staff. *International Journal of Mental Health Nursing, 11*(2), 112–120.

Gates, D. M., Fitzwater, E., & Meyer, U. (1999). Violence against caregivers in nursing homes: Expected, tolerated, and accepted. *Journal of Gerontological Nursing, 25*(4), 12–22.

Geser, A. M. (1999). Aggressionen von hospitalisierten psychisch Kranken: Eine systematische Evaluation von knapp 2000 Aggressionsfällen. Unpublished Inaugural-Dissertation zur Erlangung der Doktorwürde, Universität Zürich, Zürich.

Haller, R., & Deluthy, R. (1988). Assaults on staff by psychiatric in-patients: A critical review. *British Journal of Psychiatry, 152*, 174–179.

Hanson, R., & Balk, J. (1992). A replication study of staff injuries in a state hospital. *Hospital and Community Psychiatry, 43*(9), 836–837.

Hauck, M. (1993). *Die Wut bleibt — Gewalt von Patienten gegenüber Pflegenden (The anger remains — Patient violence towards nurses)*. Unpublished Thesis. Aarau: Kaderschule für die Krankenpflege.

Hislop, E., & Melby, V. (2003). The lived experience of violence in accident and emergency. *Accident and Emergency Nursing, 11*(1), 5–11.

Jones, J., & Lyneham, J. (2000). Violence: Part of the job for Australian nurses? *The Australian Journal of Advanced Nursing, 18*(2), 27–32.

Lanza, M. L. (1983). The reactions of nursing staff to physical assault by a patient. *Hospital and Community Psychiatry, 34*(1), 44–47.

Lanza, M. L. (1992). Nurses as patient assault victims: An update, synthesis, and recommendations. *Archives of Psychiatric Nursing, 6*(3), 163–171.

Lanza, M., Kayne, H., Hicks, C., & Milner, J. (1991). Nursing staff characteristics related to patient assault. *Issues in Mental Health Nursing, 12*(3), 253–265.

Lee, S. S., Gerberich, S. G., Waller, L. A., Anderson, A., & McGovern, P. (1999). Work-related assault injuries among nurses. *Epidemiology, 10*(6), 685–691.

Lehmann, L. S., McCormick, R. A., & Kizer, K. W. (1999). A survey of assaultive behavior in Veterans Health Administration facilities. *Psychiatric Services, 50*(3), 384–389.

Levin, P. F., Hewitt, J. B., & Misner, S. T. (1998). Insights of nurses about assault in hospital-based emergency departments. *Image–The Journal of Nursing Scholarship, 30*(3), 249–254.

May, D. D., & Grubbs, L. M. (2002). The extent, nature, and precipitating factors of nurse assault among three groups of registered nurses in a regional medical center. *Journal of Emergency Nursing, 28*(1), 11–17.

Menckel, E., & Viitasara, E. (2002). Threats and violence in Swedish care and welfare-magnitude of the problem and impact on municipal personnel. *Scandinavian Journal of Caring Sciences, 16*(4), 376–385.

Morgan, J. F., & Porter, S. (1999). Sexual harassment of psychiatric trainees: Experiences and attitudes. *Postgraduate Medical Journal, 75*(885), 410–413.

Murray, G., & Snyder, J. C. (1991). When staff are assaulted. A nursing consultation support service. *Journal of Psychosocial Nursing and Mental Health Services, 29*(7), 24–29.

Needham, I., Abderhalden, C., Meer, R., Dassen, T., Haug, H. J., Halfens, R. J. G., et al. (2004). The effectiveness of two interventions in the management of patient violence in acute mental inpatient settings: Report on a pilot study. *Journal of Psychiatric and Mental Health Nursing, 11*(5), 595–601.

Nijman, H. L. I., Muris, P., Merckelbach, H. L. G. J., Palmstierna, T., Wistedt, B., Vos, A. M., eet al. (1999). The Staff Observation Aggression Scale — Revised (SOAS-R). *Aggressive Behavior, 25*, 197–209.

Nijman, H., & Rector, G. (1999). Crowding and aggression on inpatient psychiatric wards. *Psychiatric Services, 50*(6), 831–831.

Noble, P., & Rodger, S. (1989). Violence by psychiatric in-patients. *British Journal of Psychiatry, 155*, 384–390.

Nolan, P., Dallender, J., Soares, J., Thomsen, S., & Arnetz, B. (1999). Violence in mental health care: The experiences of mental health nurses and psychiatrists. *Journal of Advanced Nursing, 30*(4), 934–941.

O'Connell, B., Young, J., Brooks, J., Hutchings, J., & Lofthouse, J. (2000). Nurses' perceptions of the nature and frequency of aggression in general ward settings and high dependency areas. *The Journal of Clinical Nursing, 9*(4), 602–610.

O'Rourke, E. M. (2002). My worst nightmare. A nurse's personal account of assault and recovery. *Journal of Psychosocial Nursing, 40*(11), 38–43.

Owen, C., Tarantello, C., Jones, M., & Tennant, C. (1998). Violence and aggression in psychiatric units. *Psychiatric Services, 49*(11), 1452–1457.

Palmstierna, T., Huitfeldt, B., & Wistedt, B. (1991). The relationship of crowding and aggressive behavior on a psychiatric intensive care unit. *Hospital and Community Psychiatry, 42*(12), 1237–1240.

Richter, D. (1998). Gewalt und Gewaltprävention in der psychiatrischen Pflege-eine Übersicht über die Literatur. In: D. Sauter & D. Richter (Eds.), *Gewalt in der psychiatrischen Pflege* (pp. 40–44). Bern: Huber.

Richter, D. (2005). Post-traumatic stress disorder in mental hospital staff following a patient assault – empirical data and prevention measures. In: T. Palmstierna, H. L. Nijman & N. Oud (Eds.), *Violence in clinical psychiatry: Proceedings of the 4th European Congress* (pp. 40–44). Amsterdam: Oud Consultancy.

Richter, D., & Berger, K. (2000). Physische und psychische Folgen bei Mitarbeitern nach einem Patientenübergriff: Eine prospektive Untersuchung in sechs psychiatrischen Kliniken. *Arbeitsmed, Sozialmed, Umweltmed, 35*(8), 357–362.

Rippon, T. J. (2000). Aggression and violence in health care professions. *Journal of Advanced Nursing, 31*(2), 452–460.

Ryan, J. A., & Poster, E. C. (1989). The assaulted nurse: Short-term and long-term responses. *Archives of Psychiatric Nursing, 3*(6), 323–331.

Sonnenberg, S. M. (1988). Victims of violence and post-traumatic stress disorder. *The Psychiatric Clinics of North America, 11*(4), 581–590.

Steinert, T., Beck, M., Vogel, W., & Wohlfahrt, A. (1995). Gewalttätige Patienten: Ein Problem für Therapeuten an psychiatrischen Kliniken? *Der Nervenarzt, 66,* 207–211.

Suserud, B. O., Blomquist, M., & Johansson, I. (2002). Experiences of threats and violence in the Swedish ambulance service. *Accident and Emergency Nursing, 10*(3), 127–135.

Tam, E., Engelsmann, F., & Fugere, R. (1996). Patterns of violent incidents by patients in a general hospital psychiatric facility. *Psychiatric Services, 47*(1), 86–88.

Vanderslott, J. (1998). A study of incidents of violence towards staff by patients in an NHS Trust hospital. *Journal of Psychiatric and Mental Health Nursing, 5*(4), 291–298.

Vincent, C., Perlt, D., Sørensen, S., & Winther, L. (2000). *Violence against trainees — A questionnaire study.* Copenhagen: Socialt Udviklingscenter SUS.

Whittington, R., & Wykes, T. (1992). Staff strain and social support in a psychiatric hospital following assault by a patient. *Journal of Advanced Nursing, 17*(4), 480–486.

Wykes, T., & Whittington, R. (1991). Coping strategies used by staff following assault by a patient: An exploratory study. *Work and Stress, 5*(1), 37–48.

Wykes, T., & Whittington, R. (1994). Reactions to Assault. In: T. Wykes (Ed.), *Violence and Health Care Professionals* (pp. 105–126). London: Chapman and Hall.

VII
CONCLUSIONS

Toward an Evidence-Based Approach in the Management of Violence in Mental Health Settings

Dirk Richter and Richard Whittington

1 INTRODUCTION

The chapters of this volume have gone a long way toward establishing the current state of research and practice relating to the understanding and management of violence in mental health care. It should be apparent that the issue of violence in psychiatry is no longer a taboo, and that many scientific and practical initiatives are underway to grapple with this problem. In many individual countries, and even on a supranational level, political concerns about the extent of this problem can also be seen (Eurogip, 2001). Research funding bodies and government institutions are investing more and more money into scientific work and into the implementation of related organizational efforts. Politically, violence in psychiatry can now be seen as only a part of the whole picture of violence in health care and, even more broadly, as part of the problem of violence at work in general (Leather, Brady, Lawrence, Beale, & Cox, 1999). Without doubt, this political reframing may facilitate the work of researchers and practitioners in the field, but movement up the political agenda can come at a cost. The UK National Health Service "Zero Tolerance" campaign, for instance, is another reflection of the new political visibility of the problem and is much discussed within psychiatry insofar as many people have concerns about the dangers of applying such politically driven efforts to mental health care (Behr, Ruddock, Benn, & Crawford, 2005).

However, the work here also demonstrates that there is still a long way to go in terms of developing a real framework for evidence-based practice in this area. Of course, in many countries of the world, health care and professional organizations have launched guidelines for the management of aggressive and violent patients. Such initiatives are known, for example, from the US, UK, Switzerland, and Germany. But a closer look at these guidelines makes clear that the recommendations are usually, and inevitably, based on weak scientific evidence. Randomized controlled trials and similar "high quality design" studies about the issues of violence and its management are usually not available. Even the risky and disturbing practice of coercing aggressive patients, among the most restrictive of measures in health care, is not based on scientific arguments but rather on national and, in many cases, local traditions, and legal guidelines. The crucial question of whether to restrain or to seclude patients simply cannot be answered scientifically because of the current lack of relevant studies and this leads to quite absurd differences in practice. For instance, the German practice of coercion depends on the region (e.g., seclusion is more often used in southern Germany, mechanical restraint more often in the north), and on the field of psychiatry (e.g., practitioners in forensic and child and adolescent psychiatry seclude, those in general psychiatry favor restraint). In a nutshell, this lack of uniformity is repeated across Europe and the rest of the western world. As Trond Hatling and his colleagues have shown in their chapter on the legal background to involuntary admissions, detentions, and treatments, there is much diversity and even contradiction between the available national guidelines. Although the social and cultural origins of many of these countries are very similar, in some states mechanical restraint is not allowed, whereas in others seclusion is forbidden or forced medication is only allowed by a judge's order. As a consequence very vulnerable patients, and involuntarily admitted patients certainly fit this description, are treated very differently all over the western world. In the light of the strong impact of national traditions it is no wonder that the rates of involuntary admissions and coercive measures against patients vary so much between different countries (Salize, Dressing, & Peitz, 2002). But in a rapidly globalizing world, where a definition of fundamental human rights is shared across many countries, it is becoming questionable why and whether such local contradictions are tolerable.

Coercion is obviously not the only field where sound studies are still lacking. Other areas of research covered here include training programs for staff, psychological consequences of assaults for staff, psychological consequences of coercion for patients, etc., and the same message is apparent: some emerging research but currently, weak evidence, much diversity, and little systematic sharing of best practice across countries. In this final chapter we will attempt to pull together some conclusions that can be drawn from the contributions to this book. We aim to answer the question of what today, to the best of our knowledge, can be done in psychiatric hospitals, wards, and services when front-line staff and managers want to improve the experience of staff and patients when trying to prevent and deal with aggressive and violent behavior.

2 MEASURING AND PREDICTING VIOLENCE

The first step is accurate measurement and description of the problem and the chapter on measuring violence in psychiatric institutions by Henk Nijman and colleagues has given several ideas on how to improve the reporting of incidents. It is widely known that many, or even most, violent incidents are not recorded if there is no form which is dedicated to capturing the relevant information on violence and aggressive behavior. Although there is a shift toward "near miss" and adverse incident reporting in some countries, in many psychiatric institutions across Europe and the US, violent incidents are only logged via injury reports. This procedure, by definition, excludes all incidents that do not lead to physical injuries and in reality, however, only major injuries are usually reported. Many psychiatric staff still subscribe to the view that minor bruises are just part of the job and, therefore, do not need to be reported, so the official information held on incidents is badly skewed. Related to this is the fact that reports usually do not lead to any changes for the staff or patient involved, so many staff end up with the feeling that nobody really cares about the incidents and their consequences.

A good place to start to investigate and to raise awareness toward violence is the implementation of a psychometrically sound reporting instrument but, of course, the implementation of such an instrument is no guarantee that all incidents will then get reported. Recent research by Henk Nijman and his colleagues has shown that there are huge differences in reported levels of incidents between countries and even between neighboring wards when you apply the same instrument (in this case the SOAS-R). Simply the introduction however, of such an instrument, is a fine opportunity to stimulate discussion and reflection on violence-related issues on the ward and to work toward a common definition or threshold of what really counts as violence on a specific ward. Similarly, another advantage of many of these instruments is that they raise staff sensitivity to "minor" aggressive expressions such as verbal threats. This reduces the skew of the organization's audit dataset and, most importantly, enables the consideration of "near miss" patterns which can inform the construction of robust risk assessment procedures.

Related to this, another problem that still awaits a real solution is the effective prediction of violence in specific situations. As Tilman Steinert has shown in his chapter, there are only a few statistical variables which may be regarded as strong predictors. As so often in psychiatry, the history determines the future, and the best variable in this regard is previous violence in the history of an individual patient. Tilman Steinert stresses the argument that most of the prediction instruments used in acute inpatient settings are no better than clinical wisdom and expertise. There is some hope that a new scale, the Brøset Violence Checklist (BVC), developed by Roger Almvik and colleagues (Almvik, Woods, & Rasmussen, 2000), is able to predict aggressive inpatient behavior more effectively. At the moment, however, the prediction of aggression and the decision to take action (e.g., close observation) cannot rely solely on instruments, and it is unlikely that it will ever be possible for this to happen anyway. The clinical wisdom of doctors and nurses must not be left out of the risk assessment equation and it is likely that clinical expertise and prediction instruments together are more accurate than either one alone. As yet this hypothesis has, to our knowledge, never been tested.

3 CAUSES OF VIOLENCE IN PSYCHIATRIC SETTINGS

A major reason for our difficulties in the prediction of violence is the often exclusive focus on patient properties alone, e.g., their history of violence, psychopathology, impaired impulsivity control. Most of the causal and prediction research isolates these attributes and attempts to build individualistic models out of them and many front-line staff do the same thing. This "internal" attribution has a long scientific and medical history. As Stal Bjørkly has argued in his chapter, prominent psychological approaches, e.g., psychoanalysis and drive theory, have also originally focused purely on internal variables. Later theoretical developments, however, have moved from an internal model of aggression toward an awareness of the patient's environment and the importance of close, interpersonal interaction with others on the ward. Thus it should now be clear that violence in psychiatric settings is not just a patients' problem. The next step is to take this theoretical insight into the real world of practice though such a process will take some time.

This argument for the importance of interaction is a central theme of our own chapter on the process of escalation preceding violent incidents. We are convinced that violence in general, and thus violence in psychiatric settings in particular, comes mainly from the interaction between patient and staff. In our chapter, we have highlighted some promising biological, psychological, and sociological approaches. Although the patient's psychopathology and biology must not be overlooked while trying to analyze causal pathways that lead to violence, there is now a huge amount of evidence from different scientific fields that suggests some relevant interaction and escalation to the final trigger when violence occurs. The scientific challenge for the next few years is to draw the "big picture" of violence in mental health, i.e., to identify and then synthesize the relevant factors from biology, psychology, and sociology. "Theory of Mind" research seems a particularly promising approach that might help to integrate the different domains.

The staff's contribution to the emergence of violence is also underlined in the chapter on the users' perspective by Chris Abderhalden and colleagues. The finding, from several reported studies, that patients and staff see different causes for the emergence of violence is most important. While staff mainly attribute violence to the patient and his or her illness, users more often identify staff behavior, and interaction conflicts as important. As researchers, we are not in a position to say who is right and who is wrong. If patients feel provoked or aversively stimulated by staff behavior, this should be an argument to think hard about this behavior. From a practical perspective, this means that staff should take a different point of view compared to how professionals have considered things in the past. Staff should be highly sensitized to their own contribution to the escalation of aggression and violence. We do not intend to blame assaulted staff for patient violence, but would encourage staff to be aware of themselves as, potentially, part of a conflict system where each party is aversively stimulating the other in the process of escalation. Such a perspective takes us to the issue and potential of prevention.

4 ORGANIZATIONAL ISSUES OF PREVENTION AND MANAGEMENT OF VIOLENCE

The roots of aggression and violence start much earlier than in the aggressive encounter itself and so should attempts to manage and the prevent the problem. As Joy Duxbury and her colleagues have shown, ward design, ward architecture, ward regime, and the whole ward atmosphere and culture should be designed to avoid as much aversive stimulation as possible. Beyond architecture, this point stresses the importance of the everyday behavior of staff in general, and of nurses in particular. The atmosphere is mainly imprinted on a ward by the regime of the nurses. Nurses and doctors should be aware of this cultural process and try to examine their professional behavior as a group on the ward. One question might be about how the necessary control of patients, e.g., in admission situations, should be carried out. Another topic might be the individualization of ward rules: should, for instance, all patients be treated alike regardless of their disorders and needs? Depending on the type and size of the ward, there are many more such questions which could be usefully examined to change the culture of the ward and thus the potential for unnecessary conflict.

Of course, every hospital and every ward must balance the need for a minimally aversive atmosphere on the one hand, and the need for safety and security on the other. Seamus Cowman has argued in his chapter that there is obviously a professional role dilemma when navigating between caring and security. This dilemma needs to be discussed by staff and sometimes with patients, too. Thorough security measures must not be dismissed as prevention efforts, e.g., in the case of weapons brought into the ward, and in many hospitals clear policies regarding safety and security are still missing. However, an over-controlling and over-sanctioning atmosphere, which may be justified by the hospital policy, will certainly increase the aversive stimulation of patients and, again, the potential for violence. As with the ward atmosphere, this balance of caring and safety must be openly discussed by all of the staff.

Training in physical and nonphysical techniques for aggression management is now a prerequisite for all mental health staff, especially those in acute care settings. In his chapter, Nico Oud has convincingly argued that aggression management training must cover all aspects of this topic. Staff have to be able to apply the appropriate technique at every point along the escalation curve. If staff are untrained or badly trained there is a real danger of ineffective or unethical behavior. Ineffectiveness, for instance, may occur when staff try to deescalate a situation that is actually no longer controllable without coercion. Conversely, unethical behavior may occur when staff use coercion when there is no real indication that it is needed. Although no figures are available, we assume that there are high rates of what might be called preventive coercion by mental health workers who feel insecure and therefore initiate force in order to protect themselves.

Nico Oud has also given ideas to psychiatric institutions on how to organize their training. In many countries of the western world there are commercial companies who offer specialized training for mental health staff but many of these companies have their origins in the criminal justice system. Psychiatric institutions, operating from a healthcare philosophy, must be aware of this. Before contracting for a training program, the compatibility between the institutions' therapeutic goals and the values espoused in the content of the training must be analyzed. A major difficulty lies in the diversity of settings within a psychiatric hospital and thus the diversity of training needs. In forensic mental health, we see different kinds of violence than in elderly care, or in child and adolescent psychiatry. One way round this problem is to train trainers in-house so they are able to adopt the training curriculum to the specific settings where it will be applied. A further advantage of such an approach, of course, is the opportunity to minimize costs.

Along with many others, the training of mental health staff is, in our view, the crucial component within an institution's aggression management policy. The chapter by Dirk Richter and colleagues on the effects of such training, however, has shown how difficult it is to measure results, and institutions which want to establish effectiveness should be aware of the methodological pitfalls. However, as this systematic review has revealed, there are clear positive effects on staff confidence and knowledge and improvements in these domains must not be undervalued. As we have already noted, with regard to other fields of research in this area, again we need more sophisticated study designs to move beyond the contradictory evidence we now possess.

It is clear though, that training can only be one part of an organizations response to this problem. As a multifactorial problem, violence requires a multifactorial solution. Kevin McKenna and Brodie Paterson have explored the issue of designing a whole-systems approach to reduction involving cognizance of workplace safety, risk management practice, and policy perspectives into which training initiatives should be embedded. Training is crucial but must not be seen as a quick fix which avoids the need for deeper level organizational change. As they conclude, management of aggression is part of patient care, not something separate and distinct.

5 IMMINENT BEHAVIOR AND AGGRESSION MANAGEMENT

Many of these issues of prediction, atmosphere, and training come together at the point when staff become aware of the potential for imminent violence by a patient. It goes almost without saying that every staff member should skillfully be able to apply deescalating behavior. Although up to now, the mental health research literature on that topic is only sparse, there are quite a lot of basic principles which can be meaningfully imported from other fields. As Dirk Richter has pointed out in his chapter on deescalation and nonphysical aggression management techniques, the requirements in mental health care are very similar to the techniques which the police, and even international organizations, have already developed. With regard to deescalation, much can be gained if the basic principles of empathy, respect, and fairness are mastered by every staff member.

It is obvious, though, that not every situation can be deescalated by nonphysical means and that some incidents require physical coercion to maintain overall safety and security. Richard Whittington and his colleagues argue, in their chapter on this topic, that coercion must always be considered as potentially harmful to patients. As mentioned before, there is currently only weak research evidence on the effectiveness and effects of physical aggression management in mental health settings. This lack of knowledge applies to the choice of procedure (i.e., physical restraint, mechanical restraint, seclusion, forced medication, or even net bed) as well as to the effects of singular or combined procedures. Today it is impossible to say which measure is effective, in terms of the safety of all the people involved, and it is also impossible to say which measures are generally preferred by patients in cases where they agree on the need for some form of coercive intervention. It is likely that different procedures will fit for different patients and these preferences can be considered as part of an advance directive. For some patients, it is certainly most horrifying to find themselves alone in a seclusion room but for others it is more horrifying to be tied down to a bed. As there is no safe knowledge on this today, one can only recommend to hospitals that they are flexible enough to be able to apply a range of different measures. As many potentially aggressive patients go through a lot of hospital admissions in their lives, we recommend that staff and patients work collaboratively where possible to develop advance directives in which the preferred procedure for coercion could be agreed upon by patients and staff well before it becomes necessary to apply.

The literature on the pharmacological management of aggression is unique in this field in that it is much larger and more advanced when compared to the other interventions here considered. Laurette Goedhard and her colleagues have clearly shown that pharmacological interventions need to be separated according to whether they have, on the one hand, acute and short-term goals, or maintenance therapy goals on the other. When faced with acute aggressive crises, the authors recommend a combination of a neuroleptic and a benzodiazepine. As far as we can oversee the practical reality across and beyond Europe, this recommendation is already implemented in most psychiatric institutions. The recommendations for maintenance therapy, however, are less robust. Up to now, no effective pharmacological treatment of chronic aggressive behavior exists. One reason might be similar to the issue of violence causation and prediction discussed above: aggressive behavior is highly dependent on situational cues which cannot be eliminated by medication.

6 POSTINCIDENT CARE

The mental well-being of psychiatric hospital staff does not receive sufficient attention from hospital management nor, more surprisingly, from staff themselves.

However, as Ian Needham has shown in his systematic review of evidence on the psychological consequences of assaults, a professional's mental health can be severely impaired after such an incident. Potential symptoms range from emotional, to cognitive and motivational, and even social responses, and these responses can be very severe. A recent study by one of the authors here (Richter & Berger 2006) has confirmed that a minority of affected staff members suffer from chronic posttraumatic stress disorder (PTSD) after an assault.

Given the high frequency of assaults on staff, posttraumatic stress becomes an occupational health issue which must be addressed through organizational efforts to minimize work-related injuries. In most psychiatric institutions, however, the organizational response to occupational health injuries is still only triggered by evidence of physical damage. The management of psychological damage and posttraumatic stress in health care institutions requires, firstly, a strategy to recognize and detect possible psychological effects. However, this can be a difficult task because of a tendency toward avoidant behavior among affected staff. Secondly, postincident management support has to be provided by the organization. Recent PTSD-management strategies developed by the US and UK military stress the importance of peer support (Jones, Roberts, & Greenberg, 2003; Keller et al., 2005), and such a strategy also offers a manageable solution for psychiatric hospitals. Experience from German hospitals reveals that assault victims do not want to be emotionally supported by their management, but do accept support from colleagues. In the home institution of Dirk Richter, a peer support program has recently been set up in which experienced mental health nurses try to keep in touch with severely assaulted staff over a period of several months. This program aims at providing psychological support, not therapy, and a crucial component of the initiative is for the support team to actively solicit and identify the needs and emotional states of the assaulted person. However, the assaulted employee retains control of the process by determining the frequency and intensity of the contacts. As indicated by current best evidence, psychological debriefing sessions are not provided. If the assaulted employee shows relevant PTSD-symptoms over several weeks, the support team suggests referral to some form of professional psychological therapy.

It is vital not to forget the postincident aftercare for the patient who has been subjected to coercion by the institution, especially when physical force has been applied. The days of restraining or secluding patients, releasing them, and just going back to everyday routines should be over. Staff must be sensitive to the potentially traumatizing effects of the use of coercion. The chapter by Chris Aberhalden and his colleagues, on the users' view, has reported the findings of several studies which support this requirement. From clinical experience we know that some patients cannot remember the initial situation that led to the outburst of violence, so sometimes they find themselves in a restraint or seclusion situation and they cannot work out why. This inevitably increases the fear and trauma of the situation. Other patients, who remember every detail of the interaction, are left with strong feelings of being treated unfairly. Obviously, if unresolved, these experiences do not encourage long-term engagement and other important therapeutic goals. Therefore, staff should make a point of discussing their reasons for the use of physical coercion after the incident with the patient and this procedure should become an obligatory standard in all institutions where such force is used.

7 CONCLUSIONS

The aim of this book has been to give an overview of current research into the problem of violence in mental health care settings and, where possible, to start translating this body of evidence into practical recommendations for front-line staff and their employing organizations. Clearly there is much activity going on among researchers around the world and we are edging towards a comprehensive picture of why violence occurs and what we can do to minimize it. Equally, there is much awareness and concern among governments in many countries about protecting both the well-being of a valuable national resource (health care professionals) and the quality of the experience of people who enter mental health settings for care and treatment. With such a complex and universal social phenomenon as violence, success in improving the working lives of staff and the humanity of wards will only be achieved through collaboration at the individual level (through advance directives, for example) and in the research domain. Collaboration across academic disciplines in affected countries drawing on multiple research methodologies, as hopefully exemplified in this book, provides the most likely path to a solution and the development of a mental health care system fit for the 21st century.

REFERENCES

Almvik, R., Woods, P., & Rasmussen, K. (2000). The Brøset Violence Checklist: Sensitivity, specificity and inter-rater reliability. *Journal of Interpersonal Violence, 15,* 1284–1296.

Behr, G. M., Ruddock, J. P., Benn, P., & Crawford, M. J. (2005). Zero tolerance of violence by users of mental health services: The need for an ethical framework. *The British Journal of Psychiatry, 187,* 7–8.

Eurogip (Ed.). (2001). *Workplace violence in Europe.* European conference (Conference proceedings). Eurogip, Paris.

Jones, N., Roberts, P., & Greenberg, N. (2003). Peer-group risk assessment: A post-traumatic management strategy for hierarchical organizations. *Occupational Medicine, 53,* 469–475.

Keller, M., Greenberg, N., Bobo, W., Roberts, P., Jones, N., & Orman, D. (2005). Soldier peer mentoring care and support: Bringing psychological awareness to the front. *Military Medicine, 170,* 355–361.

Leather, P., Brady, C., Lawrence, C., Beale, D., & Cox, T. (Eds.). (1998). *Work-related violence: Assessment and intervention.* London: Routledge.

Richter, D. & Berger K. (2006). Post-traumatic stress disorder in mental health staff following a patient assault: a prospective follow-up study. BMC Psychiatry, 6, 15. In: T. Palmstierna, H. Nijman & N. Oud (Eds.), *Violence in clinical psychiatry (Conference proceedings)* (pp. 40–44). Amsterdam: Oud consultancy.

Salize, H. J., Dressing, H., & Peitz, M. (2002). *Compulsory admission and involuntary treatment of mentally ill patients – Legislation and practice in European Union member states.* Final Report. Mannheim: Central Institute of Mental Health. Available at http://europa.eu.int/comm/health/ ph_projects/2000/ promotion/fp_promotion_2000_frep_08_en.pdf.

Index

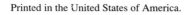